Scanning
the Pharaohs

Scanning
the Pharaohs

CT Imaging of the New Kingdom Royal Mummies

Zahi Hawass
Sahar N. Saleem

edited by
Sue D'Auria

The American University in Cairo Press
Cairo New York

This paperback edition published in 2018 by
The American University in Cairo Press
113 Sharia Kasr el Aini, Cairo, Egypt
One Rockefeller Plaza, 10th Floor, New York, NY, 10020
www.aucpress.com

First published in hardback in 2016

Dar el Kutub No. 27484/17
ISBN 978 977 416 887 1

Dar el Kutub Cataloging-Publication Data

Hawass, Zahi
        Scanning the Pharaohs: CT Imaging of the New Kingdom Royal Mummies / by Zahi
    Hawass and Sahar N. Saleem.—Cairo: The American University in Cairo Press, 2018
        p.   cm.
        ISBN 978 977 416 887 1
        Egypt—Antiquities
        Saleem, Sahar N. (Jt. auth.)
        932

    2 3 4 5   27 26 25 24 23 22

Designed by Sally Boylan
Printed in China

Dedicated to the
memory of Mark Linz

Contents

Tables

Foreword

Scanning the Pharaohs tells us a fascinating story about a landmark of twenty-first-century archaeology, involving an outstanding combination of scholarship and forensic science. Named the Egyptian Mummy Project, this initiative has often been referred to in the media, but this is the first fully comprehensive treatment to appear in print. As such, it is essential reading for both scholars and the public, as well as a book one can't put down. While it is a serious and accessible work of scholarship, Scanning the Pharaohs—like a good detective story—presents us with intriguing theories about famous pharaohs and their queens; explores a myriad of scientifically derived clues; and presents conclusions, some definitive, others honestly acknowledged to be still open to debate. At the same time, this book retells, but from new perspectives, the complicated story of the relationships between modern Egypt and these statue-like entities, the mummified and surprisingly durable bodies of most kings and some queens of the New Kingdom.

As the book's valuable historical summaries make clear, this was an age of imperial grandeur and sometimes surprising cultural innovation, including the brief imposition of monotheism under the 'heretic' king Akhenaten; and any new data, as we have here, are of great significance in historical terms. For example, were Akhenaten's innovations the product of severe physiological disabilities? The answer to this you'll find in this book, as well as those relevant to other rulers and their personalities and experiences. Yet despite the significance of these mummies, their disposition generated debate among Egyptians in recent and contemporary times. Should they be replaced in their original sepulchers; retained, but only for purposes of scientific study; or be exhibited as artifacts, and if so, only for scholarly visitors, or for Egyptian citizens and foreign tourists at large?

Scanning the Pharaohs is a superbly co-authored book. Dr. Zahi Hawass, PhD, and Dr. Sahar N. Saleem, MD, seamlessly interweave Egyptological and forensic data (based on their research studies and acknowledging by name the many Egyptian and some foreign scientists who contributed to the endeavor) as they describe the sometimes dramatic results of the project and their historical implications. At the same time, it becomes clear that this initiative would not have been undertaken without the perceptiveness and energy Dr. Hawass brought to it. In his then capacity as secretary general of the Supreme Council of Antiquities, Dr. Hawass developed a clearly articulated plan of action; recruited an outstanding team of Egyptian forensic experts, together with some from abroad; and as a skillful scholarly entrepreneur persuaded major cultural institutions (the National Geographic Society and the Discovery Channel) to facilitate the provision of equipment and the setting up of labs in Egypt.

Here, I can only provide you with some intriguing hints as to the discoveries you will make in this marvelous book. Why was a tooth so important for the identification of the unusual female pharaoh Hatshepsut? Who were the royal parents and grandparents of that famous king, Tutankhamun, whose largely unplundered tomb was discovered in 1922 and was like a thunderbolt in terms of its extraordinary richness? His lineage is now clear, his supposed murder discussed, and surprising disabilities revealed for this 'god-king.' And did Pharaoh Ramesses III come to a bloody end, as surviving texts indicate but, absent forensic evidence that is now available, could not confirm? As well as these specific issues, there is also intriguing information about new evidence regarding the technology of mummification as applied to royalty, and the listing of jewelry and amulets detectable beneath the surviving wrappings.

Interwoven with the narrative treatment by Dr. Hawass and Dr. Saleem is the dedication Dr. Hawass brought to this initiative, fired as he was not only by the need for forensic analysis and historical information, but also by respect and concern for the royal mummies,

these unique survivals of once powerful kings. The royal mummies in fact led complicated lives until most of them ended up in the Egyptian Museum in Cairo (where they are displayed in much upgraded and more respectful surroundings than before), and even now they are scheduled to be moved to another museum that hopefully will be constructed once conditions permit. For a while, some royal mummies were in Cairo, some kept at Thebes (modern Luxor), and even now Tutankhamun's mummy rests in his tomb. Perhaps most spectacularly, the mummy of King Ramesses I was discovered to have been lodged in the modest Niagara Falls Museum since 1871, and was purchased by the Michael C. Carlos Museum of Emory University in Atlanta in 1999. Dr. Hawass persuaded the Carlos Museum that Ramesses should be returned to Egypt and personally escorted the royal mummy on its flight.

But prior to this, Dr. Hawass's concern for the royal mummies was already long conceived. In part, his interest in the study of mummies was stimulated by his spectacular discoveries of the "Golden Mummies" of Bahariya Oasis, but goes back even earlier, when in 1972 he was escorting Princess Margaret of the United Kingdom through the Egyptian Museum in Cairo. Catching a glimpse of the exhibited royal mummies, the princess was upset by treatment of them that seemed to her disrespectful, a perspective that Dr. Hawass never forgot and sought to remedy—a surprising intersection of modern and ancient royalty!

Enjoy this book; there is nothing else like it.

David O'Connor
Lila Acheson Wallace Professor
of Ancient Egyptian Art
Institute of Fine Arts
New York University

Acknowledgments

We would like to thank many people who helped us in the production of this book.

First, we would like to thank David Silverman (Eckley Brinton Coxe, Jr. Professor of Egyptology, University of Pennsylvania), Ray Johnson (director of the Epigraphic Survey, University of Chicago), Nicholas Reeves (Lila Acheson Wallace Associate Curator, Metropolitan Museum of Art), and Janice Kamrin (assistant curator, Metropolitan Museum of Art), who read this book from the Egyptological point of view. We would like to thank Gerald Conlogue (codirector of the Bioanthropology Research Institute, professor of diagnostic imaging, Quinnipiac University) and Andrew Nelson (associate professor of anthropology, University of Western Ontario), who read the information on the CT scans.

We would also like to acknowledge the help of Egyptologist Tarek El Awady, who was able to search for the Egyptological photos to be used in this book, and Kallie Day, Dr. Hawass's assistant at Sierra Nevada College.

Special thanks must be given to Nigel Fletcher-Jones, director of the American University in Cairo Press, who encouraged us to write this important book that is going to be useful to both scholars and the public. Special thanks also to Neil Hewison, associate director for editorial programs at the AUC Press, who worked hard to make this book available to the readers.

Last but not least, we would like to give a very special thanks to Egyptologist Sue D'Auria, for her hard work in editing this book, and her careful look at all the information contained therein. Without Sue, this book would never have been written.

Thanks to all of you.

Chronology[1]

Tutankhaten/Tutankhamun	1336–1327
Ay	1327–1323
Horemheb	1323–1295
Dynasty 19	1295–1186
Ramesses I	1295–1294
Seti I	1294–1279
Ramesses II	1279–1213
Merenptah	1213–1203
Amenmesse	1203–1200
Seti II	1200–1194
Siptah	1194–1188
Queen Tawosret	1188–1186
Dynasty 20	1186–1069
Sethnakht	1186–1184
Ramesses III	1184–1153
Ramesses IV	1153–1147
Ramesses V	1147–1143
Ramesses VI	1143–1136
Ramesses VII	1136–1129
Ramesses VIII	1129–1126
Ramesses IX	1126–1108
Ramesses X	1108–1099
Ramesses XI	1099–1069
Third Intermediate Period (Dynasties 21–25)	1069–664
Late Period (Dynasties 26–Second Persian Period)	664–332
Ptolemaic Period	332–30
Roman Period	30 BC–AD 395

Introduction

by Zahi Hawass

My interest in the study of mummies began when I excavated the Valley of the Golden Mummies at Bahariya Oasis in 1999. The most important goal of this excavation was the preservation of the numerous mummies that were discovered. This was achieved both by conservation work on the mummies at the site, and by closing down the excavations after three seasons in order to preserve unexcavated remains.

The discovery was very important and became famous, attracting tourists from all over the world who wanted to visit the mummies. To accommodate these requests, I moved a few mummies from the site to a room in the Inspectorate of Antiquities for the tourists to see, and closed the site to the public for the preservation of the remainder of the mummies, which remain in their tombs.

My interest in mummies was reignited when I brought the so-called mummy of Ramesses I from the Michael C. Carlos Museum in Atlanta back to Egypt in 2004. This mummy's story began in the mid-nine-

teenth century when it was purchased from a family in Luxor for seven Egyptian pounds. The mummy traveled to Canada in 1871 and was exhibited in the Niagara Falls Museum, a collection of curiosities that also included the Daredevil Hall of Fame, located at that time on the Canadian side of the falls.

In the 1980s, the late Arne Eggebrecht, the German scholar who was then the director of the Hildesheim Museum, saw this mummy in the museum and suggested that it could be a royal mummy, based in part on the position of the hands on the chest and the mummy's resemblance to known Ramesside royal remains.

In 1999, the Niagara Falls Museum closed, and its Egyptian collection was offered to the Michael C. Carlos Museum at Emory University in Atlanta. Bonnie Speed, the Carlos Museum's director, and Peter Lacovara, its curator of Egyptian and Nubian art, decided to buy this collection, which included the mummy. In less than two weeks, they mounted a successful campaign, appealing to the citizens of Atlanta to procure the necessary funds to make the purchase, which was about two million dollars. The mummy was transported to the museum and exhibited there in 1999. Peter Lacovara, with a team of radiologists from Emory University, studied this mummy.[1] The position of the two hands, crossed on the chest, and the style of mummification are similar to that observed on the mummy of Seti I, the son of Ramesses I. When I went to Atlanta to give a lecture and saw the mummy, I was convinced that it is the mummy of Ramesses I. Peter and Bonnie are good people and have a cordial relationship with me. I was able to convince them that a royal mummy cannot be away from Egypt. They agreed to return the mummy, as well as fragments from the tomb of Seti I in the museum's collection.

I journeyed to Atlanta to bring the mummy back to Egypt, accompanied by two of my great friends, Mohamed Farid Khamis and Adel Hamouda. Mohamed is a businessman who owns a carpet factory in Atlanta. He threw a party at the Michael C. Carlos Museum and gave a generous donation of $100,000. My dear friend Adel, a famous writer, also came to attend this event. At the reception, I announced that my gift on behalf of Egypt to the people of Atlanta would be to bring a King Tut exhibition to the city. I kept my promise, and "Tutankhamun: The Golden King and the Great Pharaohs" opened at the Atlanta Civic Center in November 2009. During this very successful exhibit I again traveled to Atlanta and gave a lecture at the Fox Theatre to an audience of 4,500 people.

In preparation for its return to Egypt in 2004, the mummy of Ramesses I was placed in a coffin draped with the American and Egyptian flags, which was received by Bonnie and me during a ceremony in front of the museum in October of that year. At the airport, members of Congress and many young people came to pay their respects and to say goodbye to Ramesses, and a group of young students sang a song of farewell. I escorted the mummy onto an Air France flight, and the captain announced, "We have two important people on our flight today: Ramesses I and Zahi Hawass." A woman seated next to me could not sleep when she heard that there was a mummy on the flight—she was afraid of the mummy's curse.

Ramesses I returned home after 133 years away. He was received at the Cairo airport with all the fanfare befitting a king. Many reporters were there to greet him, and Bonnie Speed and I held a joint press conference at the Egyptian Museum in Cairo to welcome the pharaoh. I decided to send this mummy and that of Ahmose I, the famous Eighteenth Dynasty king who ended the Hyksos domination of Egypt, to be exhibited in the new wing of the Luxor Museum dedicated to the Golden Age of the pharaohs. I journeyed with the two kings to Luxor. Ramesses I was the star, made even more famous because he came from the States, and he was transported to the museum with great celebration. He was welcomed by the governor of Luxor amid dancing and music. Ahmose was relatively neglected, which was strange, since Ramesses I achieved very little in history and ruled for only two years, in comparison with Ahmose, the great king who expelled the Hyksos from Egypt. Both kings are still exhibited in Luxor today.

There were many doubts about the identification of Ramesses I, but recently we took DNA samples from this mummy and also from the mummies of Seti I and Ramesses II (fig. 1). The resulting analysis indicated that the former is his son and the latter his grandson. I

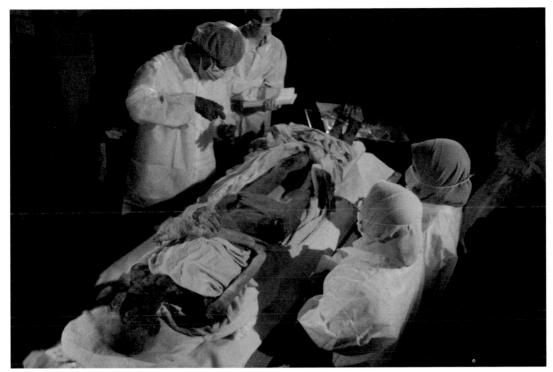

Fig. 1: The mummy of Ramesses II inside the DNA lab of the Egyptian Museum, Cairo.

always maintained our belief that it could be Ramesses I but that the final conclusions should wait until we undertook DNA analysis.

A singular event in my life opened my eyes to the way that mummies are exhibited at museums. In 1972, when I was twenty-five years old, I was asked by the head of Antiquities, Fouad el-Orabi, to give a tour to Princess Margaret of England at the Egyptian Museum in Cairo. As I was explaining the beautiful artifacts, we moved to the west side of the building on the first floor. The mummy of Ramesses II was exhibited in this hall. As we approached the mummy, suddenly Princess Margaret rushed away, covering her eyes. I was astonished and asked her directly, "Why did you do this?" She replied that it was not a good idea to display mummies this way, and that it was disrespectful to the ancient personage.

This made an impression on me, and later in my career, I began to look at this idea and see that the way mummies are exhibited in museums is contrary to the spiritual values of the pharaohs. Oftentimes, mummies are shown for a thrill and can frighten children or upset sensitive people.

During a 1979 press conference at the Egyptian Museum, President Anwar al-Sadat addressed the mummy situation. He stated that we could not leave them like this, without proper respect, and suggested either returning the mummies to their tombs or displaying them with more sensitivity. As a young man, I was so happy to see that the president of Egypt had this type of insight. The public, and children in particular, never learn from mummies when they are exposed in this manner. They do not know that mummies and mummification are science. We can exhibit them, respect them, and understand about their lives and also the achievements of the ancient Egyptians with regard to mummification. We also need to teach our children about the philosophies of life and death of the ancient Egyptians and to help visitors think of the mummies as the remains of individuals, not just as objects of horror or fascination.

In 2002, I was asked by Farouk Hosni, then minister of culture, to be the secretary general of the Supreme Council of Antiquities (SCA, formerly the Egyptian Antiquities Organization). I was not excited about this offer because I was working at the Giza pyramids, the place that I loved. However, I needed to accept the position, because I saw that the SCA was ineffective in its mission and that it was essential that we have good Egyptian archaeologists in the future to direct this council. At the time, we depended completely on foreigners. Our museums were dark and had no educational message. The pharaonic, Jewish, Coptic, and Islamic monuments were deteriorating. I am not going to explain here my overall concept and how I was able to implement it, but I would like to explain my vision concerning mummies and the methods I used to make this vision a reality.

I began by hiring an architect to create a site museum at Bahariya Oasis for the mummies chosen to explain the story of the Valley of the Golden Mummies. The plan of the museum adopted the architecture of the oasis environment. The design is finished, but the museum has not yet been built.

I decided that this was the time to take action to display the Egyptian Museum's mummies in a more respectful manner. I had both short-term and long-term plans to implement this. The short-term plan was designed to break with the old style of the Egyptian Museum and to display the mummies sensitively, with more educational information. We designed two new halls in the museum for the mummies. I also directed the conservation lab to work to preserve them, as nothing had been done prior to this to ensure that their condition did not deteriorate. The royal mummies are now displayed in specialized vitrines with controlled humidity and temperature. Thanks must be expressed to the Getty Conservation Institute for undertaking this scientific project. For the first time, we could see how well the mummies are preserved, and visitors can now understand the lives of these people by reading new information on text and illustrative panels and labels. Before visitors enter each hall, they are presented with information on the cachettes where the mummies were found, and also on death and the afterlife in ancient Egypt. (For the mummies on display, see the appendix, "List of the Royal Mummies in the Egyptian Museum, Cairo.")

For the long term, I issued an order that all the mummies of the pharaohs from Dynasties Eighteen through Twenty should be exhibited at the new National Museum of Egyptian Civilization that we have built in Old Cairo. The museum, which only requires completion of the interior design before it can be opened to the public, is part of a master plan conceived during my tenure as secretary general to construct two new museums in Cairo to complement the existing Egyptian Museum in Tahrir Square. Farouk Hosni, the former minister of culture, was a driving force behind the creation of these two museums. The first, the Grand Museum, is currently under construction next to the Giza plateau. This museum will exhibit the great collections and masterpieces of pharaonic Egypt, such as the treasures of

Tutankhamun. It will also house a conservation lab and storage magazines that will be connected to the museum by a tunnel.

The National Museum of Egyptian Civilization was built in cooperation with UNESCO and is located in a beautiful area in Fustat, Old Cairo, in front of a lake. From its vantage point, one can see the Pyramids, and the churches and mosques of Old Cairo. The museum will explain the broad sweep of Egyptian history from the Predynastic Period to modern times. The Egyptian Museum will continue to house Egyptian art, the great statues to be shown within their archaeological context through photographs and graphics.

I decided that some mummies should be shown inside the Civilization Museum, which would attract many visitors to this new building, because any tourist who comes to Egypt must see three things: the Pyramids, Tutankhamun's treasures, and mummies. The scenario for the exhibition is to display each royal mummy respectfully, with the face covered, in a special vitrine surrounded by text panels explaining all the achievements of the individual, to exhibit with the mummy statues and artifacts of their reign, and to present the results of scientific analysis of the mummy (CT scanning and DNA). In addition, one hall of the museum will be dedicated to illustrating and describing mummification and funerary beliefs through text panels and graphics.

With the two new museum projects underway, I decided to pursue a dream of mine to initiate an Egyptian mummy project, choosing the best scholars in the field of radiology, anatomy, and DNA, and bringing new technology, such as CT scanning and DNA analysis, to study the mummies. This was the first time that royal mummies were studied by CT examination, but this was not the first time that the royal mummies had been studied using modern technology. The first such study was undertaken in 1903, when an x-ray study was performed on the mummy of Thutmose IV. Subsequent studies took place in 1932 and from 1967 to 1971, when all of the royal mummies at the Egyptian Museum were x-rayed. This led to the journey of Ramesses II's mummy in 1976 to France, where it was x-rayed and conserved.

President Valéry Giscard d'Estaing of France asked President Anwar al-Sadat to allow the mummy of Ramesses II to be studied and treated in Paris, because concerns had been raised about the mummy's condition. Actually, many people believed that the reason the mummy traveled to Paris was to determine whether or not Ramesses II was the pharaoh of the Exodus. President Sadat agreed to the examination, and the Egyptian Antiquities Organization (EAO), as it was known then, gave the approval. The mummy was sent to Paris on September 26, 1976, on a French military plane, accompanied by Shawki Nakhla, an Egyptian scientist from the EAO. The mummy was greeted at Le Bourget Airport with the full military honors that a living king would receive, and studies were undertaken in a laboratory at the Musée de l'homme, with the participation of 105 scientists from many other French institutions. The mummy stayed in Paris for more than seven months.

When the mummy returned to Cairo on May 10, 1977, at the airport an Egyptian journalist asked a French scientist who had worked on the project and who had accompanied the mummy on his return to Egypt, if the mummy suffered from any diseases. The French scientist answered that they found a strange insect on the mummy. The reporter said, "Maybe it is a French insect?" Everyone laughed at his reply.

Though these events happened in 1976, I was informed in 2006 that the scientist who treated Ramesses II removed some hair from the mummy. To this day, I do not understand how he was able to do that, because the mummy was accompanied by an Egyptian official. We don't know if the official was complicit in this act or if the samples were taken illegally from this mummy in the Egyptian Museum during the 1975 study, because they did not have permission to take the samples without his knowledge. I found out about it in November 2006, when someone in France put the hair for sale on the Internet for two thousand euros. The seller was a French citizen living in Grenoble who claimed that he inherited these relics from his father, who was a member of the scientific team that examined the mummy of Ramesses II in France in 1976. I moved quickly and was able to contact French authorities through the Egyptian Ministry of Foreign Affairs and also through the efforts of the Egyptian ambassador in Paris, Nasser Kamel. I asked them to retain the pieces, and the French court ruled in our favor. We were able to retrieve remnants of hair, linen bandages, and resin used in the mummification of King Ramesses II. They arrived back in Egypt on April 1, 2007, after having been in France for thirty years. It was a crime for the scientist to secretly remove these things without the consent of the Egyptian government.

I sent Ahmed Saleh from the SCA to France to recover the hair samples. He brought back to Egypt six small samples of Ramesses II's hair along with a larger lock, linen bandages that were once used in the mummification of the king's body, and ten samples of resin from the mummies of Ramesses II and his son Merenptah, a total of forty-one samples. The samples of Merenptah's mummy came into the possession of the Frenchman because the French scientific mission also took samples from this mummy in the Egyptian Museum during a 1975 study. It seems that the French requested to take the samples but their request was rejected; nevertheless, someone from the Egyptian authority apparently allowed them to take forty-one samples from the mummies of Ramesses II and Merenptah in 1976. It is a crime that both the French scientists and the Egyptian scientists who permitted them to take the samples without permission have gone unpunished. In the future we should not permit any scientific expert to work in Egypt without the supervision of an Egyptologist from a respected institution such as a museum or a university to prevent such a thing from happening again.

Additional samples have been taken from other mummies as well. In the mid-1990s, Brigham Young University took samples from ten royal mummies. Permission to do so was given only by the director of the museum and the staff member in charge of the mummies, but permission should have been granted by the Permanent Committee of the SCA as the national antiquities authority. Sadly, any results of this work remain unpublished in a scholarly forum.

My intention was to begin our recent project with non-invasive CT scans of the mummies. Because CT scans produce three-dimensional images and show the soft tissues as well as the bones of the body, it is a much more effective research tool than x-ray examination. Before I could begin to choose the Egyptian scientists who could be members of the Egyptian Mummy Project, a problem to overcome was the acquisition of this technology. One solution was to approach major television channels that would be interested in broadcasting such a project. By funding our work, in return they could record the process, under our conditions.

I contacted Terry Garcia, the chief science and exploration officer of the National Geographic Society, and explained that we needed to have people contact Siemens, a leading company in healthcare technology, to request the donation of a CT scanning machine to the SCA. Terry is one of the most honest and helpful persons I know, and he has done more important scientific projects for Egypt and National Geographic than anyone. Someday Terry should be rewarded by both institutions. I told Terry if he could help us acquire the machine, we could give National Geographic permission to broadcast the story first, but not exclusively, and also permission to publish it in *National Geographic* magazine. The machine, after that, would belong to the SCA.

I asked Frederick DeWolfe ("Dee") Miller, who is a professor of medicine at the University of Hawaii and a specialist in tropical medicine (he was in Egypt working on a project for the prevention of hepatitis C), to follow up and write the needed proposal to Siemens for the machine. In the end, National Geographic succeeded in bringing the scanner to Cairo, which cost more than a million dollars, and arranging for Siemens to continue to maintain the machine, at the expense of National Geographic. This CT scanner is a trailer-mounted, mobile unit that was (and still is) set up outside the Egyptian Museum.

I decided that we should now, for the first time, have a wholly Egyptian team responsible for the study of the mummies, not under the direction of a foreign team. It was my opinion that we should begin with the non-royal mummies, but Saleh Bedeir, who was the dean of the Faculty of Medicine and the first member of the Egyptian Mummy Project, proposed that we should begin with the mummy of Tutankhamun, and the SCA Permanent Committee agreed. The CT scanning took place on January 5, 2005 in Luxor.

The scientific team was made up of a group of Egyptian radiologists, pathologists, and anatomists. The team that worked with me in the initial phase of this project was composed of Mervat Shafik, professor of radiology, Faculty of Medicine, Cairo University; Essam el-Sheikh, professor of radiology, Cairo University; Sherif Abdel Fatah, lecturer in radiology, also from Cairo University; Hany Abdel-Rahman Amer, professor in the Department of Animal Reproduction at the National Research Center; Fawzi Gaballa, professor of anatomy, Cairo University; and Aly Gamal Eldin, professor of forensic medicine at Cairo University. I thought that we should also have a foreign team to review the data, and we chose Frank Rühli, professor in the Institute of Anatomy at the University of Zurich; Eduard Egarter-Vigl, director of the Pathology Institute at General Hospital, Bolzano, Italy; and Paul Gostner, director of the Department of Radiology at Central Hospital, Bolzano.

The team stayed almost one month to examine the CT results. Before they completely finished the examination of the data, I heard about a great professor of radiology from Cairo University, Professor Ashraf Selim. In one day, he examined the data from Tutankhamun's mummy and was able to confirm all of the team's findings. He is a genius and a very straightforward person, and we decided that he should be the head of the team and work with Dr. Amer of the National Research Center and CT specialist, Siemens, Ltd., Egypt, who was in charge of the operation of the machine. The technician was Salah Mohamed Ali.

I believe that, in this introduction, I should explain in more detail Ashraf Selim's role in the Egyptian Mummy Project. He began, as mentioned, in the CT project to scan King Tutankhamun's mummy. Later, he was the sole radiologist involved in the discovery of Hatshepsut's mummy: he recognized the existence of the tooth in the box and collaborated with Dr. el-Behiry to identify the mummy. He continued on to become the head of the CT scanning project of the family of Tutankhamun as well as Ramesses III. I sincerely believe that he deserves full credit for making our project successful.

Our second project was the search for the mummy of Queen Hatshepsut, and we began to think that we should also have a DNA lab to do our own analyses. What is DNA? Deoxyribonucleic acid is a chemical in each cell that carries the genetic instructions for making living organisms. The mitochondria of each cell contain mtDNA, which is passed down from mother to daughter to daughter to daughter. Mitochondrial DNA is also passed down to each son from his mother, but a son cannot pass mtDNA to his children. The nucleus of some cells contains Y-DNA. There is much less Y-DNA than mtDNA in each cell, because Y-DNA is found only in the nucleus. This means it is much more difficult to study. Y-DNA is passed from father to son to son to son, but it is not passed to daughters.

The decision to employ DNA analysis was a difficult one, because I was always skeptical of DNA results. Until recently, it was not possible to get long enough sequences to consider results reliable. Scholars doing this type of analysis in modern labs work with live patients, and contamination of the samples could result. Labs dedicated solely to working with DNA of mummies would bring more accurate results. I realized that the only way to achieve this was again to approach television channels for financial support. We needed to establish two DNA labs and hire the scientists to conduct the studies. Discovery Channel made the best offer, agreeing in return to shoot the result of our work without interfering in the scientific process, and to broadcast their program free of charge on Egyptian TV.

We opened two labs, one at the Egyptian Museum and one at the Faculty of Medicine, Kasr Al-Ainy Hospital, so that each could work independently and confirm the other's results; this is standard in the field. We established an Egyptian team headed by two great scientists, Yahia Gad, professor of medical molecular genetics at the National Research Center and the overall head of the team, and Dr. Somaia Ismail from the same institute. They brought a group of Egyptian scientists consisting of Naglaa Hasan, Rabab Khairat, and Tarek Abdel Aala. The second lab employed three scientists, Abdel Hamid el-Zoheiry and Mohamed Fateen, assistants at the Faculty of Medicine, Cairo University, and Sally Wasef, a scientist from the SCA. I have to thank Ahmed Sameh Farid, dean of the Faculty of Medicine at Cairo University, who helped us establish the second lab at Kasr Al-Ainy Hospital. I would like to emphasize the great work done on the DNA project by Dr. Gad and Dr. Ismail. I went to Luxor with them twice, and I observed how careful they were in extracting samples from the mummies. The scientific work done by these two scholars was excellent, and they have proved to the world that it is possible to successfully retrieve DNA from ancient mummies.

On April 24, 2007, Dr. Gad did the first sampling on an unidentified mummy. This was executed as a preliminary experiment for testing the DNA sampling procedure before its application to any royal mummy, in addition to providing samples for establishing the lab assays for ancient DNA testing later on. The sampling technique, as Yahia Gad explained in his report, relied mainly on using a bone-marrow biopsy needle to take samples from the deep layers of the mummy through gentle manual burrowing, instead of using automated drilling equipment that may cause considerable damage. Dr. Gad added in his report that trials were made to get more than one sample from the same puncture hole, through the same point of entry but with different angles, thus limiting the number of puncture holes in the mummy.

The scientific team followed the nine criteria for authenticity established by Alan Cooper and Hendrik Poinar to avoid sample contamination and adhere to proper scientific procedure. The samples of DNA were taken first to Lab 1 and then to Lab 2. The results have been studied by the Egyptian team, reviewed by the group of foreign scientists, and published in scientific journals. Carsten Pusch of the University of Tübingen deserves credit for his dedication to the project and his ability to work so well with the Egyptian team. I want to recognize also Albert Zink of the EURAC Institute for Mummies and The Iceman, Bolzano, Italy, for his hard work with us and for his excellent preparation for the publication of the Ramesses III project.

The third major project with the same teams was the study by CT scan of all the mummies that are thought to be connected by familial ties to Tutankhamun, and an attempt to identify family members using DNA analysis. This was followed by another project to discern how Ramesses III died, and to identify the mummy of Unknown Man E (thought to be his son Pentawere) through CT and DNA analyses. Finally, we looked at other Ramesside kings, studying their mummies with the CT scanner alone.

I first met Sahar Saleem, professor of radiology at Cairo University, in early 2007 at a medical conference in Cairo where I gave the keynote lecture. Dr. Saleem had just arrived from Canada, where she was involved in CT studies of mummies as a member of the paleopathology research group at the University of Western Ontario. I invited Dr. Saleem to join the Egyptian Mummy Project, as I anticipated her valuable contribution. Dr. Saleem studied all of the CT scans of the royal mummies of the Eighteenth to Twentieth Dynasties, and provided comprehensive, accurate, systematic analysis of the individual mummies as well as intensive research studies. In addition to her scientific knowledge, Dr. Saleem uses her computer skills in reconstruction and preparation of the CT images. Her input helped in solving mysteries of the feet of King Tutankhamun and the diseases related to his family, and she added new evidence that supports the success of the harem conspiracy against King Ramesses III. Together, we completed and published several CT mummy studies on topics such as the fetuses in the tomb of King Tut, the discovery of new mummification techniques, amulets and jewelry, the spinal diseases of the mummies, and more. For her extensive contribution, I invited her to be the second author of this book.

Unless stated otherwise, all of the information written about the CT scans is the research done by Dr. Sahar Saleem. The chapters to which she contributed are as follows: chapter 1 (all); chapter 3 (examination of the mummy of Hatshepsut); chapter 4 (examination of the mummies); chapter 5 (scanning and conclusions; the sidelight was written by both of us); chapter 6 (x-ray and CT scans of the fetuses); chapter 7 (Marfan's Disease); chapter 8 (CT scans of KV21 A and B; the conclusion was written by both of us); chapter 9 (CT examination of the mummies and Merenptah sidelight; the Exodus sidelight was written by both of us); chapter 10 (examination of the mummies and Ramesses III sidelight); chapters 11 and 12 (all); and chapter 13 (all except Tutankhamun's facial reconstruction).

Egyptologist Sue D'Auria edited this book. She is familiar with the mummies because she was a coauthor of the book *Mummies and Magic*, an exhibit at the Museum of Fine Arts, Boston, where she worked for nearly twenty years. She was involved in one of the earliest CT scanning projects, an investigation of the mummies at the MFA. I have to say that she not only worked very hard in editing the English, but also tried to be very accurate regarding references and information. I always accepted her suggestions, and I really have to credit Sue because she was keen to see this book succeed.

I would like to say that the Egyptian team for both the CT scanning and the DNA project, as well as the foreign consultants, worked beautifully together, and with their contributions we were able to make some important discoveries recounted in the book.

This book is just the beginning. With the completion of this first project of CT and DNA analysis, we still have many additional things to do in our second phase, our future line of research. We need to include the study of the mummies of Amenhotep II and Thutmose IV, to compare them to the Thutmosid family. Also, regarding the search for the mummy of Queen Nefertiti, we need to further study the DNA of the two fetuses of Tutankhamun in comparison with the KV21 A mummy, because the primary study indicated that the latter could be Ankhesenamun. If this can be corroborated, then it would be essential to compare the DNA of KV21 A and the mummy KV21 B. At the same time, it will be vital to locate the bones of Queen Mutnodjmet. Finally, we also need in the future to do more DNA analysis on the Ramesside mummies, to gather more information about their lives and deaths.

I hope that you will enjoy reading this new information on the royal mummies, published here for the first time.

1

Radiographic Imaging of Royal Egyptian Mummies: Previous and Current Studies

Introduction

Mummy research has focused on studying embalming techniques, possible anatomic abnormalities, diseases, or the cause of death of an individual. For the purpose of studies in the past, mummies that were found unwrapped and in poor condition were studied with anthropologic and paleopathologic methods,[1] including dissection and tissue sampling; others have been unwrapped specifically for this purpose. Nevertheless, there are still many well-preserved mummies in the Egyptian Museum in Cairo (some of which have never been on public display) that can be examined with noninvasive methods. Finding an ideal compromise between investigating a mummy and not destroying it encouraged the use of noninvasive methods.

Radiology represents an accurate, noninvasive method of evaluation, and its application in mummies' studies has been used since the introduction of x-rays in the late 1800s. Soon after the discovery of x-rays by Wilhelm Roentgen in November 1895, x-ray study was used to evaluate mummies of both humans and animals without performing dissection.[2] In 1896, a book was published containing fourteen x-rays of an Egyptian mummy.[3] Radiography using plain x-ray is used to make the contents of mummies visible, to distinguish authentic mummies from fakes, to evaluate bone age, to detect skeletal diseases, and to search for burial goods.[4]

The royal mummies at the Egyptian Museum in Cairo are a unique and important resource for our knowledge of ancient Egyptian culture (plates 1 and 2; fig. 2).[5] As would be expected, the collection of royal mummies was subjected to several radiological investigations through the years. The first x-ray study of a royal Egyptian mummy was performed on Thutmose IV in 1903 by an Egyptian radiologist.[6] The mummy of Thutmose IV was brought by horse-drawn taxi to a hospital in Cairo, where the x-rays were then taken. No significant findings resulted from this study. In February of 1932, an x-ray examination of Amenhotep I was done at the Egyptian Museum after the removal of the mummy from its coffin and cartonnage mask. Douglas Derry, an anatomist and professor at the Faculty of Medicine (Kasr Al-Ainy) in Cairo, who worked with Howard Carter on the mummy of Tutankhamun, assessed the age of the mummy using the x-ray findings.[7]

In 1965, extensive x-ray examination of the skulls of ancient Nubian populations was carried out by Alexandria University in Egypt in collaboration with a team from the University of Michigan School of Dentistry.[8] The study was mainly on teeth (etiology of malocclusion, or causes of misalignment of upper and lower teeth) and changes in human faces

through history. This encouraged the Egyptian Antiquities Organization (EAO) in December 1967 to invite James E. Harris from the University of Michigan to study the royal mummies. The study resulted in complete x-ray examination of all the royal mummies at the Egyptian Museum in the years between 1967 and 1971 (fig. 3). The mummy of Tutankhamun, which remains in his tomb, was x-rayed on site in 1968. At the beginning of the study, only the skulls of the mummies were x-rayed using an isotope source of x-ray (ytterbium). The mummies were x-rayed while they were still lying within their glass cases to prevent any damage. However, the glass contained lead, which caused severe degradation of the x-ray images. Later, permission was given to x-ray the mummies out of their glass cases, though

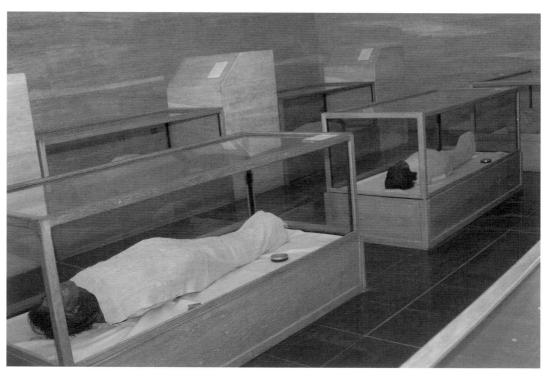

Fig. 2: The so-called new mummies room in the Egyptian Museum, Cairo.

still in their wooden coffins; this resulted in a better quality of the x-ray images. At this time, the ytterbium source was replaced with a conventional x-ray machine using 90 kV, and the whole mummy was imaged. The x-ray protocol included examination of the entire body of the mummy as well as zoom (more localized) films on regions such as the skull (lateral and frontal), chest, pelvis, and lower limbs. In the following years, the Michigan project x-rayed not only the royal collection, but also other mummies in the museum from the Middle Kingdom through the Greco-Roman Period. Two publications originated from this study: *X-Raying the Pharaohs*[9] and *An X-Ray Atlas of the Royal Mummies*,[10] which focused primarily on variations in the skull, face, and teeth.

During this project, scholars became concerned about the condition of the mummy of Ramesses II. In preparation for conserving this mummy, it was moved to France on September 26, 1976, becoming the subject of intensive research through May 10, 1977. The resulting x-rays showed Ramesses II to have reached the age of eighty, which corresponds with our historical knowledge.[11]

The mummy of Tutankhamun was x-rayed again in 1978, and in 1988, twelve royal mummies were selected for x-ray studies for disease detection, a study that was published in a peer-reviewed journal.[12]

In the plain x-ray method, the three-dimensional information about the mummy is projected onto a two-dimensional x-ray film. This makes the characterization of wrappings, contents, mummification techniques, and other findings less satisfactory.[13] Mummy research has benefited from the advancement in radiology technology and the development of modern medical imaging methods, namely computed tomography (CT).[14]

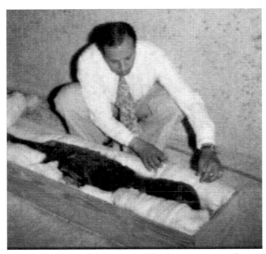

Fig. 3: Ibrahim al-Nawawi with the mummy of Tutankhamun during the research and x-rays carried out in 1968.

CT scanning represents a significant advance from x-rays. Instead of producing one image at a time, the CT machine takes hundreds of images of individual thin sections of the body (slices). These slices can be taken at multiple angles, and then combined into a complete, three-dimensional image of the body. CT can provide much more detailed information than x-ray films, generating images of soft tissues as well as bones.[15]

Multi-Detector Computed Tomography (MDCT) is a recent advancement in CT technology.[16] The chief advantage of MDCT is its capability to perform a large-volume examination in a short time during a single acquisition using thin scans (1.25 mm). As a result, a complete examination of the body of the mummy may be performed with great accuracy (plates 3–4). The advent of graphics workstations and image-processing software packages, multiplanar projections, and three-dimensional (3D) reconstructions produced the research tools for analyzing volume data sets (data in three dimensions).[17]

The volumetric reconstructions can render information about surface details that are not depicted on axial images (transverse plane). Surface CT imaging can show how the mummified humans looked in life and the degree of success of the art of embalming (plate 5).

This chapter will discuss the technique of MDCT imaging for the mummies and CT image analysis. We will also include a scheme for CT image interpretation of the mummies.

MDCT Scanning Technique

All of the royal mummies in the study, except for two fetuses at the Faculty of Medicine of Cairo University (see below), were scanned using an MDCT unit[18] installed on a truck at the Egyptian Museum in Cairo. (The two mummified royal fetuses were examined using MDCT[19] at the radiology department of Cairo University with a technique discussed in chapter 6, "The Two Fetuses Found in the Tomb of Tutankhamun.") The mummies were removed from their coffins for CT examination. The number of linen wrappings on the mummies varied significantly.

The typically used scanning parameters of mummies were: KV=130 effective MAS range from 23 to 63; pitch range from 0.83 to 1.8; FOV from 350 to 500; slice thickness from 0.6 to 1.25 mm; and reconstruction from 0.4 to 0.8 mm.[20] The total number of images generated per mummy varied significantly, from 700 for the five-month-old fetal specimen (mummy numbered 317a by Howard Carter) to about 3,000 for a large adult male such as Ramesses III.

MDCT Image Analysis and Reconstruction (figs. 4a–g)

In addition to the workstations provided by the CT machine's manufacturer,[21] we used other special reconstruction software programs.[22]

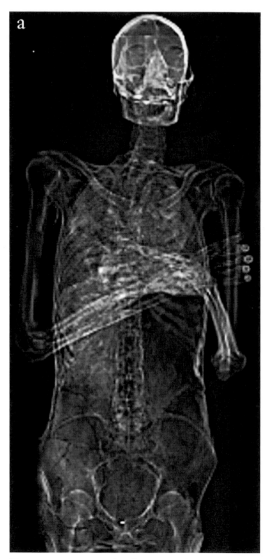

Figs. 4a–g: An example of image analysis and reconstruction in the CT study is given for the mummy of King Ramesses II. CT scout view in anteroposterior (AP) projection of the mummy (a): a scout view is a preliminary image obtained prior to performing the CT study. It permits overall evaluation of the preservation status of the mummy and is used to plot the locations where the subsequent slice images will be obtained.

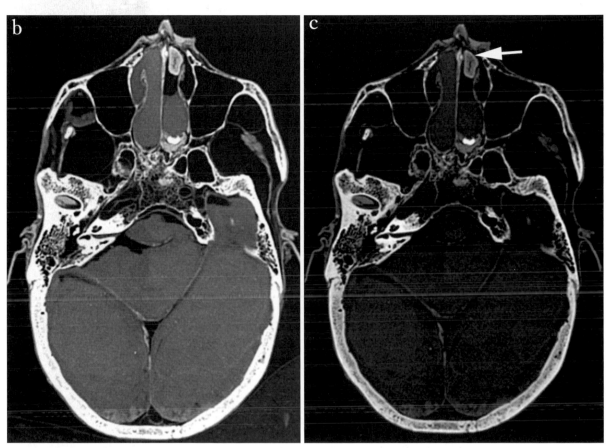

The produced axial images of a region (for example, the head) can be visualized in different window settings for evaluation of soft tissues (b) and bones (c). The bone window setting in this particular example enabled better evaluation of a small animal bone placed within the left nasal opening of the mummy (arrow).

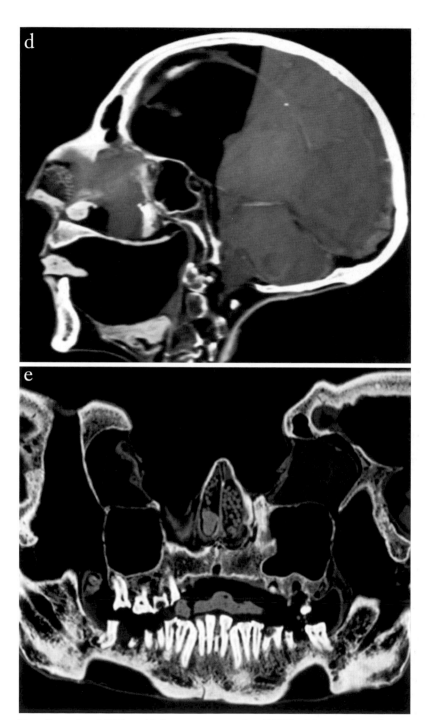

Two-dimensional (2D) multiplanar reconstruction (MPR) of the raw data of a region is possible in any plane, such as (in this example of the head) sagittal plane (d), and curved plane, as in dental arcades (teeth panorama) (e).

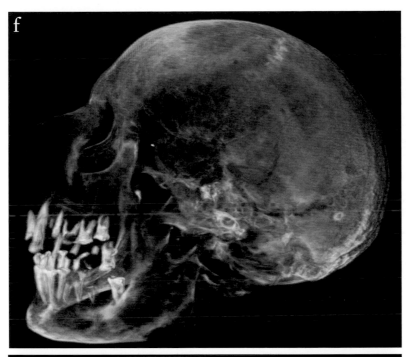

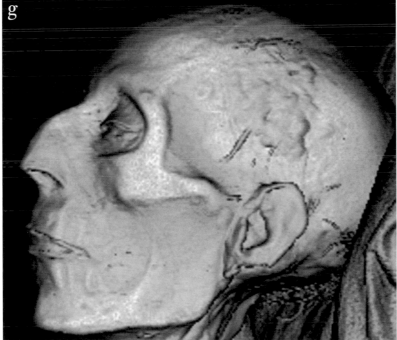

Three-dimensional reconstruction of the region using Maximum Intensity Projection (MIP) (f) shows the features of bones and teeth, and Shaded Surface Display (SSD) (g) shows the surface features of the face.

Image analysis includes anatomical evaluation, and metric and attenuation (radiodensity) measurements. In the case of the presence of metal streaking artifacts, we used Metal Deletion Technique (MDT).[23]

We first visualized the axial images in cineview to obtain a general idea of a mummy's preservation condition, anatomy of body parts, and presence of any foreign bodies.

The improvement of MDCT increases the overall amount of information in terms of raw data. The raw data can thus be reconstructed in two dimensions (multiplanar reconstruction, MPR) and three dimensions (3D reconstruction) (see below). The reconstructed images can reveal more information about the relationships between structures, shape, and orientation within the scan plane.

Multiplanar Reconstruction (MPR)

The raw data produced by thin CT images can be reformatted in coronal (a vertical plane that divides the body into ventral [front] and dorsal [rear] sections), sagittal (a vertical plane that passes from front to rear, dividing the body into right and left halves), or oblique (inclined in direction) planes. MPR images can offer varying perspectives on the anatomy, as well as the changes in the body created by mummification. For example, sagittal plane can show the skull-base defects created for brain removal better than axial imaging can do alone. Coronal plane can detect the location of the heart. Reformatting of images can also be done in curved planes, as in dental arcades to produce orthopantomographic-like images (panorama for teeth).

The superior contrast and spatial resolution inherent in MPR are helpful in anatomical evaluation of the mummy, as well as in accurate metric and attenuation measurements.

Measurements of CT densities in Hounsfield Units (HU) of various structures in the mummy aid in the detection of residual or atrophied body organs and in revealing the nature of the embalming materials used and artifacts included within the wrappings. This knowledge improves our understanding of the mummification process.

Three-dimensional reconstruction (3D reconstruction)

Three-dimensional reconstruction is accomplished by using established reconstruction algorithms for soft tissues and bones with varying window-width parameters. The volume can be rotated to obtain different projection views and to exclude overlapping structures.[24] Post-processing 3D techniques include:

- Volume MPR: This is accomplished through using thick-slab MPR to produce pictures similar to conventional x-ray films.

- Maximum Intensity Projection (MIP): MIP is a 3D visualization technique that is achieved by evaluating each voxel value along an imaginary projection ray within a particular volume of interest and then representing only the highest value as the display value. Voxel intensities below the chosen threshold are eliminated. MIPs can be very useful in locating intrinsically high-density structures in the mummy, such as the skeleton and teeth, as well as dense foreign objects, such as amulets. A drawback in this type of image is that the low-density structures within an object are masked, because only dense points are shown. To control the objects seen, it is possible to adjust the value the ray follows as it penetrates the volume.

- Three-dimensional Volume Rendering (VR): Volume rendering refers to techniques that allow the visualization of 3D data by selective display of density of the grayscale level of the voxels. This means that only voxels with values that lie within a selected interval are seen, while those outside this interval are not. VR can provide accurate representation of the osseous anatomy of the mummy with minimal inclusion of soft tissue (or noise).
- Shaded Surface Display (SSD): This technique represents the surface of a structure.[25] For example, facial features of a mummy can be studied by rotating the head around multiple axes. Location, length, and curvature of mummification incisions can be clearly displayed using SSD, as can external male genitalia.

Other Methods of CT Image Reconstruction
Virtual unwrapping of the mummy

Virtual unwrapping can be done by manual selection of the bandages on the circumference of the body on axial images, then excluding the layers from reconstruction. A similar effect can be achieved by using preset reconstruction algorithms for soft tissues with varying window-width parameters to obtain progressive elimination of external layers with a density less than that of the dried skin.[26] However, presets established for clinical examinations often do a poor job on mummified tissues. Manual selection of a structure, to reconstruct it and exclude all other structures, is used for studying amulets and other foreign objects.

Virtual fly-through endoscopy

Virtual navigation through the inside of the body and hollow structures, for example the skull, trachea, or chest, can be done by using special software installed on the workstation. This technique eliminates the necessity for invasive techniques used in the past for exploring mummies.[27]

Image Interpretation

We adopt the following scheme in the interpretation of CT study of royal ancient Egyptian mummies.[28] The first five will be discussed here, and the remainder in subsequent chapters.

- Preservation status
- Determination of gender
- Estimation of age at death
- Anthropometrical data
- Body and arm position
- Mummification style (see chapter 11, "CT Findings on the Mummification Process")
- Presence of amulets and other foreign bodies (see chapter 12, "Amulets, Funerary Figures, and Other Objects Found on the Mummies")
- Royal faces (see chapter 13, "Faces of the Royal Mummies")
- Examination of individual regions of the body for findings, diseases, and possible cause of death (see chapters on individual mummies)

Preservation status

Although the royal mummies presumably received the most advanced level of treatment with the aim of preserving their bodies, some are currently in poor physical condition. This could be due to mutilation by tomb robbers in antiquity, physical damage by underground water in the tomb, careless handling or intentional invasion by early archaeologists or investigators, or poor environmental conditions of storage at the archaeological or early display sites.[29]

CT can show accurately and noninvasively the current preservation status of the mummy through determining any missing anatomical part, as well as recording skeletal and soft-tissue alterations. The preservation status of the mummy is assigned subjectively as well, fairly, or poorly preserved. Assignment of the preservation status of a mummy can be achieved at a glance in the scout (preliminary) full-body images, as well as by inspecting the 2D and 3D reconstructed images[30] (figs. 5a–b).

Determination of gender

The gender of the mummy can be determined from the morphology of the external genitalia (if preserved), as well as from its skeleton. In general, the female bones are smaller with less prominent ridges; however, secondary sex characteristics are most evident in the pelvis (table 1) and the skull (table 2). MDCT is capable of obtaining 2D and 3D images of the skeleton of the mummy (virtual skeleton) (figs. 6a–d). A feasibility study by

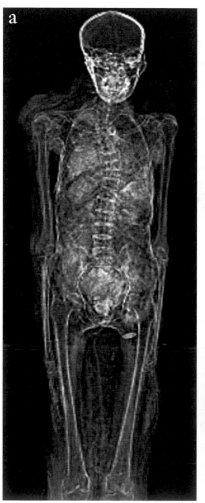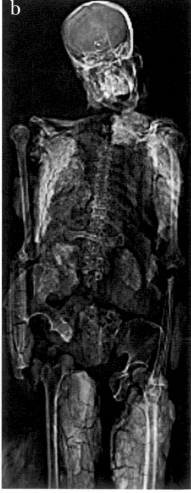

Figs. 5a–b: Full-body scout helps in rapid estimation of the preservation status of a mummy. CT scouts show a well-preserved, mummified Thuya (a) while revealing the poor status of Amenhotep III (b).

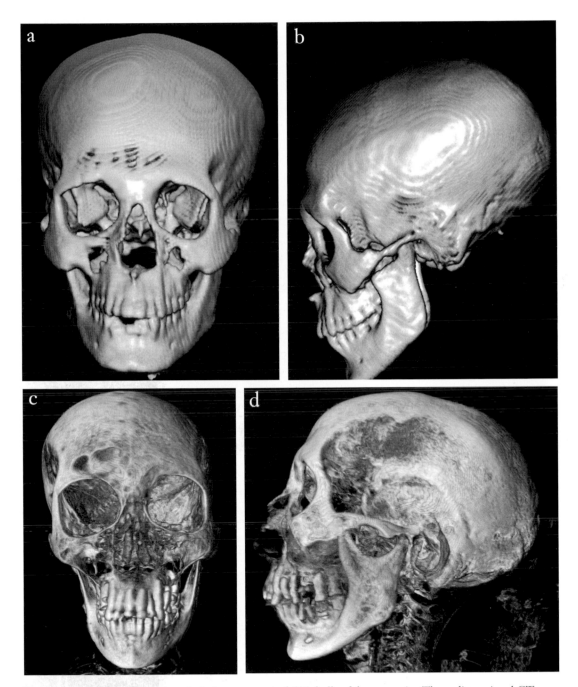

Figs. 6a–d: Secondary sex characteristics in reconstructed CT skulls of the mummies. Three-dimensional CT images in frontal and lateral projections of the skull of the KV55 mummy (a and b) show the masculine characteristics of large size and rugged, prominent bones when compared to feminine smaller, smooth bones in corresponding 3D CT images of the skull of Thuya (c and d).

Table 1. Secondary sex characteristics in male and female pelvic bones

Pelvis	Male	Female
Morphology of the symphysis	Smooth	Roughness of the anterior surface of pubis
Pubic bone body width	25–30 mm	40 mm
Sub-pubic angle	<90	>90
Obturator foramen	Long and rounded	Broad and triangular
Femoral head diameter	>51 mm	<45 mm

Sources: Grabherr et al., "Estimation"; Phenice, "A Newly Developed Visual Method."

Silke Grabherr and colleagues in 2008 demonstrated that MDCT is capable of facilitating the estimation of skeletal sex and age of a deceased person. The study proved that the different parts of the virtual skeleton can be visualized by MDCT in a quality that allows examinations as they are performed on real skeletons. However, sex-related differences between skeletons have such a large overlap between the sexes that in the middle of the range no sexual distinction can be made.[31]

Estimation of age at death

In each mummy, determination of age is based on assessment of features of the body and skeletal system. These include a combination of the following attributes: teeth eruption, epiphyseal union, closure of skull sutures, pubic symphyseal face morphology, changes in the sternal rib end, age-related degenerative changes, and occlusal wear.[32]

The age of subadult individuals can be accurately estimated, as it depends primarily upon observed developmental changes such as teeth eruption and epiphyseal union. In adult individuals, where age estimates are more often accomplished via the observation of degenerative changes, age estimation has a larger margin of error of about a decade.

Determination of age using these morphological methods relies on the assessment of the physiological age of the skeleton, as opposed to the chronological age of the individual. The physiological age depends on environment, nutrition, and diseases; these stresses can cause changes in the skeleton that may mask the true age of the individual.[33] In MDCT studies of the mummies, the absence of degenerative changes, osteophytes, and advanced ossification of epiphyses, sutures, and cartilages is usually indicative of a younger age, while their presence points toward a mature age.[34]

Teeth eruption

Dental age is a major indicator of maturity in the juvenile, especially in ancient remains, as the teeth may be the least damaged of any body part. Dental age is more reliable than skeletal, as it is less affected than bone formation by nutrition or endocrine disturbances. Deciduous (baby) teeth begin to form at about six weeks in utero, and the last permanent tooth completes in early adult life. The third molar (wisdom tooth) is so variable in age of eruption, if it erupts at all, that it is not a reliable age indicator.[35] Dental age can be estimated in children and juveniles according

Table 2. Secondary sex characteristics in male and female skulls

Feature	Male	Female
General size	Large	Small
Architecture	Rugged	Smooth
Supraorbital margin	Rounded	Sharp
Mastoid process	Large	Small
Occipital bone	Marked muscle lines	Muscle lines not marked
Glabella	Bony	Flat
Gonial angle	Squared	Wide angle
Morphology of chin	Broad	Pointed
Occipital condyles	Large	Small

Sources: Buikstra and Ubelaker, *Standards for Data Collection*; Grabherr et al., "Estimation."

to developmental traits of the teeth: eruption, and mineralization of the crowns and roots.[36]

MDCT can detect dental eruption well through study of 2D MPR (orthopantomographic-like) as well as 3D images of the maxilla and mandible. There are several charts and figures that can be used for dental age estimation in child and juvenile subjects, including that of Schour and Massler and others.[37]

Table 3 gives a general idea of dental age according to the eruption of the deciduous and permanent teeth.

Epiphyseal unions

The ends of the long bones (epiphyses) are separated from their main bones by layers of cartilage that gradually ossify along a growth algorithm that can be used to estimate age. For example, the distal ulnar epiphysis appears at 5.5–7 years, and fusion occurs at 15–17 years in females and 17–20 in males.[38] Epiphyseal union is considered the most important characteristic for age determination of adolescents. Union or non-union of the epiphyses can be detected on coronal and sagittal MDCT images (figs. 7a–b). Based on the degree of fusion of the epiphyses, for example, MDCT indicated that Tutankhamun died at the age of nineteen.[39]

Cranial suture closure

This method bases age upon the degree of closure, union, or ossification of the cranial sutures; progressive fusion of sutures occurs with advancing age. Studies have indicated that parietal ectocranial sutures are reliable indicators of age over forty years.[40] The cranial sutures can be examined using a 3D model of the skull in different views.[41]

Pubic symphyseal face morphology

The pubic symphyseal face in the young is characterized by an undulating surface; this surface becomes smoother with age.[42] The pubic bones can be examined on 3D MDCT

Table 3. Chronological appearance of deciduous and permanent teeth in males and females

	Eruption of maxillary teeth	Eruption of mandibular teeth
Deciduous teeth		
Central incisor	8–12 months	6–10 months
Lateral incisor	9–13 months	10–16 months
Canine	16–22 months	17–23 months
Molar 1	13–19 months	14–18 months
Molar 2	25–33 months	23–31 months
Permanent teeth		
Central incisor	7–8 years	6–7 years
Lateral incisor	8–9 years	7–8 years
Canine	11–12 years	9–10 years
Premolar 1	10–11 years	10–12 years
Premolar 2	10–12 years	11–12 years
Molar 1	6–7 years	6–7 years
Molar 2	12–13 years	11–13 years
Molar 3 (wisdom tooth)	17–21 years	17–21 years

Source: American Dental Association, "Eruption Charts."

images. By the use of the virtual cut tool, the symphysis can be cut in the midline and the symphyseal surface of each pubic bone can be shown[43] (figs. 8a–d).

Age-related degenerative changes

There are conditions that become more pronounced in old age and can provide evidence of advanced age, such as degenerative joint diseases, presence of osteophytes (bone spurs), ossification of the rib and laryngeal cartilage, and degeneration of the spine.[44]

MDCT images in multiple planes can detect accurately the degenerative changes, such as the presence of osteophytes, that may help in estimation of age at death[45] (fig. 9).

Occlusal wear

Occlusal wear has been proposed as an indicator of age.[46] However, it has been shown to be highly inaccurate in archaeological contexts where high-grit-content diets can wear down the occlusal surface of the tooth at an early age, especially in ancient Egypt (see figs. 4e–f).

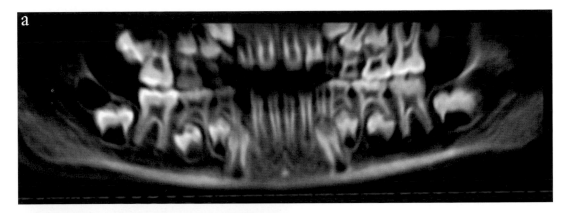

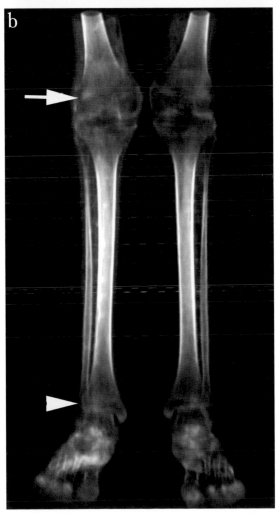

Figs. 7a–b: Estimation of the age of juvenile mummies, using data about teeth eruption and epiphyseal union. Two-dimensional CT curved reconstruction along dental arcades (teeth panorama) of a child mummy found in the tomb of Thutmose IV (KV 43) (a) shows deciduous and multiple nonerupted permanent teeth. Dental age can be calculated on the basis of tooth eruption using the tables. 3D CT image of the legs in frontal projection (using x-ray mode) (b) shows separation of the ends of the long bones around the knees (arrow) and ankle (arrowhead). Estimation of age can be done based on the degree of fusion of the epiphyses.

The structure of spongiosa of the proximal humerus and proximal femur

The internal trabecular structure of the long bones is dense and has regular internal patterning after the maturation of bone. With aging, there is marked loss of internal bone mass and breakup of the trabecular structure. Bone density can be assessed by x-rays. Two-dimensional reconstruction coronal images of the femora and the humeri, viewed in MIP, allows the production of images similar to conventional x-ray images.[47]

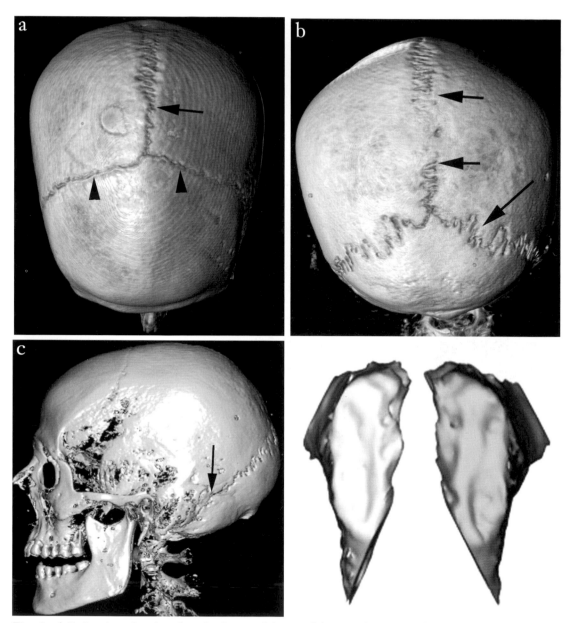

Figs. 8a–d: Estimation of age based on the degree of closure of the cranial sutures and pubic symphyseal face morphology in adult mummies. Three-dimensional (SSD) reconstructed CT images of skull sutures (a–c) and pubic symphyseal face (d) of Ramesses III. The degree of union of the cranial sutures indicates an age over fifty years. The front of the skull's top (a) coronal suture (arrowheads) and sagittal suture (arrow); back of the skull (b) lambdoid suture (long arrow) and sagittal suture (short arrows); and left lateral skull (c) parietomastoid suture (arrow). Three-dimensional CT image (d) of the symphyseal surface of the pubic bones of Ramesses III after applying a virtual midline cut tool. The symphyseal face is completely rimmed with a slight depression of the face itself relative to the rim, with moderate lipping on the dorsal border and prominent ligamentous outgrowths on the ventral border. Changes indicate the estimated age at death is 25–83 years (average 45.6 years).

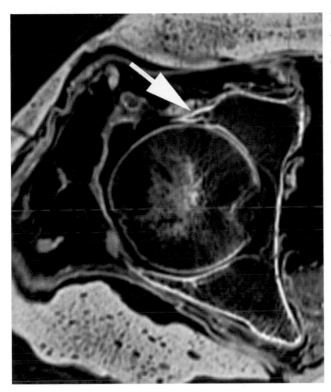

Fig. 9: Age-related degenerative changes. Axial MDCT image of the right hip of Ramesses II shows osteophytic lipping (arrow), indicative of old age at death.

Anthropometric data

Anthropometry is the science of measurement of the size, weight, and proportions of the human body. MDCT studies can establish accurate measurements of the mummified bodies by providing images in multiple planes.

The stature of a complete mummy (or skeletonized mummy) can be measured directly using an MIP midsagittal reconstructed image from vertex (top of skull) to tarsus (heel). For an incomplete or severed mummy, height cannot be measured directly, but estimation of stature can be inferred from a single extremity bone (the femur, for example), using simple regression equations. Such equations can be more specific when the gender and ethnicity are considered.[48]

Stature estimation equations for ancient Egyptians based on long-bone lengths:

Females: (2.340 x femur length) + 56.99 = stature ± 2.517 cm

Males: (2.257 x femur length) + 63.93 ± 3.218 cm[49]

Anthropometry also includes measurements of the skull and face (craniofacial), which will be discussed later with evaluation of the faces of the royal mummies (see chapter 13).

Body and arm position

The position of the arms of ancient Egyptian mummies varied according to the fashion of the time (dynasty), gender, and royal status.

Predynastic mummies had flexed arms with their hands in front of their faces, while Old Kingdom and many Middle Kingdom mummies tended to have their arms beside their bodies. From the Seventeenth into the Eighteenth Dynasty, the arms were laid along the sides, with the hands often placed on the front of the thighs for women, and over the genitals for men. As the New Kingdom progressed, both men's and women's arms lay along their sides, with their hands over their genitalia. In the Nineteenth and Twentieth Dynasties, the 'royal' crossed-arm position over the chest was the norm for the royal mummies. In the Twenty-first Dynasty, the arms of both royal and non-royal mummies returned to their sides, with hands over or near the pubic area.[50]

Conclusion

This chapter highlights the importance of studying ancient mummies and the role of CT as a noninvasive tool. The optimum technique of CT imaging and systematic image analysis facilitates assessment of forensic, anthropological, and radiological aspects of royal ancient Egyptian mummies. We applied this knowledge in our studies of the mummies, and it aided in solving several mysteries, which will be presented for the first time in this book.

2

The Story of the Royal Caches

Historical Introduction

We owe the priests of Dynasties Twenty-one and Twenty-two a great debt for preserving the royal mummies. They transferred the mummies from their original tombs to caches in order to hide them away from tomb robbers. Thus far, two caches have been discovered. The first was found at Deir al-Bahari and is known as DB320. The second was found in the tomb of Amenhotep II, KV35 in the Valley of the Kings, and it is believed that KV57 (the tomb of Horemheb) may have contained a third cache.[1] It is possible that there are more still hidden under the sands of Egypt. Many of the Eighteenth Dynasty queens, for instance, are unaccounted for.

If the priests had not saved the mummies and moved them to a safe location, it is unlikely that they would have survived until the present because of tomb robberies that took place at the end of the New Kingdom.

They saw what had happened to the royal tombs at that time and took action to save them for the future. The Valley of the Kings was plagued by multiple tomb robberies, and most of its tombs were broken into. The tomb of Tutankhamun was the only one found intact, though it had been entered in ancient times by tomb robbers and resealed, and another few tombs were found semi-intact, such as the tombs of Amenhotep II (KV35), Yuya and Thuya (KV46), and Maiherperi (KV36). There are many papyri that tell us about the destruction of the tombs and the court proceedings that followed, most notably the Abbott and Amherst papyri. The records indicate that the tombs began to be violated during the reigns of Ramesses IX and Ramesses XI. The poverty of the people during the reign of Ramesses IX, caused by unstable political and economic conditions, was a factor that led them to contemplate the gold and treasures inside the royal tombs.

They began to break the seals of the tombs and steal the objects that were valuable.

The two main papyri that tell us the story are dated to the reign of Ramesses IX.[2] The tale began when the mayor of the east bank of Luxor, called Paser, received a report that the tomb of Amenhotep I had been robbed. It seems that there was jealousy or hatred between him and Paweraa, the mayor of the west bank, where the tomb was located. The tomb of Amenhotep I was important to the workmen at Deir al-Medina who cut and decorated the royal tombs because they worshiped him as their patron under whose reign the village was established. Paser wanted to make the vizier, to whom he reported the violation, take action when he heard the name of this sacred king. It seems also that Paser wanted to suggest that Paweraa, who was responsible for the protection of the tombs in the west bank, was corrupt, but that Paser could be trusted by the vizier.

The thieves had begun by stealing from private tombs in the necropolis of the west bank and later began to enter the royal tombs in the Valley of the Kings. They were confident that the authorities were closing their eyes because they took a share of the pillage, but the report of Paser was unexpected. The vizier appointed a committee to investigate, with Paweraa and the chief of the police as members. Their report indicated that the thieves entered some tombs, including that of the Seventeenth Dynasty king Sobekemsaf, but that the tomb of Amenhotep I was safe. Paweraa had several people arrested, and one suspect confessed to having entered the tomb of Queen Iset, wife of Ramesses III. The vizier, Khaemwaset, decided to go to the Valley of the Queens to see the situation for himself. However, the suspect, when brought to the scene in the presence of the vizier and Paweraa, was unable to identify the location of the tomb, even after a brutal beating.

Court proceedings began in the vizier's presence, and Paser himself served on this court. The vizier confirmed his findings that the tombs were safe after a personal inspection of the valley. It is possible that the vizier was a part of the plot and was supportive of Paweraa. He issued an order after the court decision to drop the charges, and the court decreed that Paser was a liar.

Paweraa was presumably happy with the results, and he gathered a group of his supporters and crossed the Nile to the east bank and began to celebrate in front of Paser's house. The two parties of Paweraa and Paser became involved in an argument, with the result that Paweraa sent a report to the vizier against Paser.

The investigation continued, eventually implicating tomb workers who lived in Deir al-Medina. Much important information was extracted from the tomb robbers during vicious interrogations. The tomb of Iset, the queen of Ramesses III, had actually been attacked through the rear of the tomb, and the tombs of Seti I and Ramesses II had been robbed.

The priests of the succeeding Twenty-first and Twenty-second Dynasties made it their task to preserve the mummies after all the destruction that came to pass during the reigns of Ramesses IX and Ramesses XI. The high priest Pinudjem was primarily responsible for the safety of the royal mummies and also those of his priestly ancestors. Some scholars believe that these Twenty-first Dynasty priests were themselves looking for the treasures and the gold.[3] In the opinion of this author, this is unlikely, because if they were simply searching for gold, they would never have hidden the mummies in the secret locations they chose.

They began to transfer the royal mummies from one tomb to another. We have evidence, for example, that they moved the mummy of Ramesses I to the tomb of his son Seti I, and then selected hidden locations that fortunately remained undisturbed until modern times.

The Cache of Deir al-Bahari (DB320)

The date and circumstances of the discovery of this cache of royal mummies in the nineteenth century are uncertain, because the finders of the tomb, the Abdel Rasoul family, were very secretive and never revealed the correct information. To this day, it is the habit of the people of Upper Egypt in general not to talk a lot, keeping all of their secrets inside. The story of the discovery has achieved mythic proportions over the years, and even the names of the perpetrators vary in different accounts (see sidelight, "The Abdel Rasoul Family").

The villains in this story are the members of the Abdel Rasoul family, headed by Mohamed Abdel Rasoul and his two brothers, Ahmed and Hussein. Some stories say that in a span of ten years, they entered the tomb three times, but others say four times.[4] Large objects such as coffins would have been difficult to remove, but they were able to take papyri, linen from the top of the mummies, small boxes full of *shawabti*s, scarabs, and statues of Osiris. They entered surreptitiously at night to remove objects, which they began to sell to the antiquities market in Europe in 1874.

Upon hearing rumors of important objects appearing on the market, Auguste Mariette Pasha, the head of the Antiquities Service, began to investigate, but he died at the beginning of 1881. Mariette's successor, Gaston Maspero, continued the inquiry and went to Luxor on April 3, 1881, accompanied by the Egyptologists Victor Loret, Emile Brugsch, and others.

Maspero had received information that the Abdel Rasoul family were suspects in a possible royal tomb robbery and were conspiring with Mustafa Agha Ayad, the vice consul of England, Belgium, and Russia, to sell the objects. It was impossible to search the house of Ayad, which was located in front of the temple of Luxor, because of his diplomatic status.[5]

On April 14, Maspero sent a letter to the chief of the Luxor police to arrest Ahmed Abdel Rasoul, and he sent a telegram to Daoud Pasha,[6] the governor of the provincial capital at Qena, and the minister of public works, Fakhry Pasha, who was in charge of antiquities, to undertake an investigation with the leaders of the village of Sheikh Abd al-Qurna.

The police arrested Ahmed Abdel Rasoul when he was coming back from his work in the mountain and took him across the Nile to the east bank. Emile Brugsch, who was assistant curator at the Bulaq Museum, and Mohamed Bialy, the vice deputy of the governorate, interrogated him in Maspero's presence. They accused him of selling papyri, statues, and *shawabti*s from a secret tomb, but Abdel Rasoul denied everything. They also searched his house and found little. Despite this, Ahmed and his brothers Mohamed and Hussein were taken to prison for questioning before their trial. They were subjected to all sorts of methods of interrogation, from beating and threats to promises that they would receive a reward if they revealed any information. The investigation was unable to produce any evidence against them, and all the witnesses were on their side. The sheikhs of the villages swore that the Abdel Rasouls were honest men and would never steal anything or hide antiquities.

Mustafa Agha, the vice consul, did not come to the aid of the Abdel Rasouls, and Ahmed Abdel Rasoul believed that he would not help his faithful friends.[7] Ahmed, along with his brother Hussein, was held for two months in prison and he suffered a lot, but due to the lack of evidence, the police freed him under the recognizance of two people from Qurna, Ahmed Serour and Ismail Sayed Naguib. He arrived at the village "bearing the weapon of honesty"[8] (though he certainly had not been honest!) in the middle of May, but he could not forget the hardships that he had faced in prison and the betrayal of Mustafa Agha.

A rift cleaved the family because Ahmed Abdel Rasoul requested half of the share in the cache due to his sufferings in prison, and he threatened that if they did not agree, he would reveal the secret tomb to the antiquities authorities. After a month of fighting and discussion among the family members, they were all suspicious of each other, and each of the brothers was afraid that one of them would disclose the secret to the police.

Their fears were not in vain, because Mohamed, the elder brother, went secretly to Qena on June 25 and informed the director that he would lead them to the location of the cache. Daoud Pasha heard the news and informed the minister of the interior, who in turn informed the khedive.

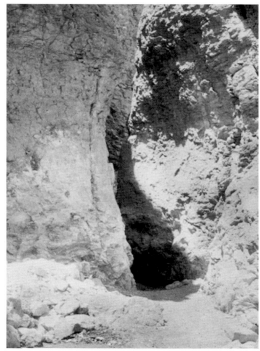

Fig. 10: View of DB320.

Daoud Pasha went in the company of Mohamed to the cache and viewed all the treasures of the tomb, including the mummies and coffins. A message to Brugsch concerning the tomb and its contents was translated from Arabic to French by Ahmed Pasha Kamal, the first Egyptian scholar of Egyptology, on June 28, 1881. Maspero was in Europe, but the khedive ordered Emile Brugsch, Ahmed Pasha Kamal, and others to travel to Luxor. They began the boat trip to Luxor on July 1.

On July 6, Mohamed Abdel Rasoul led them to the cache. It was the perfect place to hide the royal mummies due to its inaccessibility (fig. 10). The tomb shaft was twelve meters deep and two meters wide. On the western wall, there was a doorway. Spread through a long corridor and side chamber were the mummies, coffins, and funerary goods.

It was a great shock to all the Egyptologists who entered the tomb to encounter the great pharaohs, such as Seqenenre, Ahmose, Thutmose III, Seti I, and Ramesses II.[9] It took them forty-eight hours to take everything out of the shaft, and the coffins were so heavy that they required a large group of men to carry them. The transportation of the objects was a challenge also because there were many small artifacts that could be easily stolen, but the police secured the mission. Unfortunately, no proper recording of the tomb's contents in situ was done because the operation was undertaken in such haste for security reasons.

All the objects and the mummies were stored in a boat called *Le Menshieh*, owned by the Antiquities Department, for their journey to Cairo. The people of Qurna were unhappy that their ancestors were leaving them. Men, women, and children came to the west bank of the Nile and lamented tearfully.[10] The best re-creation of this scene is by a famous film director, the late Shadi Abdel Salam, in the 1969 film *al-Mummia*, "The Mummy," also known as "The Night of Counting the Years."

Three days later, *Le Menshieh* arrived in Cairo. When the boat reached the customs office in Bulaq, the customs officer declared that these mummies could not enter Cairo because in the customs book there was no item called "mummy." But the officer permitted the mummies to enter under the category of "salted fish." The mummies were removed to the Bulaq Museum, and the tomb in Deir al-Bahari was sealed but reopened again in January 1882 for a final investigation.

Maspero was able to analyze hieratic inscriptions found on the wall near the entrance door to the cache recording the burial of the high priest Pinudjem II, whose mummy and coffin were found in the tomb.[11] Hieratic dockets (inscriptions) found inked onto the coffins and wrappings of the mummies provided further information and allowed for the identification of individual mummies.

In November 1882, Ismail Pasha Ayoub was able to raise funds to build more rooms in the Bulaq Museum that would provide better lighting. In the same year, Mahmoud Pasha Fahmy, the new minister of public works, issued an order to install the mummies in glass vitrines. However, because of flooding at the Bulaq Museum, the objects and mummies were eventually transferred to the palace of Ismail Pasha at Giza (Giza Museum) until the opening of the Egyptian Museum in Tahrir Square in 1902.

A new extension to the Egyptian Museum was built and the mummies were exhibited in one room in 1958, the first time that they were shown to the public in this museum. In 1980, President Sadat ordered the closing of the room, which reopened in 1989 with a better display than before. It was upgraded in 2002, and a second room was also prepared for the royal mummies. The mummies of the kings will be transferred to the new Civilization Museum, which was scheduled to open in 2012, but due to unrest in Egypt, its opening has been postponed.

The Second Royal Cache: The Tomb of Amenhotep II (KV35)

A second cache of royal mummies was discovered hidden inside the tomb of Amenhotep II, KV35 in the Valley of the Kings (plate 6), by Victor Loret.

Loret (fig. 12) was appointed as the head of antiquities in 1897, and his dream was to excavate in the Valley of the Kings. He was excavating at Saqqara in August 1897, but he redirected his work to the Valley of the Kings,

SIDELIGHT:
The Abdel Rasoul Family

Two dates, 1871 and 1875, for the discovery of the cache by Abdel Rasoul's family have been cited in the literature through the years. I believe that 1871 is possible, because I heard this from older-generation Egyptian Egyptologists. But it may have been even earlier, with the objects secreted from the tomb over a period of many years. The discovery occurred, as many people have explained it, when one of the members of the family was leading his goats on the west bank, and one goat ran away up the valley from Deir al-Bahari. He ran after the goat and while trying to catch it stumbled upon the shaft to the tomb. This is the story that is depicted in Shadi Abdel Salam's 1969 film mentioned in this chapter.

I believe that, though this makes for a good tale, the real story is that members of the Abdel Rasoul family, who knew the west bank as they knew the lines on their hands, were in touch with antiquities dealers. They were searching for hidden tombs and found this cache by accident.

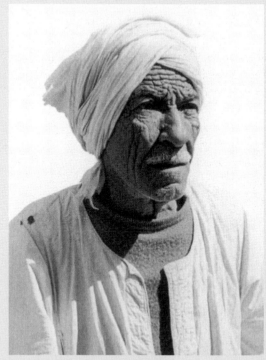

Fig. 11: Sheikh Ali Abdel Rasoul.

The names of the family members also became a legend, and everyone had his own version. Gaston Maspero wrote of the circumstances surrounding the discovery in 1889, though he was not present for the opening of the tomb, and named Abderrassoul Ahmed [sic], Mohammed Abderrasoul, and Husséïn-Ahmed as the culprits.[12] Selim Hassan, who was a friend of most of the people involved with this discovery, wrote in 1951 that the family of Abdel Rasoul consisted of Abdel Rasoul Ahmed and his brothers Mohamed and Hussein, and that Abdel Rasoul Ahmed was the one arrested.[13] Ahmed Fakhry, another member of Hassan's generation, also mentioned three brothers, and named Mohamed as the one who led the police to the cache.[14] More recently, Salima Ikram and Aidan Dodson name Ahmed Abdel Rasoul and his brother Mohamed,[15] and Dennis Forbes, following Maspero, names Ahmed and Hussein.[16]

In order to clarify the situation, I called Sayed Abdel Rasoul, the son of Sheikh Ali Abdel Rasoul (fig. 11), who is known for his search for the end of the tunnel inside the tomb of Seti I in 1960.[17] Sayed, who lives now on the west bank and owns the al-Marsam Hotel, told me that at that time, the family was headed by his great-grandfather Abdel Rasoul. His elder son, Mohamed, who led the police to the cache, had two brothers, one called Abdel Rasoul Abdel Rasoul, and the second Abdel Rahman Abdel Rasoul. It is also important to note that the correct spelling of the family name is Abdel Rasoul.

The story of the mummies' cache had the trappings of a myth and seems destined to remain one.

Z.H.

possibly because he heard the gossip of tourists in Luxor. Apparently Mohamed Abdel Rasoul, who had been given a position as *rais* (overseer) of Theban excavations, was telling the visitors that he knew the location of an undiscovered tomb, and Loret remembered Mohamed Abdel Rasoul's part in the discovery of the Deir al-Bahari cache.[18]

Loret arrived at Luxor on January 30, 1898. He issued an order the next day to Hassan Effendi Hosni, inspector of Qurna, to do a survey in the southernmost end of the Valley of the Kings, in the area between the tombs of Ramesses III and Seti II.

Loret's workmen informed him on February 12, 1898, while he was in Aswan, that they had found the entrance of a tomb, which proved to be KV34, the tomb of Thutmose III. Loret returned to Thebes, and while the excavation of the tomb was underway, he also began sondages, or trial trenches, in the center of the valley. On the evening of March 8, the entrance of another tomb was found. Upon exploring it, he discerned that this tomb belonged to Amenhotep II, the son and successor of Thutmose III, and he hoped that the mummy of the king would be resting inside, because the mummy of Amenhotep II had not been found in the DB320 cache of mummies in 1881.[19]

In a side room (no. 1, to the right off the burial chamber), he found three mummies (figs. 13a–c). The first is known as the mummy of the 'Elder Lady.'[20] Her left arm was on her chest, and her long hair was visible. There has long been speculation that this mummy is that of Queen Tiye, the wife of Amenhotep III. The mummy was examined by CT during our mummy project and DNA samples were taken in an attempt to confirm its identity (see chapter 7, "Investigations into King Tutankhamun's Family").

The second mummy belonged to a young boy with a shaved head displaying the side-lock of youth. It was Loret's opinion that he died at the age of fifteen and could be Prince Webensenu, son of Amenhotep II.

The third mummy is known as the 'Younger Lady.' The head is shaved. The right hand is lost, and the left arm extends downward. The lower part of the face is severely damaged. Loret said when he examined the mummy that she appeared to have "died choking on a gag" because of a plug of linen stuffed into the lower part of the face.[21] This mummy has been identified in the past as the mummy of Queen Nefertiti without any accurate evidence. The Egyptian Mummy Project included the mummy in its investigations (see chapters 7, "Investigations into King Tutankhamun's Family," and 8, "The Search for the Mummy of Queen Nefertiti").

Loret also found a mummy in the antechamber inside a wooden model barque.[22] This mummy has been tentatively identified as the mummy of King Sethnakht,[23] also without any solid evidence.

On March 31, Loret began to open another sealed room off the burial chamber that he designated no. 4. It had been blocked with narrow blocks of stone in antiquity, but a small hole in the top allowed him to peer in. He was surprised to discover nine coffins

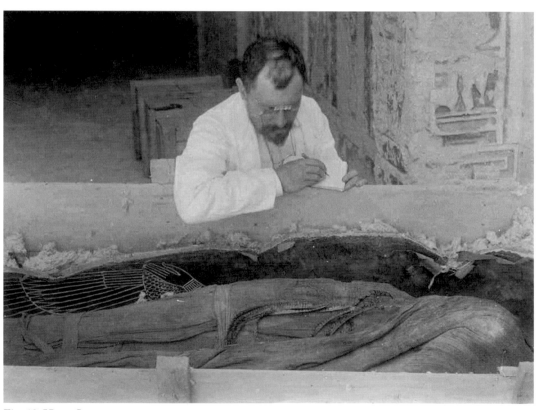

Fig. 12: Victor Loret.

set in two rows on the floor of the room, which was 3 meters by 4 meters. There were six in the back and three in the front; five coffins had their lids and four were without them. Loret thought before he examined them that they could be relatives of Amenhotep II, similar to what he found in the tomb of Thutmose III, but the mummies in that tomb were eventually determined to belong to a later period.

Loret commenced studying the coffins, taking their measurements, describing each coffin in detail, and recording the hieratic inscriptions found on the bandages of the mummies. He was able to identify the following mummies: Thutmose IV; his son and successor Amenhotep III, found inside a coffin base inscribed for Ramesses III with the lid for Seti II; Merenptah, who was placed inside the coffin base of Sethnakht; Seti II; his successor Siptah, in a reused coffin, inscribed but illegible; Ramesses IV, found in a reused coffin made originally for the *wab*-priest Aha-aa; Ramesses V; Ramesses VI, found in a reused coffin made originally for the First Prophet of Amun, Ray; and an unknown woman, who was lying on the overturned lid of the coffin of Sethnakht. This mummy is thought to be that of Queen Tawosret, but also without conclusive evidence.[24]

The last mummy found was that of Amenhotep II, inside his quartzite sarcophagus in the burial chamber (fig. 14). This was the first mummy of a king to be found intact in his tomb. (The mummy of Tutankhamun was the second.)

Victor Loret found more than two thousand objects in the tomb, and we know that Howard Carter found in the intact tomb KV62 of Tutankhamun 5,398 objects.

The voyage of the mummies

Loret thought that it was best for the security of the mummies to move them to Cairo, because the tomb was not safe. He submitted all the necessary applications and wrote letters to Fakhry Pasha, who was the minister of public works, since antiquities fell under this ministry. He removed the top four layers of stones blocking the room off the burial chamber, put all the mummies in boxes, and prepared to sail on a cargo boat to Cairo. After he set sail, he received an unwelcome surprise in the form of a message sent from the minister ordering him to return the mummies to the tomb.[25] Apparently Sir Flinders Petrie, the British archaeologist who is known as the father of Egyptology, was not on good terms with Loret. The reasons are unclear; perhaps it was jealousy between Egyptologists that we sometimes see today. At any rate, he succeeded in inciting public opinion, which concluded that it was not good for the mummies to be removed from the tomb.[26]

This was a shock to Loret. He wrote to other authorities from Nag' Hammadi on April 7, 1898 that he could not return to the south against the Nile current because this would be dangerous for the mummies. Loret wrote that he had moved the mummies based on a written agreement and that he needed to travel to Cairo to meet the minister. But he had no luck and was ordered to bring the mummies back to the tomb.

Loret was right that the mummies should have gone to Cairo to be exhibited at the Bulaq Museum. The mummies were, after all, not found in their original tombs. Most of these tombs are open to the public, which could place the mummies in danger, a concern that proved all too true. Also, the tomb of Amenhotep II would be an unsuitable place

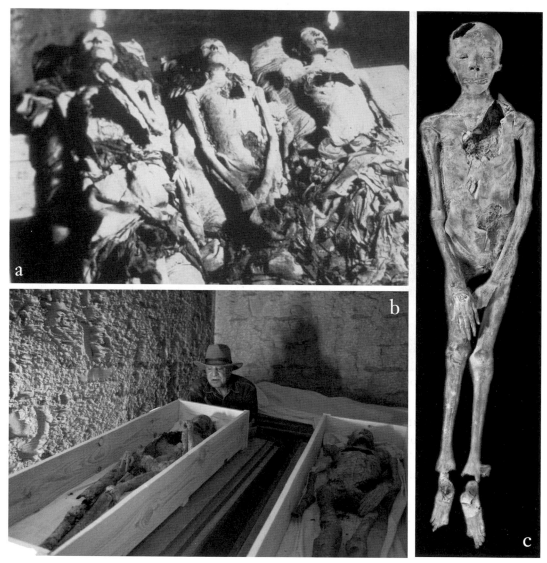

Figs. 13a–c: Three mummies found in the tomb of Amenhotep II (a). The two mummies known as the Elder Lady (left) and Younger Lady (right) before their transfer to the Egyptian Museum in Cairo for examination (b). The unidentified young male mummy (c).

for the preservation of the mummies due to the changes in temperature and humidity caused by large numbers of visitors.

Loret was forced to comply with the minister's wishes, but he continued his excavation in the Valley of the Kings in 1899. He found the tomb of Maiherperi (KV36), who was a close companion to the king and royal fan bearer, on March 30, 1899. He also discovered KV37, an Eighteenth Dynasty tomb

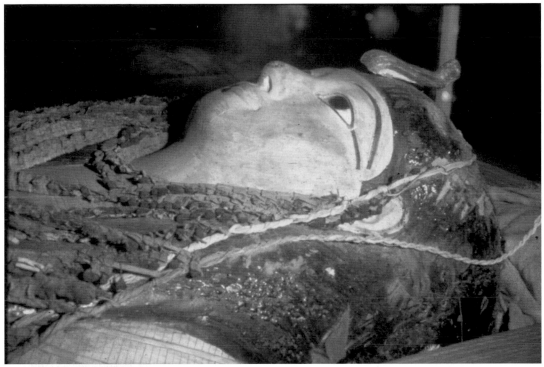

Fig. 14: Archival photograph of the mummy of Amenhotep II in the Egyptian Museum, Cairo.

whose original occupant is unknown, on April 6, and KV38, which housed the sarcophagus of Thutmose I and may have been prepared for his reburial, on April 11. At the end of that year, however, he was forced to resign. He returned to his native France and took with him all the records of his work in Egypt, intending to take the needed time to publish all of his amazing discoveries. Unfortunately, he never did.[27]

In January 1890, Maspero became the director of the Antiquities Department for the second time. He ordered Howard Carter, who was then an antiquities inspector in Luxor, to send the mummies found in KV35 back to Cairo, in response to a request from Carter that all the identified mummies should be transferred. All nine mummies found in room 4 inside KV35 were moved to Cairo.

What was then left in the tomb were the mummy of Amenhotep II inside the sarcophagus, the mummy found atop the barque, and the three unidentified mummies, which Carter also placed in side room no. 1 off the burial chamber. Disastrously, in November 1901, tomb robbers entered the tomb of Amenhotep II. They stole the barque that was holding the mummy, which they shattered to pieces. The thieves rifled inside the mummy of Amenhotep II, searching for amulets and gold, damaging the mummy in the process.

Carter suspected that the Abdel Rasoul family was responsible, and he sent Mohamed Abdel Rasoul and his brothers to prison after he found evidence of Mohamed's footprint on the dust of the tomb. But the evidence did not hold up, and the brothers once again were freed. Despite the depredation, the mummy of Amenhotep II remained on view in the tomb until 1931, when it was sent to Cairo by first class in a sleeper train, which left the three unidentified mummies in room no. 1.[28]

When we recently established the identities of the Elder and Younger Ladies (see chapters 7 and 8), these two mummies were moved to the Egyptian Museum, where they are exhibited now outside the second mummy room. Only the mummy of the unknown young boy remains inside the tomb.

The Mummies in the Valley of the Kings

The mummy of Tutankhamun could be the only mummy to be discovered in situ and never moved from his tomb since he was buried. And it is the only identified mummy now in the Valley of the Kings. The other mummy found in situ, that of Amenhotep II, discovered by Victor Loret, was damaged in antiquity, and the priests of the Twenty-first Dynasty moved the mummy, rewrapped it, and replaced it in his sarcophagus.

Howard Carter was keen to move all the identified mummies to Cairo and leave the unidentified mummies inside the tombs, but it is strange that he did not move the mummy of Tutankhamun to Cairo as the other mummies had been. When we embarked on our first mummy-scanning project and saw the mummy of King Tut, the reason was apparent. Its condition was so poor that Carter could not risk showing it to the public. When he opened the sarcophagus inside the tomb in 1925 and found the golden mask that was placed over the head and chest of the mummy (plate 7), he tried to remove the mask, but could not because of the resin that was applied to the mummy and coffins, which had

adhered the mask to the mummy. Thinking that heat would soften the resin, he took the mummy outside the tomb and exposed it to the sun. This did not work. Thereupon he moved the mummy to the tomb of Seti II, which he used as a lab, and employed hot knives to take off the mask. In doing so, Carter badly damaged the mummy. After removing the mask and the amulets found on the body, he transferred the mummy to a tray filled with sand and replaced it inside the sarcophagus.

When our mummy project came to the Valley of the Kings, we found many unidentified mummies, such as one of two female mummies that Carter found in 1903 in KV60. He moved the other one, identified as Sitre-In, the wet nurse of Queen Hatshepsut, to Cairo, and left the unidentified mummy in the tomb. This mummy was designated for study during our project (see chapter 3, "The Discovery of the Mummy of Queen Hatshepsut, and Examination of the Mummies of Her Family"); it is now at the Egyptian Museum.

The project recovered two more female mummies, one of them without a head. Donald Ryan rediscovered them in 1989 in KV21, a tomb probably of the Eighteenth Dynasty, and restored them and placed them in boxes (figs. 58a–b). We moved them to the Egyptian Museum when we began to search for the mummies of Ankhesenamun and Nefertiti (see chapter 8).

We also moved another unidentified mummy that was found in 1904–1905, in the debris outside the tomb of Seti II, first to a storage magazine in 2007, and later to the Egyptian Museum.

Besides Tutankhamun, the Valley of the Kings now houses only the mummy of the boy inside KV35 and another mummy of a boy found in a storeroom off the burial chamber of the tomb of Thutmose IV (KV43).

The Egyptian Mummy Project is determined to identify all the royal mummies. We still have many mummies whose identities are unknown, including 'Unknown Man C' and 'Unknown Women A, B, and C.' As we will see below (chapter 10, "Dynasty Twenty: Ramesses III, Pentawere, and the Harem Conspiracy"), we were able to ascertain the identity of 'Unknown Man E.' Through our studies, we can also answer most of the questions that have been raised by James Harris, Edward Wente, and Dennis Forbes in their previous studies, for example their observation that the mummy of Seti II is more similar to the Thutmosid than the Ramesside kings. The Egyptian Mummy Project, with the aid of the new technologies of CT scanning and DNA analysis, can solve the mystery of the royal mummies.

3

The Discovery of the Mummy of Queen Hatshepsut, and Examination of the Mummies of Her Family

Historical Introduction

It seems important for this chapter to shed a brief light on the historical record of this great queen who ruled Egypt under excellent political and economic circumstances, the opposite of other queens who ruled in less stable periods.[1]

Hatshepsut (plate 8) was the daughter of Thutmose I, who ruled during the early Eighteenth Dynasty. She married her half-brother, Thutmose II, who came to the throne after the death of her father. Hatshepsut's titles during this time included King's Daughter, King's Sister, Great Royal Wife, and God's Wife of Amun. She bore a daughter called Neferure, and Thutmose II also had a son, Thutmose III (plate 9), by a secondary wife, Iset. Thutmose II had a brief reign of only a few years. After his death, Thutmose III, who was probably a young child, took the throne with Hatshepsut serving as his regent. By the time that seven years had passed in their joint reign, Hatshepsut began to assume masculine, kingly titles and effectively became the sole ruler. To legitimize her rule, she created a legendary religious story stating that the oracle of the god Amun had declared her pharaoh. She also emphasized her descent through the royal line of her father, depicting herself as the offspring of Amun in the guise of Thutmose I. However, Thutmose III is still depicted beside her as coregent, his name inscribed beside hers in a cartouche in the Red Chapel at Karnak,[2] which housed the barque of the god Amun.

Hatshepsut raised Thutmose III as a king and probably sent him for military training in Memphis, the primary royal residence and the Egyptian administrative capital, with the goal of leading the Egyptian army and expanding the empire. It was the custom for the children of New Kingdom kings to receive their education and military training in Memphis. It is possible that Thutmose III led military campaigns late in their core-gency; if he was entrusted with military power, it suggests that he was not viewed as a threat to her reign.[3]

Hatshepsut gave her daughter to Thutmose III as a wife.[4] She appears with the title Great Royal Wife in the temple of Thutmose III at Qurna[5] and had the title Mistress of the Two Lands, a title only given to a ruler, on the walls of the mortuary temple of her mother at Deir al-Bahari.[6] Neferure was shown as a royal wife, wearing the vulture crown of the goddess Nekhbet, which was the crown that the royal wives had worn since the Old Kingdom. Her name was placed in a cartouche, as were the names of some other queens of the New Kingdom, such as Queen Nefertari of the Nineteenth Dynasty. The image of Princess Neferure on the walls of the temple of her mother is an official recognition by Hatshepsut that Thutmose III was the one who would suc-ceed her as king. This could be taken as evidence that no conflict existed between Hatshepsut and Thutmose III.

There were many officials[7] who played a prominent role in the life of Queen Hatshepsut, such as the two viziers Ahmose and User. The vizier Hapuseneb also served as the High Priest of Amun and directed Hatshepsut's ambitious building program at Karnak temple. The treasurer Nehesy was responsible for Hatshepsut's renowned trading expedition to the land of Punt, whose location is debated by scholars, but which may have been adjacent to the Red Sea in east Africa. The chief steward Amenhotep arranged her royal jubilee in Year 16, which included the erection of two obelisks in front of the main entrance to

Karnak temple, of which only one is still in situ.[8] It is the tallest in Egypt, at 29.5 meters, and weighs 323 tons. The most prominent official of her reign, who has often been cited as her architect and intimate, was the royal steward Senenmut,[9] who oversaw the building of her mortuary temple at Deir al-Bahari (plate 10) and also built a small tem-ple for the god Pakhet at Establ Antar in Middle Egypt. At the Aswan granite quar-ries, Senenmut left an inscription indicating his responsibility for the cutting of two obelisks that Hatshepsut had ordered for the temple at Karnak, and the transport of these is illustrated on the walls of her Deir al-Bahari temple.

Two tombs are attributed to Hatshepsut. The first is a cliff tomb at Wadi Sikket Taqa al-Zeide, which was documented by Howard Carter in 1916[10] after he was informed that tomb robbers had located it. This tomb was prepared for Hatshepsut before she assumed power as king. The second is number KV20 in the Valley of the Kings. James Burton par-tially cleared it in 1824, and Howard Carter continued the work in 1903 for Theodore Davis.[11] He believed that it was a double tomb built for Hatshepsut and her father before she became the queen of Egypt. However, it is now generally accepted that the tomb, the first in the Valley of the Kings, was begun by Thutmose I and finished by Hatshepsut to house both burials. Thutmose I was later moved to KV38, a tomb prepared for him by his grandson, Thutmose III.[12]

The mummy of the queen was never found. Some scholars believed that she was buried in her south tomb in Wadi Sikket Taqa al-Zeide. Others believed that she was buried in her tomb at the Valley of the Kings.[13]

The Search for the Queen

We began the search for the mummy of the queen by investigating the following relevant sites and objects:

A. Tomb KV20
B. Mummies of women from the cache of royal mummies at Deir al-Bahari (DB320): Unknown Women A and B
C. Mummies from cache KV35
  1. The Elder Lady
  2. The Younger Lady
  3. Unknown Woman D
D. Hatshepsut's family members:
  1. The mummy of Thutmose I
  2. The mummy of Thutmose II
  3. The mummy of Thutmose III
E. Objects associated with the queen: the wooden box from DB320
F. Mummies and objects from KV60
  1. Mummy KV60 A
  2. Mummy KV60 B

A. Tomb KV20

KV20 was first recorded by Napoleon's expedition to Egypt in 1799, and in 1817 Belzoni again recorded its location. The entrance (fig. 15) and a small area inside were cleared by James Burton in 1824, but in 1903, Howard Carter was able to completely excavate and clear the tomb on behalf of Theodore Davis. KV20 consists of three tunnel-like passageways connected by stairwells, extending more than 200 meters (nearly 700 feet), where they reach an antechamber and burial chamber at a depth of over 100 meters (300 feet) below the entrance. It is very difficult to enter or to walk within it because the incline is steep and the ground is slippery. It is believed that the original intention was to locate the burial chamber directly under the holy of holies of the mortuary temple of Queen Hatshepsut at Deir al-Bahari, but that this had proven impossible due to the poor quality of the limestone. Therefore,

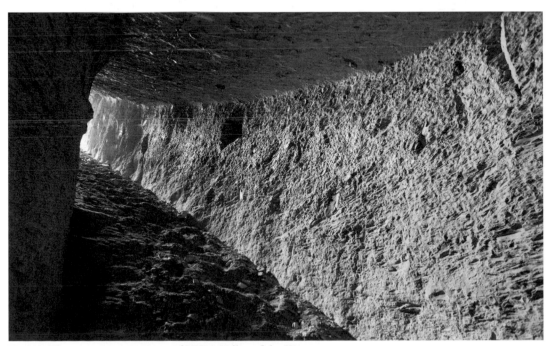

Fig. 15: The entrance passageway of KV20, Valley of the Kings.

over the course of their length, the passageways bend to form a half circle. The tomb, however, was never completely finished.[14]

Carter and Davis found a quartzite sarcophagus in the burial chamber, now in the Egyptian Museum in Cairo,[15] belonging to Hatshepsut as pharaoh, and another one, now in the Museum of Fine Arts, Boston,[16] originally made for Hatshepsut but reinscribed for her father.[17] Funerary furnishings discovered in the tomb included a canopic chest inscribed for Hatshepsut; fifteen slabs of limestone with red and black drawings and inscriptions from the Book of Amduat ("That Which Is in the Underworld"), which would have been placed on the walls of the tomb, since the stone of the walls was of inadequate quality for decoration; fragments of a blue-glazed *shawabti* coffin; remains of stone vessels with the names of Ahmose-Nefertari, Thutmose I, Queen Ahmose, Thutmose II, and Hatshepsut; fragments of faience; part of a head and foot of a large wooden statue; and remains from the mummification process.[18]

Carter believed that this double burial chamber was originally built for Thutmose I, and that Hatshepsut was later buried in the tomb, using the discovery of their two sarcophagi as proof. But others, including this author, believe that Queen Hatshepsut cut this tomb and ordered that her father should be reburied with her. The other tomb that was cut in Wadi Sikket Taqa al-Zeide was made for her when she was a queen, and would have been deemed unsuitable for the burial of a pharaoh.

B. The cache of royal mummies at Deir al-Bahari (DB320)

For this investigation, it was a priority to visit most of the important places that were connected with Queen Hatshepsut. (See sidelight,

"Adventure in the Valley.") The second such site was the cache of the mummies at Deir al-Bahari, because there were two female mummies in the cache that we thought should be examined, as well as a wooden box inscribed for Hatshepsut.

The mummy of an elderly woman from the cache is known as Unknown Woman B.[19] Some scholars believe that this mummy belongs to Queen Tetisheri of the Seventeenth Dynasty, the wife of Seqenenre Tao I and the mother of both Seqenenre Tao II and his queen Ahhotep. This lady was not of royal origin. She lived at a time when the Egyptians were beginning their struggle for independence against the Hyksos invaders. The mummy was found inside a coffin dated to Dynasty Twenty-one that had been inscribed with the name of Ramesses I. (For the mummy of Ramesses I, see the introduction). The length of the mummy of Unknown Woman B is 157 cm. Her head is bald in front, with the remaining white hair in curls with false black locks attached. Her ears are pierced for earrings, a common style of the New Kingdom. The face is oval in shape, short, and with a pointed chin. When it was discovered, the mummy was covered with black resin, the residue from the funeral and burial ceremonies. The head and the right arm of the mummy are broken. Previous x-ray studies of this mummy focused only on her mouth and teeth.

The second mummy from DB320 relevant to our study is another elderly woman, Unknown Woman A.[20] This mummy was poorly preserved, and the mummification was not of the highest quality. The upper teeth are lost, and there is no hair. Though the docket on the mummy's wrappings identified her as the "king's daughter and king's sister,

Merytamun," of the late Seventeenth or early Eighteenth Dynasty, Maspero studied the mummification style and thought that it was not of royal origin, dating it to the Middle Kingdom. However, Elliott Smith, who also studied this mummy, found nothing that would warrant a date outside the New Kingdom. He remarked that the position of the body was unusual: the head bends to the side, and the two legs are crossed below the knees. The mouth is wide open as well. It may be that she suffered some kind of trauma before death. The left leg is broken in the front and the two arms were cut off, possibly by thieves or maybe by the priests who moved this mummy from its original place to DB320.[21]

These two mummies from DB320 were designated for examination by CT scan during our search for the mummy of Hatshepsut.[22]

C. Mummies from cache KV35 (see figs. 13a–b)

It was decided to include in the investigation three mummies found in this tomb:

1. The Elder Lady
2. The Younger Lady
3. Unknown Woman D

A full analysis of both the Elder Lady and the Younger Lady appears in chapter 7, "Investigations into King Tutankhamun's Family." The scanning of Unknown Woman D was abandoned as the project began to assign identities to the other mummies in the study.

D. Hatshepsut's family members

Let us concentrate here on the result of the scans of the mummies belonging to Hatshepsut's close relatives. We begin with the mummy that in the past has been identified as the queen's father, Thutmose I, although this conclusion had been questioned by many scholars.

1. The mummy of so-called Thutmose I
Genealogy of Thutmose I
Father: uncertain, perhaps Ahmose-Sipairi
Mother: Senisoneb

Identification of the mummy
The mummy was discovered in the Deir al-Bahari cache in 1881, inside a pair of nested coffins, one dated to the Eighteenth Dynasty and the other to the Twenty-first Dynasty. Both coffins had been severely damaged but were inscribed with the name of Pinudjem I, high priest and claimant to the kingship in the Twenty-first Dynasty. The presence of these cartouches led Gaston Maspero to identify the mummy as Pinudjem at first, but in 1896 he changed his mind and reidentified the mummy as Thutmose I.[23] Maspero also expressed the opinion that the facial features of this mummy were very similar to those of Thutmose II and III. The mummy was the proper age to be Thutmose I, Maspero also conjectured, because that king should have been over fifty years old when he died. G. Elliot Smith corroborated these conclusions and went on to suggest that the positioning of the mummy's arms and the mummification technique placed the mummy in line with the Eighteenth Dynasty pharaohs.[24] However, later studies by the Egyptian Mummy Project questioned this identification.

Table 4. General CT findings for the mummy of 'Thutmose I'[25]

Preservation Status	Very good
Age	About 20 years
Gender	Male
Stature	157 cm

SIDELIGHT:
Adventure in the Valley

When I went to the Valley of the Kings to search for the mummy of Queen Hatshepsut, I did not have any idea if I would succeed in finding the mummy, but I thought that it would be appropriate for me as an archaeologist to visit the sites connected with the queen that I had not previously visited. I started with KV20. I read Howard Carter's report of his clearance of the tomb in 1903 and learned that it was very difficult work to clear the tomb.

The guards came and opened the tomb. I entered for a few meters, but the surface of the floor was extremely slippery, and I found myself down on the ground. I was unable to continue, and had back pain for a month from this accident. Rais Ali Farouk, who was the *rais* in my excavations at the Valley of the Kings, was my right-hand man in all of my work in the valley. He is the last of the great people from Qift, a village north of Luxor whose residents for many years worked with archaeologists, both foreign and Egyptian, and became experts at excavation techniques. He came up with the idea to tie a long rope to a beam at the entrance, and by clutching it, I was able to ease into the tomb. That was a great help. When I approached the entrance to the burial chamber, I discovered it was closed off with debris and I had to excavate the entrance to reach the inside. The tomb had been completely cleared, and nothing remained.

I then went down to the smaller KV60, which I now believe belonged to the wet nurse of Hatshepsut. Entering the tomb was no easier than KV20, because the entrance was very steep and I had to enter from above (plate 11). There was a tunnel to the entrance, and then a jump down to the burial chamber. There I found the good work that Donald Ryan had done to preserve the KV60 A mummy by placing it in a box, which was still in the tomb, as well as recording all of the objects found in the tomb. When I removed the lid of the box and looked at the mummy, I could see that the left arm was on the chest, symbolizing royalty. We moved this mummy to the Egyptian Museum for scanning.

Great care was taken in the move; it was done very slowly by workmen under my supervision in order to avoid any disturbance to the mummy.

The next day, I entered DB320. I entered this cache on two separate occasions. The descent to the tomb was difficult. The first time I entered down the long shaft (about 12 meters down), the procedure was to use a pulley tied to a beam at the top, with the pulley connected to a basket. I climbed into the basket and was let down slowly. It was not easy. Then I asked myself a question: How did the members of the Abdel Rasoul family descend and enter the tomb three times in ten years? It was difficult, and it would have been impossible for them to remove a coffin because it was too heavy. This could explain why they entered the cache only a few times and removed only smaller objects.

We found that the entrance was sealed with chunks of limestone and cement, which were removed with the help of Rais Ali Farouk. We then entered the tomb but could only imagine the treasures that were once stored inside, since everything had been removed after the tomb's existence was revealed. I was able to explore this place in which the wooden canopic box, as well as other female mummies, had been found.

Back in Cairo, I searched for the mummy of the wet nurse Sitre-In, KV60 B, in the Egyptian Museum. The curators did not know its location. It was discovered that since the mummy was moved to Cairo in 1908, it had been neglected in a storeroom in the third-floor attic of the museum, and there were no photographs available. I was able to locate the mummy, which still lay in its coffin. At that time, I thought that this mummy could be Queen Hatshepsut.[26]

Z. H.

General position

Both upper limbs are extended. The hands are broken off and missing, but would have been placed in front of the genital area.

CT findings in different regions
Head

Brain extraction was not performed. The brain is intact, shrunken, with both hemispheres, and appearing well preserved.[27] The eyes were left in place within the orbits. There was no CT evidence of packs or embalming materials within the orbits, nose, oral cavity, or throat.

Teeth

Apart from several broken teeth, the rest appear intact and erupted. Some of the broken teeth are separated and lying loose within the oropharynx (two on the right side and one on the left side).

Spine

The spine is healthy with no sign of degeneration or disease.

Torso

The heart is present and within the right hemithorax; no other organs are identifiable within the torso. The right side of the chest is filled with concentric layers of variable CT densities that ranged between 300 HU in the outer to 705 HU in the more central parts. A thin marginal layer of lower density is observed all around this homogeneous filling.

A very dense, triangular metallic object (fig. 16) that measures about 3000 HU in density and 20 mm in length was first recognized by Hany Abdel-Rahman within the right hemithorax; it was further examined by Ashraf Selim, who determined that the shape of this object resembles the head of an arrow with a pointed tip and two wings.[28] The object was clearly shown by 3D reconstruction of the CT images done by Sahar Saleem (see chapter 12, "Amulets, Funerary Figures, and Other Objects Found on the Mummies"). A few smaller, dense metallic objects are also observed around it, and another, measuring 1 cm in length, lies just below the head of the left eleventh rib. The chest wall on the right side, particularly along the side and back, appears significantly thickened. A substance of moderate to high CT density (300–700 HU) is seen in the lower hemithorax, and the adjacent upper abdomen measures 145–675 HU. Linen fibers measuring –500 HU are seen within the left hemithorax and the abdomen.

An embalming incision measures 44 mm x 20 mm and extends obliquely in the left inguinal region. A resin-treated pack is seen at the lower margin of the embalming incision. The phallus could be identified.

Cause of Death
The presence of a metallic object within the right thoracic cavity surrounded by unusual multilayered fillings may suggest that death was due to an arrowhead that penetrated the right chest wall.[29]

Conclusions
The CT scan results were compared to previous examinations of the mummy by Maspero and Smith. Since many scholars had cast doubt on the identification of the mummy itself, the team wanted to see if the CT scans support the conclusion that this mummy is not Thutmose I. The scans show that this man died at a young age (around twenty years), whereas historical records indicate that Thutmose I died around the age of fifty. The epiphyses of the long

bones at the shoulders (proximal humerus), knees (distal femur, proximal tibia and fibula), and ankles (distal tibia and fibula) are not fused with their shafts. These findings have also been reported by plain x-rays study and helped in estimation of the age of the mummy at death.[30] In addition, the arms of the mummy are extended, rather than crossed over the chest, as is typical of the New Kingdom royal mummies. It is a fact that every known mummy of the Eighteenth Dynasty kings beginning with Amenhotep I has its arms crossed. Another important discovery is the metallic objects that can be seen in the mummy's torso, especially the arrowhead just below the eleventh rib. There are no historical records that indicate that Thutmose I died in battle; therefore the presence of the arrowhead casts even more doubt on the identification of this mummy.

In conclusion, this new evidence can be summarized as follows:

1. The mummy is too young to be King Thutmose I.
2. There is no evidence that Thutmose I died in battle, but the 'Thutmose I' mummy in our study likely died from damage inflicted by an arrowhead, which is lodged in the right upper thorax.
3. The position of the arms suggests that the mummy is not a king. Thus we can confirm that the mummy labeled at the Egyptian Museum as Thutmose I is not actually this king.

However, based on the date of the mummification (said to be early Eighteenth Dynasty), and the fact that it was included in a royal cache, it is possible that it is the mummy of some other member of the Thutmosid family.

It is conceivable that a male mummy found in front of the entrance to the tomb of Seti II is that of Thutmose I. This mummy was taken to the Egyptian Museum but has not yet been examined. Donald Ryan has proposed yet another identification for the mummy of Thutmose I. In 1906, Edward Ayrton, working for Theodore Davis, discovered KV48, an undecorated tomb consisting of a shaft and a single rectangular room. (The tomb is located in the vicinity of KV35, the tomb of Amenhotep II.) In the published report, the following is noted: "The mummy, that of a man, tall and well-built, had been unwrapped and thrown on one side."[31] A few inscribed objects in the tomb indicate that it belonged to Amenemopet, a vizier of Amenhotep II, who

also has a tomb chapel in Sheikh Abd al-Qurna (TT29). In *The Royal Necropoleis of Thebes*,[32] Elizabeth Thomas wrote, regarding the mummy, that "We are not told whether it was left in the tomb or whether it has been professionally examined." During our 2008 season in the Valley of the Kings, we opened KV48 and in 2009 finished clearing the tomb, which contained many large broken pots and their contents (linen, embalming materials, etc.) along with fragments of many other objects.[33] However, the mummy reported by Davis was not inside, and there are no known records of it ever being taken to Cairo during the early twentieth century. Could the unknown mummy called Thutmose I be that of Amenemopet from KV48?

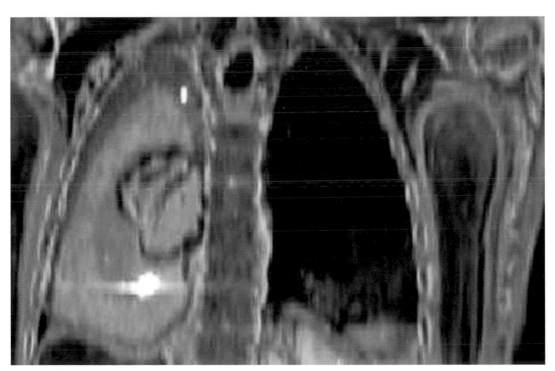

Fig. 16: CT of chest of the mummy alleged to be Thutmose I. A coronal image shows a very dense, small metallic object (the head of an arrow) in the lower right chest cavity surrounded by dense material, while the left chest cavity is almost empty.

2. The mummy of Thutmose II[34]
Genealogy
Father: Thutmose I
Mother: Mutnefret

Identification of the mummy
Found in a private coffin, which was altered with an added inscription for Thutmose II, in the Deir al-Bahari cache; the mummy had dockets identifying this king.

General position
The arms are crossed over the chest, right over left. The left hand is clenched over the right shoulder, while the right hand is flat over the chest.

CT findings in different regions
Head
Brain extraction was not performed. The nasal cavity and floor of the cranium are intact. The brain is shrunken and intact. The orbits contain dry eyes without evidence of packs. The mouth cavity and upper throat contain linen packs and linen tampons treated with resin.

Teeth
The teeth are in good condition, with minimal attrition. Both upper wisdom teeth are mesially impacted. This might have caused the king significant pain during his life. There

is no surrounding bone rarefaction to suggest superadded inflammatory changes.

Spine
The spine is in good condition; there are no fractures or congenital anomalies.

Torso
Many postmortem fractures are seen involving the right clavicle and ribs. Some of the broken bones are seen within the chest and abdominal cavities, where a large gap is noted in the front of the chest and abdominal walls. A very enlarged heart is present within the left side. The pelvic girdle is fractured in many areas. A fracture of the left sacroiliac joint has caused enfolding of the pelvis and separation of the head of the femur, resulting in a discrepancy in the length of the lower limbs, the right being longer. The embalming incision could not be identified because of the mutilated anterior wall of the torso. However, the torso is stuffed with both resin-treated and untreated linen packs. The phallus was identified.

Limbs
Both upper limbs are broken at multiple places and detached from the body, but were restored in antiquity to their original crossed-arm position. Both forearms are fractured at the elbows and bent across the chest, right over left. The palm of the right hand is flat, resting in front of the left shoulder. The thumb of the left hand is extended, while the rest of the fingers are broken and appear flexed over the right shoulder.

Cause of Death
The cause of death cannot be identified, although the large size of the heart may point to the possibility of heart disease.[35]

Table 5. General CT findings for the mummy of Thutmose II

Preservation Status	Good
Age	Around 30 years*
Gender	Male
Stature	173 cm

* In adults, age estimation has a margin of error of about a decade; see p. 22.

3. The mummy of Thutmose III[36]

Genealogy

Father: Thutmose II

Mother: Iset

Identification of the mummy

The mummy was found in its original coffin in the Deir al-Bahari cache, DB320.

General position

The body was badly mutilated by tomb robbers in antiquity. It was unwrapped in 1881 by Emile Brugsch without permission from Maspero, who ordered it rebandaged. It was then publicly unwrapped by Maspero in 1886.[37] The neck is broken at the lower border of the fourth vertebra and detached from the body. Both upper limbs are broken and detached from the body but were restored in antiquity to their original 'royal position.' The left forearm is bent at the elbow across the chest to reach the right shoulder. The right forearm was placed in front of the left. The palm of the hand is resting in front of the left shoulder. The right hand is flat, and the left is flexed with the thumb extended. The pelvic bone is broken, and most of the left foot is missing.

The height cannot be accurately estimated because of multiple postmortem fractures. However, it has been extrapolated from the femur length to be 167 cm.

CT Findings in different regions

Head

Brain extraction was not performed. The brain is shrunken at the back of the skull and intact. The floor of the cranium is intact. Both orbits contain linen packs impregnated with resin that are placed in front of the dry eye globes. Packs of linen treated with resin are placed in the anterior oral cavity; solidified resin is placed at

Table 6. General CT findings for the mummy of Thutmose III

Preservation Status	Poor
Age	Around 40 years +
Gender	Male
Stature	167 cm

the floor of the mouth, as well as the posterior of the oropharynx.

Teeth

All teeth were erupted, and none are missing. There was mild to moderate attrition that corresponds to the age at death.

Spine

Multiple postmortem fractures. The neck is fractured at the lower border of the fourth vertebra, and the lower cervical vertebrae from fifth to seventh are missing. There are mild to moderate anterior lumbar osteophytes with reduced height of the intervertebral discs, and mild to moderate osteoarthritis of uncovertebral facets and costovertebral joints.

Torso

A defect is seen on the anterior and superior part of the chest. The heart is present and shows calcification within (fig. 17). An embalming incision extends obliquely at the left inguinal region and measures 11 mm x 10 mm. The torso is stuffed with nontreated linen packs and resin-impregnated linen.

Limbs

Both arms are crossed over the chest. The left arm is disarticulated at the shoulder. The right hand is broken and disarticulated at the wrist. A thick, metallic bracelet and a thinner one are

SIDELIGHT:
Hatshepsut's Box

We began to work at night to scan the mummies. I told Brando Quilici, the director of the Discovery Channel film, that I would ask my assistant, Hisham el-Leithy, to bring the canopic box so that we could see what the liver of Queen Hatshepsut looked like. The box was under the scanner when Hany Abdel-Rahman, who operated the machine, and Ashraf Selim cried out in surprise, "There is a tooth inside the box!"

This was astonishing to me. I asked myself, Why the tooth in the box? Who put it there and why? I asked Ashraf Selim and Dr. Galal El Behiri, professor of dentistry at Cairo University, to look at this tooth and also to study all of the teeth of mummies examined for the project.

Though this is not a traditional canopic box, it is likely that the contents had become separated from the rest of the body during or after mummification, and placed here for safekeeping.

Z.H.

seen surrounding the distal forearm. Both lower limbs are disarticulated at the hips. In the left foot, only the talus and calcaneus bones are present. Through 2D and 3D reconstruction of the CT images, Sahar Saleem reported that a metallic wire was looped in place of the missing mid- and forefoot and was wrapped by linen bands. This is a modern restoration of the mummy, done in 1993 by Nasr Iskander, the director of the Egyptian Museum at that time.

Cause of death
No cause of death could be identified.[38]

Comments: The mummies of Thutmose II and III were found in the Deir al-Bahari cache, but their identities are far less ambiguous than that of 'Thutmose I.' Thutmose II was found in a private Eighteenth Dynasty coffin that had been decorated with bands of text inscribed with the name of the king. The mummy was unwrapped by Maspero in 1886 and found to be severely damaged. Fortunately, Elliot Smith was able to restore the king's limbs to their appropriate places during his examination of the mummy in 1906.

Thutmose III was found in his original wooden coffin and wrapped in his burial shroud that bore his name. He was the first mummy from the Deir al-Bahari cache to be unwrapped in 1881 by Emile Brugsch. Sadly, the great warrior king was completely dismembered. So disturbing was his appearance that unwrapping of the mummies was discontinued until 1886.

E. Objects associated with Queen Hatshepsut
A wooden, shrine-shaped box with an ivory knob was found inside the cache DB320. It is inscribed with two cartouches of Hatshepsut and contained a bundle that was said to be a liver or spleen, possibly of the queen,[39] though it was not a traditional canopic container (fig. 18).

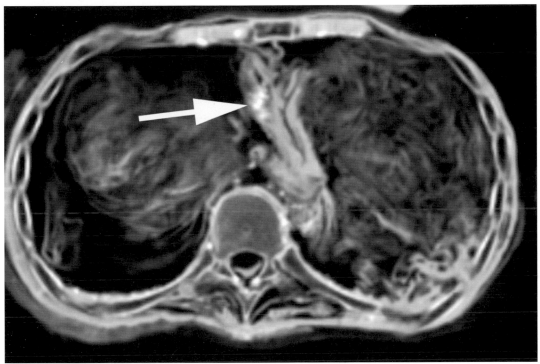

Fig. 17: Axial CT image of the chest of mummy of Thutmose III shows dense calcifications in the desiccated heart (arrow).

CT report on the wooden box

The small wooden box[40] was scanned by Ashraf Selim and Hany Abdel-Rahman (plates 12a–b). The side walls of the box are painted with resin. The box contains an oval smooth structure that is lying freely within. It measures 17.6 cm x 5.5 cm x 7 cm in length, depth, and width, respectively. It has the same density as the resin. Inside this resin structure we could identify three major items; each of them has its own coat of resin.

The largest appears as a broad, elongated, thin structure measuring 10.7 cm x 6.3 cm x 0.7 cm in length, width, and thickness respectively. It has a somewhat high CT density compared to the resin. Using different projections and computer processing, we obtained an image that could match that of a liver (fig. 19).

It is worth mentioning here that nobody has ever scanned a three-thousand-year-old shrunken liver to know how it would appear on a CT image. Without suspecting that the bundle within the box contained viscera, we might not have been able to identify it.

The second item that appeared is a long, rather thin, ribbon-like structure with an undulated surface. This could represent part or all of the intestine. The third item is formed of a few very dense small objects lying within the outer coat of the resin (fig. 20). Using different processing techniques, the longest of these appeared as a molar tooth lacking one of its roots. It measured 1.8 cm along its whole length, with the crown width of 1.1 cm, and the length of the root is 1 cm (fig. 21).

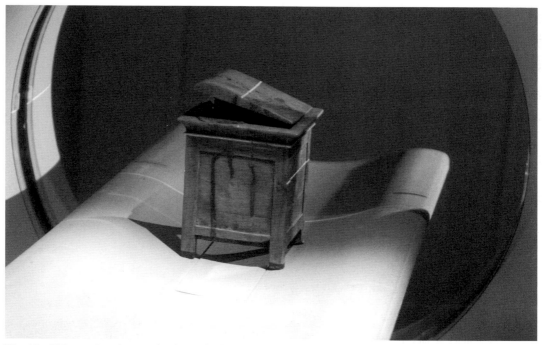

Fig. 18: CT scanning the wooden box, which bears the name of Queen Hatshepsut and is believed to hold part of the queen's viscera. Egyptian Museum, Cairo.

F. Mummies and objects from KV60

KV60 was an important tomb for our search, because two interesting female mummies were found there.

KV60 is a small undecorated tomb located in front of KV20 of Hatshepsut. KV60 is actually a perfect cache for the reburial of mummies because of its well-hidden entrance. Carter excavated this tomb in 1903[41] and found two mummies there; one, a small woman, was found inside an Eighteenth Dynasty coffin inscribed for a royal nurse, In, derived from the name Sitre-In, the wet nurse of the queen;[42] the other was a hugely obese woman (figs. 22a–b), discovered on the floor next to In's coffin. KV60 had been re-explored in 1906 by Edward Ayrton and then left alone until 1989, when Donald Ryan recleared the

tomb. When he began his work, only the mummy of the obese woman (KV60 A) was present in the tomb, and he placed this mummy in a wooden box. The mummy KV60 B (plate 13), found in the coffin with the name of the wet nurse, had been moved by Ayrton to the Egyptian Museum in 1908.[13]

The tomb is very small and is uninscribed. Its entrance is located directly in front of KV19, the Twentieth Dynasty tomb of Prince Mentuherkhepeshef. KV60 had clearly been robbed in antiquity. Apart from the mummies, many miscellaneous scattered remains were found inside, including the lid of a wooden coffin, ancient tools, the remains of pottery vessels, jewelry, scarabs, and seals.

Ryan described numerous fragments of a destroyed coffin that had been covered with

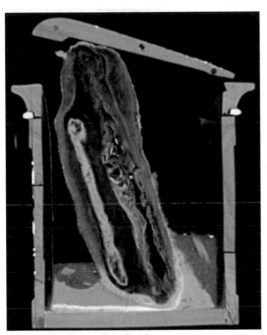

Fig. 19: Two-dimensional CT image of the box shows the liver of Hatshepsut wrapped in a linen pack.

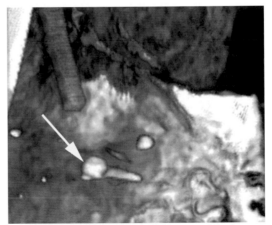

Fig. 20: Three-dimensional CT image of the box shows part of a tooth (arrow) within its contents.

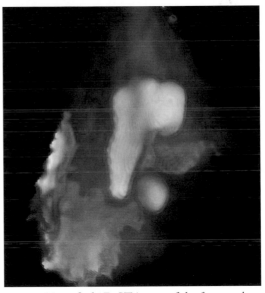

Fig. 21: Magnified 3D CT image of the fractured tooth with its single root.

a black substance.[44] The fragments consisted of pieces of wood of various sizes along with numerous pieces of cartonnage from the coffin's surface. The largest of these fragments is a sizeable curved piece from the head end of a coffin. Although it was mostly covered with the black substance, some yellow and blue/green stripes from a painted headdress were visible. In 2008, Ryan added that upon further examination, he noticed what appeared to be a hieroglyph. An SCA conservator was able to carefully remove the black substance, and it was a surprise to find that this piece was beautifully decorated and contained a text with a name.

The decoration depicts the goddess Nephthys with upraised arms standing on a colorful basket. The texts are funerary inscriptions spoken by the goddess to the deceased, who is a woman, a (temple) singer with the name "Ty." The hieroglypyhs in the name and the title are a bit blurred and crowded and give the appearance of being added over an earlier inscription. The funerary inscription also seems to be written for a male, with uses of the male k suffix and the

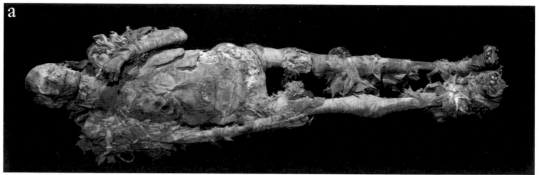

Fig. 22a: The mummy KV60 A before its transfer to the Egyptian Museum, Cairo.

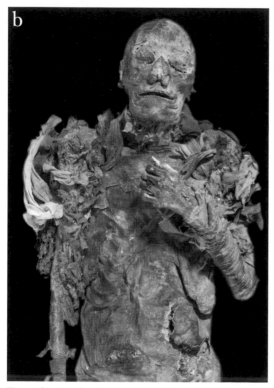

Fig. 22b: Detail of the mummy KV60 A.

Ryan also found on the floor of the tomb some hair near the head of the mummy KV60 A, the obese mummy, and also a false beard. In 1966, Elizabeth Thomas suggested that KV60 A was the mummy of Queen Hatshepsut,[45] based on the royal symbols found inside the tomb. The coffin fragments, and part of a mask with an indentation under the chin from which a false beard could have jutted, were indications that a royal burial might have lain in the tomb. Ryan, however, suggests that KV60 could be a cache with an assortment of objects, with the mummies originating from different places.[46]

The mummy KV60 A was moved to the Egyptian Museum for CT scanning (plate 14).

In addition, we searched for the mummy of the wet nurse of Hatshepsut (KV60 B), who is also known to us from a sandstone statue found at Deir al-Bahari and now in the Egyptian Museum.[47] The wet nurse's mummy was located (see sidelight, "Adventure in the Valley"), and the mummy and coffin were examined. The badly damaged coffin base in which it lies is typical of the Eighteenth Dynasty. Among the few remaining inscriptions is *wr šdt nfrw nswt 'In*, "Great Royal Nurse, In." The mummy is about 1.5 meters tall (less than five feet), but the coffin is 2.13 meters (some seven feet) long, suggesting that

word *sn·i*, "my brother." In other words, it is possible that this coffin might have been originally made for a man but was reused for a woman. Another piece from the foot end of the coffin was also cleaned, and it bears the depiction of the goddess Isis.

it was not originally intended for this person. The obese mummy that we moved to the Egyptian Museum is significantly taller, and would be a much better fit for the coffin.

The KV60 B mummy (plate 15) has her right arm extended by her side and her left forearm resting across her abdomen, with the hand closed as if it was originally holding something. She was well mummified and wrapped with fine linen, the fingers bandaged individually. The toes were evidently wrapped together; this bandaging has been torn away, as if the robbers were looking for gold. The woman was eviscerated through a V-shaped incision in the abdomen. She has long wavy red hair remaining on her head. There is also a mass of linen at the bottom of the coffin.

6. The mummy KV60 A (plates 16a–b)
CT findings in different regions
Head
Brain removal was not performed. The brain looks well preserved, shrunken, lying within the right hemisphere.

Teeth
The teeth are in very poor condition as a result of bad hygiene. Many teeth are broken and missing. The right upper second molar is absent, with one of its roots embedded within the upper jaw. Most of the teeth suffered from caries and some had broken crowns. The left upper second molar is disfigured and broken, with a large soft-tissue mass surrounding it, mimicking a pack. The root of this tooth (floor of the maxillary sinus) appeared rarefied yet with no sign of an oroantral fistula (free communication between the two). The remaining teeth show variable degrees of rarefaction and resorption

Table 7. General CT findings for the KV60 A mummy

Preservation Status	Fair
Age	50–60 years
Gender	Female
Stature	159 cm

around their roots. The extraordinarily poor state of the mummy's oral hygiene, along with her obesity, indicates that she may have suffered from diabetes mellitus.

Spine
Multiple vertebral areas of bone rarefaction support the theory of metastatic disease.[48] There is pressure erosion on the left side of the L5 vertebra.

Torso
The torso is eviscerated, except for the heart, which is present, and stuffed with linen packs.

Limbs
The left arm is crossed over the chest.

Cause of death
Death may be attributed to a malignant tumor that had spread to the bones, or due to complicated diabetes mellitus.

The Discovery
Two teams worked independently in the attempt to identify the mummy of Hatshepsut. The Egyptian team consisted of Ashraf Selim and Galal El Behiri, a professor of dentistry at Cairo University. The foreign team was headed by Paul Gostner. Both teams took measurements of the size of the tooth in the wooden box, measured the bone density, and then examined carefully the other teeth in the

mouth of the mummy of KV60 A. Both teams concluded that this tooth belongs to the mouth of the KV60 A mummy because it matches perfectly in shape, proportion, and bone density the other teeth in the mouth of this mummy. They discussed the issue of the number of roots in the tooth. In a personal communication Gostner wrote[49] that the tooth is the second upper molar, and this tooth, on the left or right, can have either two or three roots, as sometimes the two lateral roots join together, becoming one root; thus the fact that this tooth has two roots and not three is an entirely normal anatomical variation. Even in the case that this tooth did have three roots, it is quite possible that the third root is broken and among the many tiny loose bone fragments that are in the bottom of the box. Neither team was concerned about this issue, because they know that there are always some exceptions to the number of roots that a tooth can have. The bottom line is that, due to the dimensions, shape, and bone density, we can be sure that the tooth is definitely from the mouth of the KV60 A mummy.[50]

In conclusion: The tooth in Hatshepsut's box is a molar with one root missing. And in the mummy's mouth, there is a gap for a molar with one root still in place. A perfect match.

Also noteworthy is that in the area of the mouth with the missing molar, there are visible signs of inflammation due to an abscess, which started in the soft tissue around the tooth area and also in the upper maxillary bone. In the area of the extracted tooth, there are signs of medical treatment. Therefore the medical intervention (extraction) on the tooth had to have been done just before death. Considering that the person was suffering

from progressive neoplasia (tumors), in advanced stage, an abscess of this type without antibiotic protection could easily have been the cause of death.

The most important conclusion that all the above evidence suggests is that the mummy found in KV60 and distinguished by the letter A is indeed Queen Hatshepsut.

Very significant is the fact that she might have suffered from a malignant tumor (cancer), as suggested by Ashraf Selim. There is a very clear tumor of a couple of centimeters in the left part of her hip with a vast area of destroyed bone, compromising the tissue and muscles surrounding the left gluteal region. A secondary center of the same disease is evident in a lumbar vertebra.

There are two probable explanations for how Hatshepsut came to be buried in KV60. As stated above, it is thought that Hatshepsut intended for her mummy to be interred in KV20 with her father, Thutmose I. In this tomb were found two sarcophagi, one for Hatshepsut and one originally inscribed for Hatshepsut but modified for Thutmose I. The latter was moved to KV38 by Thutmose III. Hatshepsut's mummy may have been moved at the same time. It is known that toward the end of Thutmose III's reign, the monuments of Hatshepsut were defaced, and some have used this as evidence of a coup or assassination of the queen by Thutmose III. The attempts to blot out evidence of Hatshepsut holding the traditionally male role as a pharaoh may have required Hatshepsut to be removed from a kingly tomb to something more appropriate for her in KV60. The fact that her wet nurse, In, a woman no doubt very close to her in life, was in the tomb would no doubt have influenced the choice of location.[51]

There is a second possibility. Most of the mummies of the pharaohs from the Valley of the Kings were moved by priests from their tombs in the Twenty-first or the Twenty-second Dynasties, an unstable period that presumably saw looting and desecration of the tombs. This was how the mummies came to be placed in the caches in DB320 and KV35. The mummy of Hatshepsut may also have been moved at that time as well. It is possible that the mummy of Hatshepsut was intended to be moved to the cache DB320 and her wooden box was first moved, but later, for reasons yet to be explored, the decision for the mummy to be moved to DB320 was reconsidered, and the mummy was moved to KV60.

The radiologists in our investigation found that Hatshepsut suffered from diseases, possibly diabetes mellitus and cancer, that might have caused her death. This information has historical significance. It suggests that she died of diseases contracted during her lifetime and was not assassinated by her stepson, Thutmose III.

DNA Testing

A DNA laboratory was constructed in the basement of the Egyptian Museum as a scientific facility dedicated to the study of Egyptian mummies. Some sampling of mummies had been done for previous DNA analysis of the royal mummies; for example, the current team found nine 3-mm drill holes in the mummy of 'Thutmose I' from previous sampling.

The new study, under Drs. Yahia Zakaria and Somaia Ismail, relied on a much less invasive sampling procedure, which used a narrow bone biopsy needle to retrieve multiple samples from the same puncture hole. Samples were taken from the mummy of Hatshepsut (fig. 23), Sitre-In (the wet nurse), 'Thutmose I,' Thutmose II, Thutmose III, and Ahmose-Nefertari. The latter was the matriarch of the Thutmosid family and theoretically the great-grandmother of Hatshepsut through a direct female line.

Despite the well-recognized difficulty of working with highly degraded ancient DNA, the team was able to retrieve and amplify mitochondrial DNA, the type of DNA that is carried from mother to daughter, from the mummies of Hatshepsut and Ahmose-Nefertari. The very preliminary results that have emerged from this analysis so far seem to show significant similarity between the two women, but it is too early to draw definite conclusions. It will take the scientists more time to amplify the fragile nuclear DNA, but it is hoped that this may yield more data about Hatshepsut and her male relatives.

The DNA study will continue with more analysis of the samples in the DNA laboratory in the Egyptian Museum, and comparison samples will be analyzed by a second laboratory to check the results, which will appear in a later publication.[52]

Conclusions

This project was able to obtain valuable information on several royal mummies through CT scan analysis. While the primary focus was to identify the mummy of Queen Hatshepsut, the test results provided the team with new information on the male members of Hatshepsut's family. The most important discovery pertained to the mummy of 'Thutmose I'; it now seems certain that, as many scholars have previously suggested, this mummy has in fact been misidentified, for the three reasons cited above.

The team also indicated that Thutmose II may have died from an enlarged heart. This may suggest possible areas for study regarding heart disease in royal mummies. Physical inspection and CT examination of the mummy of Hatshepsut suggested that the queen was obese. As recent medical studies show that obesity may be linked with diabetes and cancer,[53] it is possible that Queen Hatshepsut may have suffered from these ailments. These results can be used in future medical studies. It was also interesting to note that most of the mummies scanned had not had their brains extracted during the mummification process, as would be expected in high-status burials. (See "Head

mummification and excerebration" in chapter 11.)

Of course, the highlight of the project was the successful identification of Queen Hatshepsut. The finding of diseases that may have contributed to Hatshepsut's death also challenges any rumors that the queen's stepson, Thutmose III, had had her murdered because she appropriated the throne for herself. It is now possible, likewise, that Hatshepsut's monuments were not defaced by a jealous and angry Thutmose III. It can be confirmed that most of the queen's monuments were destroyed at the end of the reign of Thutmose III and early in the reign of his son, Amenhotep II. The evidence suggests that

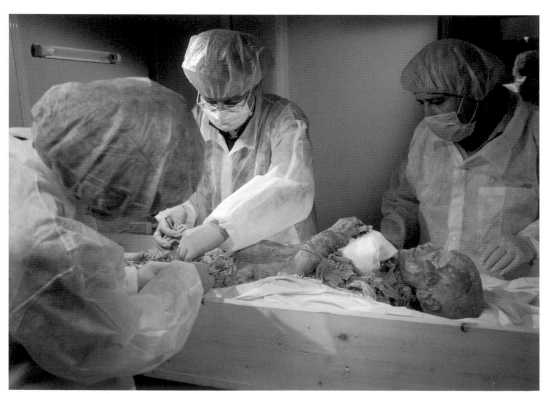

Fig. 23: Extracting samples for DNA analysis from the queen's mummy.

this destruction was performed by those who saw a female ruler to be contrary to the prevailing world view, which necessitated a male ruler on the throne of Egypt. The concept of the divine kingship had its roots in very ancient religious mythology. The Old Kingdom pyramid complex was dedicated to the triad of Re, Horus, and Hathor. This defined the roles of both king, as the son of the god Re and the living embodiment of the god Horus, and queen, associated with Hathor (who was in turn linked with the goddess Wadjet, the "eyes of Re" who protected the pharaoh[54]), the goddess who suckled the infant Horus. The queen was further associated with Nekhbet, the goddess of Upper Egypt. For a queen to take the role of a king was anathema to this entire concept. Hatshepsut broke this religious rule, and this is why her monuments were defaced, not by Thutmose III, but by the Egyptian people, who found her actions an affront to the divine order.[55]

4

CT Examination of Selected Mid- to Late Eighteenth Dynasty Mummies

Historical Introduction: The Reign of Amenhotep II to the Amarna Period

If we want to understand the golden age of Egypt in which many of Egypt's greatest kings lived, we should start with Amenhotep II. He was a celebrated warrior (plate 17), like his father Thutmose III, whose legacy for his son was a country with a great empire extending south to the Fourth Cataract of the Nile in Nubia and eastward to Syria. Amenhotep II continued to build the empire and also left substantial monuments throughout Egypt, the best known of which is the temple to the northeast of the Sphinx in Giza. He is known to have fathered about nine sons, but none of his wives took the title 'Great Royal Wife.' A prince named Thutmose, son of Tiia, a lesser queen, took the throne upon his father's death. Ancient damage to the names of other princes that appear on the 'dream stela,' erected between the paws of the Sphinx by Thutmose IV, may be an indi-

cation that there was a struggle for the throne among the family.[1]

Thutmose IV inherited a kingdom at peace. In his reign, the sun cult gained importance, and the king began to identify himself with Re and to emphasize the divinity of his kingship in his own lifetime. Statues from his reign show him with almond-shaped eyes that lend his face an eerie, unearthly quality that may be associated with cultic change. Recent theory suggests that this shift in royal dogma, which would come to fruition in the following reigns, was the result of a number of factors. The rise of the sun cult can be seen by some as an attempt to curb the power of the god Amun. In addition, we can see the growth of personal piety during the first part of this dynasty. Perhaps by being a god himself, the king could be a part of the pantheon worshiped by the populace and thus bring power back to the royal house. The rise of the empire is another point of the evidence: by becoming one with the sun, always the most important Egyptian god, the king could watch over all of the Egyptian lands from his vantage point in the sky.

Amenhotep III, son of Thutmose IV, came to the throne at the height of Egypt's wealth and power. His ancestors had built a great empire that now extended from the Euphrates in the north to the Fourth Cataract in the south.[2] He has been known as the "pasha" because he lived an extravagant lifestyle. The recent excavations of the German Archaeological Institute's expedition under Hourig Sourouzian (plate 18) have unearthed a plethora of statuary at his funerary temple (plate 19).[3] The great quantity of Sekhmet statues may indicate that he suffered from illness that he hoped would be cured by this goddess of healing. An Egyptian team under Zahi Hawass has excavated at the north entrance of the temple and found many statues of Amenhotep III with different gods and goddesses as well.[4]

Amenhotep III married a woman named Tiye (plate 21), who was the daughter of Yuya, the Master of the Horse, Commander of Chariotry, and Overseer of the Cattle of the god Min, and Thuya, a priestess of Amun. Though Tiye, whose parents were from the town of Akhmim, was of nonroyal birth, she became the Great Royal Wife of Amenhotep III, who bestowed upon her parents the privilege of burial in the Valley of the Kings. The tomb was found by Quibell and Davis in 1905[5] and was almost intact. It was richly provisioned. The best-known treasures of the tomb are the anthropoid coffin of Yuya (plate 20), covered in gold and silver foil and glass inlays; a wooden and gilded gesso chair inscribed for Sitamun, daughter of Amenhotep III; a wooden jewelry box on four legs inscribed with the cartouches

of Amenhotep III; the gilded cartonnage funerary mask of Thuya (plate 22; the wooden canopic box inscribed for Yuya and four calcite canopic jars, as well as the wooden canopic box and canopic jars of Thuya; two *shawabti* boxes; and three vessels with stoppers.[6]

The sarcophagus of Yuya was found on the northern side and that of Thuya on the south. It is interesting to note that the outer, rectangular sarcophagus of Yuya was similar to the outer sarcophagus of Tutankhamun. Yuya was provided with three anthropoid coffins and Thuya with two.

Though the mummies had been disturbed, their heads were covered with fabulous gilded cartonnage masks. In the tomb were also found amulets, necklaces, and heart scarabs. Yuya was provided with four *shawabti*s, and Thuya with fourteen. A group of furniture and wooden and stone vessels was found in front of and beside the coffins.

Their daughter, Queen Tiye, became quite powerful and was mentioned frequently on the monuments of her husband (plate 23).[7]

Egypt during the reign of Amenhotep III was wealthy beyond imagining, the golden age of the New Kingdom. This can be seen in the words of the king of Mitanni, who wrote, "Gold is like dust in your country." It was also a period of important developments in religion, including the deification of the living king as the sun god.[8] Amenhotep III stressed his identification with Amun-Re, who ruled over all the lands touched by his rays. The king ruled for thirty-eight years, celebrating three jubilee festivals, the first one in the thirtieth year of his reign, at which he reenacted his coronation and was magically rejuvenated.

King Amenhotep III and Queen Tiye had at least two sons and five daughters whose names are known. Daughters included

Sitamun, Iset C, Henuttaneb, Beketaten, and Nebetiah. Amenhotep III is shown with eight unnamed daughters in the tomb of Kheruef. Some of these may be identical to known daughters of Amenhotep III and Tiye.[9] Prince Thutmose, their eldest son, seems to have died young, and the throne passed to Amenhotep IV, who may have begun his reign as his father's coregent.[10] The length of this coregency is much disputed, with a length as great as twelve years having been suggested. Soon after the coronation of Amenhotep IV, he turned away from the worship of Amun-Re, for whom he had been named, and elevated the disk of the sun, known as Aten, to the top of the Egyptian pantheon. He changed his name to Akhenaten and founded a new city on virgin soil in Middle Egypt, called Akhetaten ('The Horizon of Aten'), Amarna today, to which he relocated the royal court (plate 25). Akhenaten and his queen, Nefertiti, served as the high priests of the new cult, as well as deified members of a new holy family (plate 24). They lived in the city and had six daughters (plate 26).[11]

From early in his reign, the royal family was shown in a new art style. The pharaoh had himself depicted with small eyes, elongated visage, thick lips, narrow nose, long prominent chin, and a swollen body with spindly limbs (plate 28). This was a dramatic departure from the traditional portrayal of kings with youthful, muscular bodies and idealized faces.

Perhaps the most interesting aspect of the Amarna years is the depiction of the royal family in intimate interactions, with the parents kissing and caressing their children, all under the rays of the sun (plate 27). Akhenaten also married a woman named Kiya; it has been theorized that she was the mother of Tutankhamun and died giving him birth.[12] Our recent DNA studies have suggested otherwise (see chapter 7, "Investigations into King Tutankhamun's Family").

There is a possibility that Amenhotep III died in Year 12 of Akhenaten's reign. This year was marked by the celebration of the festival known as Durbar, which included the reception of tribute from foreign lands and is mentioned in Amarna tombs.[13] According to those who believe that there was a coregency of Amenhotep III and Akhenaten, this festival was intended to mark the beginning of the junior king's promotion to senior king. To those who believe in a short coregency, or the consecutive rules of Amenhotep III and his son, this was simply a normal ceremony of tribute that might have occurred at regular intervals.

It has been suggested that about the same time, Nefertiti either disappeared or became her husband's coregent as Neferneferuaten or Ankh(et)kheperure.[14] The recent discovery of a graffito near Amarna, however, indicates that Nefertiti was alive, as chief queen, in Year 16 of Akhenaten's rule.[15] Akhenaten died in the following year and was followed by a mysterious king called Smenkhkare, which some have suggested could be a throne name of Nefertiti or a son of Akhenaten. Queen Tiye was buried in the tomb of her son at Amarna and was later moved to the Valley of the Kings.[16]

Examination of the Mummies

The CT examinations of the mummies of this period were done by Drs. Ashraf Selim and Hany Abdel-Rahman, who operated the machine and has expertise in CT scanners. The detailed CT analysis, reporting, and mummy researches were provided by Sahar Saleem. The following mummies of this period were examined:

A. 1. Yuya
   2. Thuya
B. Amenhotep III
C. The Elder Lady of KV35
D. The Younger Lady of KV35
E. The skeleton from KV55

A. The mummies of Yuya and Thuya
Identification of the mummies

Yuya and his wife Thuya were buried in a private tomb in the Valley of the Kings (KV46). There was no doubt of the identity of the pair, who were found resting among their torn linen wrappings, within their nests of coffins. The male mummy was identified as Yuya, and the female mummy was identified as Thuya.[17]

CT findings for the mummy of Yuya
General CT findings

The mummy is in good condition and is well preserved. The morphological appearances of the skull and hip support the known gender of a male.

Based on the epiphyseal union of all bones, the mummy has a mature skeleton. The degree of union of the sutures at the outer surface of the skull (ectocranial sutures) indicates that the age was over forty years at the time of death. The presence of moderate degenerative changes of the spine and knees, as well as tooth wear and attrition, all support an age at death of about fifty to sixty years.

Table 8. General CT findings for the mummy of Yuya

Preservation status	Well preserved
Age	50–60 years
Gender	Male
Stature (vertex–heel)	166 cm

Electronic CT measurements indicate the lengths of the humerus (right: 30 cm, left: 30 cm), femur (right: 44.9 cm, left: 45.1 cm), and tibia (right: 36.5 cm, left: 36.6 cm). The stature of the mummy measured from vertex to heel is 166 cm.

CT findings in different regions
Head (figs. 24a–b)

A defect is detected at the base of the ACF, indicating removal of the brain via transnasal route (transnasal excerebration). The skull defect measures 129.5 mm² in area, 11 mm in transverse, and 15 mm from front to back. There is partial interruption of the bony walls of the right ethmoidal air cells, and deviation of the nasal septum to the left. The posterior half of the skull contains desiccated brain impregnated with material of resin or resin-like CT features. There are two perpendicular levels of resin. One level is at the back of the skull parallel to the forehead, which may suggest that the fluid was introduced inside the skull while the head was in a resting, supine position. The other level is at the mid third of the skull base parallel to its vault; the fluid was likely introduced inside the skull, and then the body was placed in a sitting position while the resin was in the liquid state.[18]

The orbits contain atrophic eye globes and are filled with linen impregnated with resin, as well as a small amount of resin at the lower orbit. Both auricles are preserved and show no ear piercings. The nasal cavity is partially filled with resin. The mouth and oropharynx are stuffed with amorphous low-density embalming material. The deep lower part of the pharynx (hypopharynx) contains material of higher CT density, likely linen impregnated with resin.[19]

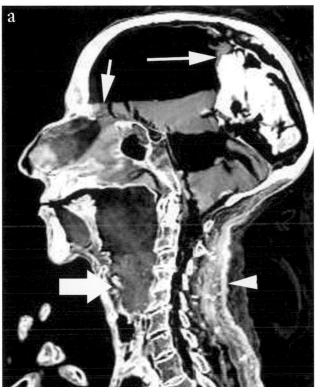

Figs. 24a–b: CT imaging of head and neck of Yuya. CT image in sagittal plane (a) shows a small defect in the anterior cranial fossa (ACF). A desiccated brain residue impregnated with dense resin occupies the back of the skull (long arrow); the resin was likely introduced while the head was in the recumbent, supine position. Another level of resin occupies the middle cranial fossa parallel to the skull vault (short arrow); it was probably introduced while the head was in the sitting position. The embalmers enhanced the contours of the neck by filling the mouth and throat with heterogeneous embalming materials (thick arrow) as well as with packs inserted under the skin (arrowhead).

Axial CT image of the neck of Yuya (b) shows well the multiple discrete, heterogeneous packs underneath the skin of the anterior and posterior neck walls (arrows). Note also that the skin was likely thickened by painting it with resin (arrowhead).

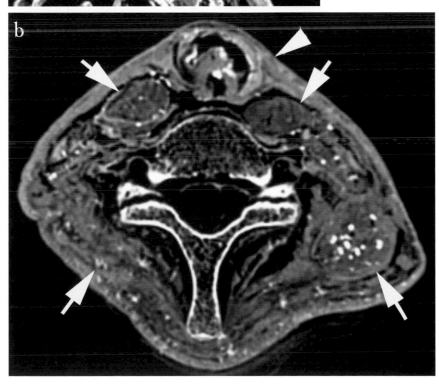

Teeth

The dental condition of the mummy of Yuya is generally poor. There is moderate tooth wear, alveolar resorption, attrition, and poor periodontal health. There are also multiple missing teeth, likely antemortem. Changes are consistent with the estimated age at time of death.

Spine

The vertebrae are intact, with moderate degeneration in the form of marginal osteophytic lippings in cervical and lumbar regions.

Torso (chest and abdomen)

A mummification incision extends obliquely above the left inguinal region. It is 99 mm in length and gaping open for 34 mm, without covering metallic plates or amulets, though at the time of the excavation, a gold embalming plate was noted.[20] There is CT evidence that the viscera had been removed (evisceration), except the heart, as thin tissue remnants are seen in the chest at the heart location.

The torso cavity is almost totally filled with resin-treated and untreated linen folds. The phallus is in its normal position, deviated more to the right side. It measures 105 mm in length and 14 mm in width, and its CT density is moderately high (300 HU). A central low-density cavity (–730 HU), 3 mm in diameter, is seen within; this could be an air-filled penile urethra. Behind the penis is a sac filled with heterogeneous material of mixed densities (–300 to 150 HU) and measuring 51 mm x 53 mm x 57 mm in maximum transverse, anteroposterior, and craniocaudal dimensions. The base of the sac is continuous with the skin of the perineum, suggesting that a small cut was induced and the scrotum was filled with embalming materials, rather than a pack placed by the embalmers for protection of the penis.

Upper limbs

The arms, flexed at the elbows and the forearms, extend over the chest, with the hands crossed under the chin. The fingers of the right hand are extended, while those of the left hand are flexed.

Lower limbs

The lower-limb bones are intact. There are moderate degenerative changes of the hip and knee joint bilaterally. The left big toe is missing, likely postmortem, marked with a large soft-tissue gap.

Comments on mummification

The mummification process is of an excellent quality, as expected for a nobleman in the Eighteenth Dynasty. Visceral removal was through an oblique left inguinal incision, and there is evidence of cranial embalming. However, there are unique mummification findings in the mummy of Yuya.

1. The crossed hands under the chin: this position is not seen in other royal mummies. It could be unique for Yuya, a nonroyal but powerful Egyptian courtier of his time.

2. Unique cranial mummification: the relatively small-sized skull-base defect that was used in cranial mummification and the double levels of intracranial resin, one parallel to the forehead and the other perpendicular to it, parallel to the skull's vault. This is unlike what is commonly seen, as there is usually just a single level of resin located at the back of the skull, perpendicular to the skull base. The location and leveling of

the solidified resin suggest a change in the position of the body during pouring of the hot resin.

3. Excellent subcutaneous packing of the face, neck, and torso enhanced the mummy's contours and gave it a lifelike appearance. The smooth bilateral and symmetrical filling of the mid and lower face around the nose and mouth was likely responsible for the delicate smile. The mummy's full neck resulted from combination effects of filling the throat as well as subcutaneous packing of the neck and thoracic inlet regions. The subcutaneous fillings are multiple packs with heterogeneous CT densities likely formed of bits of linen soaked in resin (see fig. 24b).[21]

4. Well-preserved genital region and filling of the scrotum with embalming material.

Manner and cause of death

The mummy offers no definite explanation for the manner or cause of death of Yuya.

CT findings for the mummy of Thuya
General CT findings

The mummy of Thuya is one of the best-preserved royal mummies; there is no CT evidence of significant bone or soft-tissue injuries.

The morphological appearances of the skull support the known gender of a female.

CT findings support an age at death of about fifty to sixty years. This is based on the epiphyseal union of all bones, the degree of union of the ectocranial sutures, the presence of moderate degenerative changes of the spine and knees, thin humeral cortex, and moderate tooth wear and attrition.[22]

Table 9. General CT findings for the mummy of Thuya

Preservation status	Well preserved
Age	50–60 years
Gender	Female
Stature (vertex–heel)	145 cm

The CT measurements of bone length include: right humerus 30.6 cm, left humerus 30.6 cm, right femur 44.1 cm, left femur 44.5 cm, right tibia 36.5 cm, and left tibia 36.6 cm.

When assessed by direct measurement from vertex to heel, the height of the mummy measured 145 cm. However, when extrapolated from bone length using equations, the height was 17 cm longer (161.8 cm ±4 cm). (See below under "Spine" for an explanation.)

CT findings in different regions
Head (fig. 25)

A defect that measures 24 mm in transverse and 16 mm from front to back in the skull base (ACF) was used by the embalmers to completely empty the skull of its contents, except for a few dural remains (transnasal excerebration). The embalmers did not introduce any material into the skull.[23]

The nasal cavities on both sides were filled with convoluted linen packs impregnated with resin. The nasal septum shows smooth curvature and is deviated to the right. Nasal turbinates are interrupted on both sides; this may indicate that both nares were utilized for excerebration.

The embalmers packed both orbits with pieces of linen soaked with resin in front of the dried eye globes.

Both auricles are preserved. The right lobule exhibits one ear piercing, while the left has two. Possible piercings are suspected in the

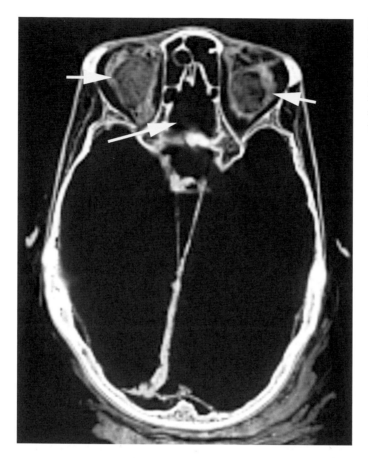

Fig. 25: Axial CT image of the brain of Thuya shows the empty skull cavity and the bony defect (long arrow) that was used by the embalmers to remove the brain. Pieces of linen impregnated with resin (short arrows) were placed inside the orbits to hide the sunken eyes.

upper part of both ear auricles. This was probably in vogue at that time.

A subcutaneous heterogeneous filling (–300 to –11 HU) is placed in the mid and lower face. The packs are of comparable widths bilaterally, producing reasonable symmetry and enhancement of facial contours.

The mouth and upper throat of the mummy (oropharynx) are filled with low-CT-density embalming material (–500 HU), likely representing linen.

Teeth

There are notable attrition changes in the dental arc and jawbone with multiple missing teeth, likely premortem. In the maxillary teeth,

the right premolar, right first molar, and left first molar teeth are missing, while only part of the left second molar tooth is present. In the mandible, the right first molar is absent, and only parts of the left first and second molars are present. Dental changes in general are consistent with the estimated age at time of death.

Spine

The spine in the lower thoracic region shows a smooth lateral curve, with its convexity to the left (thoraco-lumbar scoliosis). The upper limit of the curve is between the seventh and eighth thoracic vertebrae, its lower limit between the first and second lumbar vertebrae, and it is centered to the tenth thoracic vertebra. The angle of the curve, as measured with the Cobb method, is twenty-five degrees; angles greater than twenty degrees denote a severe degree of scoliosis.[24] There are no structural abnormalities seen in the vertebrae, such as fractures or congenital anomalies. The presence of this severe scoliosis explains the significant reduction of height of the mummy when measured from vertex to heel in relation to the estimation using equations employing bone length.

Torso (chest and abdomen) (fig. 26)
A mummification incision extends slightly vertically above the left inguinal region for 75 mm and gapes open for 30 mm. A resin-treated pack is seen at the base of the incision; however, no covering metallic plates or amulets are visible. All the viscera, except for the heart, had been removed. The torso cavity is almost totally filled with embalming materials of different CT densities and appearances that likely include resin-treated and untreated linen folds, as well as heterogeneous sawdust or soil that possibly contains small dense particles (sand or stones). A highly dense (1200 HU) embalming material of unknown nature is seen in the rectum. There is also a homogeneous layer of solidified resin lining the back (posterior) of the body cavity. Layers of linen treated with moderately dense resin are seen superficially lodged on the back of the mummy.

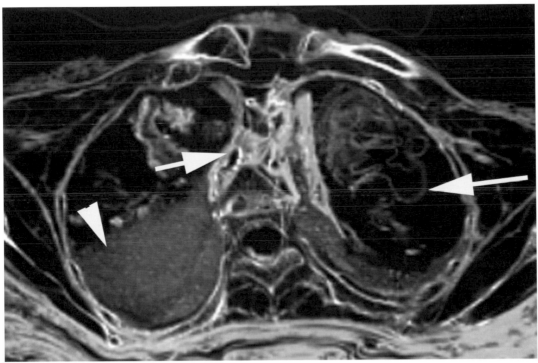

Fig. 26: Axial CT image shows the torso of Thuya. All the viscera were removed apart from the heart, which is preserved (short arrow) (probably wrapped in linen soaked with resin). The chest cavity is filled with free linen fibers (long arrow), as well as a moderately dense substance (likely solidified resin) along the dependent posterior chest wall (arrowhead).

Upper limbs

Both arms reside alongside the body with the hands flat.

Lower limbs

The lower-limb bones are mostly intact. The left forefoot shows postmortem fractures with missing distal parts of all the toes. Metallic footware (likely gold) is seen on both feet (see chapter 12, "Amulets, Funerary Figures, and Other Objects Found on the Mummies").

Comments on mummification

The mummy is well preserved and exhibits an excellent embalming job that conforms with that commonly seen in the Eighteenth Dynasty royal family, such as the transnasal removal of the brain and evisceration through an inguinal incision. The special aspects of the mummification of Thuya are:

1. Unlike the other royal mummies that we studied, the skull of mummified Thuya is empty, without evidence of any intracranial embalming materials.
2. The left inguinal incision is slightly more vertically aligned.
3. There has been subcutaneous packing of the face.

Manner and cause of death

The mummy offers no definite evidence for the manner or cause of death of Thuya.

Table 10. General CT findings for the mummy of Amenhotep III

Preservation status	Poor
Age	50 years
Gender	Male
Stature	154 ± 4.4 cm

B. The mummy of Amenhotep III
Genealogy
Father: Thutmose IV
Mother: Mutemwiya

Identification of the mummy

The mummy was found in 1898 in a side chamber of KV35, along with several other mummies.[25] The body was identified as this king by dockets on the mummy's wrappings and coffin.[26]

CT findings for the mummy of Amenhotep III
General CT findings

The mummy was badly damaged, likely by robbers in antiquity. The head and neck are detached from the body, the limbs are disarticulated, the pelvis is disrupted, and a large amount of soft tissue of the body and face is missing.

The morphological appearances of the skull support the known gender of a male.

Based on the epiphyseal union of all bones, the mummy has a mature skeleton. The degree of union of the ectocranial sutures indicates that the age was about fifty years at the time of death. The presence of moderate degenerative changes of the lumbar spine, the mild lippings of the knee, thin humeral cortex, and moderate tooth wear and attrition all likewise support an age of about fifty years.

Because the body was dismantled, we could not assess the stature by vertex–heel measurement. Alternatively, we estimated the stature to be about 154 cm (± 4.4 cm) from the length of the humerus (28.2 cm) using the following equation:

Stature (cm) = 3.26 x (length of humerus: 28.2 cm) + 62.1= 154 cm ± 4.4 cm.

In his 1912 book, Grafton Elliot Smith estimated the height of Amenhotep III to be 156 cm, and his age at death between forty and fifty years; however, it was not mentioned upon what evidence this estimate was based.[27]

CT findings in different regions
Head
The head is badly preserved and was probably subjected to violent treatment by tomb robbers in antiquity. Many of the bones of the face were broken postmortem; these include the left zygomatic arch, medial walls of both maxillary antra, and front part of the alveolar maxilla.

A large defect (34 mm in transverse and 44 mm front to back) is detected at the base of the ACF, indicating removal of the brain via transnasal excerebration. The posterior two-fifths of the skull is filled with resin-like material.[28] No packs are seen in the nose.

The orbits contain atrophic eye globes and are filled with heterogeneous material, likely linen impregnated with resin. The orbital packs are placed above and behind the dried globes. The mouth cavity and oropharynx are filled with resin. There is subcutaneous, homogeneous, moderate-density packing of comparable widths seen in the neck and a small reserved part in the lower face overlying the jaws bilaterally.

Teeth
There are multiple missing teeth, likely postmortem, as a tooth is seen fallen in the throat (oropharynx). There is generally moderate tooth wear and alveolar resorption; changes are consistent with the estimated age of the king at time of death.

Spine
The head and neck are disarticulated at the level of the fifth cervical vertebra (C5). There are multiple postmortem pathological fractures and missing vertebrae (C6, C7, L3, and L4). Flowing ossification and bony growths are observed along the right anterolateral aspect of the thoracic spine (fourth to ninth vertebrae) without involvement of discs or facet joints. There is evidence of osteoarthritic bony growths at multiple costovertebral joints; calcifications of interspinous and supraspinous ligaments; and multiple enthesopathies at the joints of the lower limbs. The disrupted sacroiliac joints indicate that they are not ankylosed. Findings are suggestive of DISH (diffuse idiopathic skeletal hyperostosis).

Torso (chest and abdomen) (fig. 27)
The wall of the right upper part of the chest is missing. The heart cannot be detected within the chest. The cavity of the torso is partially stuffed with resin-treated and untreated linen packs. There is also a homogeneous layer of solidified resin lining the posterior of the body cavity.

The pelvis is disrupted. The right hip bone is disarticulated and displaced upwards. The external genital organs could not be visualized.

Upper limbs
The right upper limb is disarticulated at the shoulder and elbow, and is missing the hand. The left arm is present. The right clavicle is disarticulated and is seen within the abdominal cavity. The left clavicle is in place and shows an oblique fracture at its proximal end.

Lower limbs
The right lower limb is disarticulated at the hip and the knee joints. There is an irregular fracture of the lateral aspect of the lower femur near the knee joint. Most of the bones of the mid and forefoot are missing; the

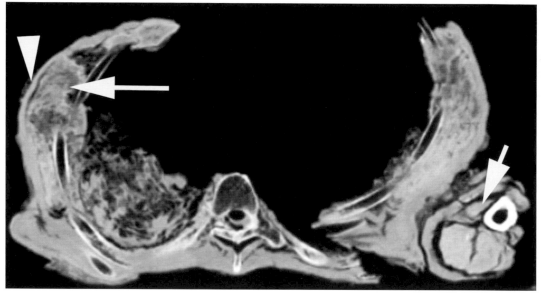

Fig. 27: Axial CT image of the torso of the mummy of Amenhotep III shows interrupted anterior and posterior walls. Thick layers of linen soaked in resin are placed beneath the skin of the torso (long arrow). The thick dense skin (arrowhead) was likely painted with a layer of resin. The skin is separate from the packs underneath. The short arrow points to subcutaneous resin fillings in the left arm.

remaining foot bones are the talus, calcaneus, navicular, cuboid, and part of the lateral cuneiform. The left lower limb shows mild displacement of the femoral head from the acetabulum. The middle shaft of the fibula is fractured and missing. The bones of the forefoot are also missing.

The embalmers placed thick diffuse layers of resin beneath the skin of the limbs to enhance their contour.

Comments on mummification
The mummification style of Amenhotep III is comparable to that commonly seen in the Eighteenth Dynasty: transnasal removal of the brain, resin placed inside the skull, evisceration with presence of visceral packs. The presence of carefully placed subcutaneous packing in the body is also a remarkable mummification feature in Amenhotep III.[29]

Manner and cause of death
The mummy offers no definite evidence for manner or cause of death. All the detected bony and soft-tissue injuries were likely induced postmortem.

C. The mummy of the Elder Lady from KV35 (Queen Tiye)
Genealogy
Father: Yuya
Mother: Thuya

Identification of the mummy
This mummy of an 'elder lady' was found in tomb KV35 beside a younger woman and a boy. The mummies did not have coffins or linen dockets to identify them. However, a lock of hair was found in Tutankhamun's tomb, placed in a nest of miniature coffins inscribed with Tiye's names.[30] Analysis of

the hair by electron probe in the 1970s matched it to that of the Elder Lady of KV35.[31] Our recent DNA analysis confirmed her identity as Queen Tiye (see chapter 7, "Investigations into King Tutankhamun's Family").[32]

G.E. Smith described the mummy as that of a small (1.46 m), middle-aged woman whose hair was brown and lustrous.[33] The mummy's age has been estimated at thirty by Wilton Krogman and Melvyn Baer.[34]

In February 2003, the Elder Lady was studied again by a group from York University, who performed x-ray examinations of all three KV35 mummies. The Elder Lady was found to be in the same condition that Smith described in 1912. The team estimated the mummy's age at thirty-five to forty-five years at death.[35]

CT findings for the mummy of the Elder Lady
General CT findings

The CT study shows that the mummy is well preserved overall, despite the presence of a large defect in the anterior wall of the torso and disarticulation of both feet. These mutilations were likely the result of an act of theft in antiquity.

The morphological appearances of the skull support the known gender of a female.

Based on the epiphyseal union of all bones, the mummy has a mature skeleton. The degree of union of the ectocranial sutures indicates that the age was over forty years at the time of death. The presence of minimal degenerative changes of the lumbar spine and moderate tooth wear and attrition support an age at death of about forty to fifty years. This range of age matches the estimated age of the queen from historical resources.[36]

The stature of the skeleton is 145 cm. The length of the right femur is 38.87 cm and the right tibia 34.26 cm.

CT Findings in different regions
Head (fig. 28)

A large defect detected at the base of the ACF indicates removal of the brain via transnasal excerebration. The skull defect measures 18 mm in transverse view and 37 mm from front to back. There is some interruption of the bony walls of the ethmoidal air cells, which are partially filled with resin. The posterior half of the skull is occupied by desiccated brain; no evidence of embalming materials was detected within the skull.[37] No nasal packs are present. The backs of the orbits contain high-density resin (75 to 100 HU) that was likely poured in a liquid state and solidified in the dependent part of the orbits, escaping through the optic foramina. In addition, small linen packs (–400 HU) were placed in front of the dried eye globes to hide their sunken appearance. The oral cavity and oropharynx contain resin-impregnated linen. The ears are unpierced.

A low-density (–300 HU) linen pack with dense resin outline (250 HU) is placed beneath the skin of the midline of the lower neck and above the sternum (suprasternal). The subcutaneous neck pack measures about 43 mm x 21 mm x 41 mm in its maximum width, depth, and height.

Table 11. General CT findings for the mummy of the Elder Lady

Preservation status	Fair
Age	40–50 years
Gender	Female
Stature (vertex–heel)	145 cm

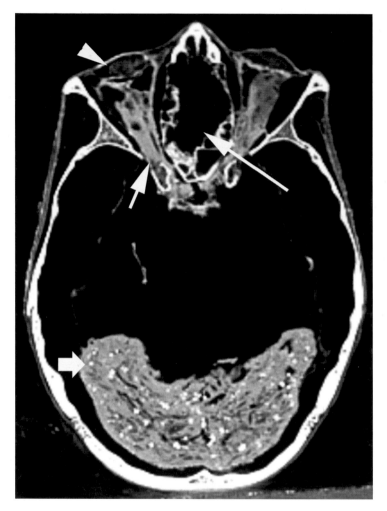

Fig. 28: Axial CT of the brain of the Elder Lady (Tiye) shows evidence of an embalming skull defect (long thin arrow). However, the brain was not removed and shows as a low-density lump at the back of the skull (thick arrow). A linen pack (arrowhead) is placed in front of the desiccated eye. Solidified resin is seen within the orbits, tracking through the optic foramina and smearing the adjacent meninges inside the skull cavity (short thin arrow).

Teeth

Generally, the dental condition of the mummy of the Elder Lady is good. There is moderate tooth wear and slight to moderate alveolar resorption consistent with the estimated age of the queen at time of death. The right maxillary canine is partially broken (medial border). All of the wisdom teeth are missing except the right maxillary one, which shows a fractured root. There is a space for the other three missing wisdom teeth in the jaws, which denotes that they were present at one time during life (fig. 29).

Spine

The spine is well preserved. There are well-defined hypodense lesions with mildly sclerotic margins seen within the vertebral body, close to the disc at multiple levels in the thoraco-lumbar region (Schmorl's nodes). There is minimal osteophytic lipping.

Torso (chest and abdomen)

There is a large defect at the right aspect of the chest wall that extends to the abdomen and pelvis. No viscera are detected except an

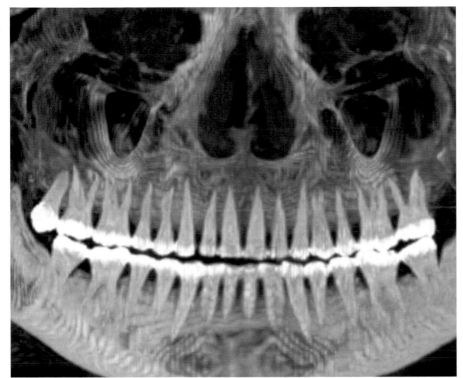

Fig. 29: CT panorama for teeth (curved multiplanar reformatted images) of Tiye shows good dental condition in general, with mild resorption and moderate wear.

atrophic heart in the chest. The cavity of the torso is only partially stuffed with resin-treated and untreated linen packs. There are multiple rounded stones in the right side of the chest; they measure about 20 mm in length, 8 mm in width, and 2052 HU density. A smaller stone (10 mm in length, 1728 HU density) is seen at the left side of the pelvis.

Upper limbs

The right upper limb is preserved. It extends alongside the body with the hand over the right groin region. There are no fractures; however, the middle finger is missing, likely disarticulated in an act of postmortem vandalism. The left arm is crossed over the chest, and the left hand is tightly clenched, with raised thumb, as though it was originally holding something.

Lower limbs

The two legs are separated from the body. The left iliac blade shows an oblique fracture with no evidence of sclerosis. The right foot is disarticulated at the ankle joint and is missing. The left is present but disarticulated at the ankle. There is a fracture at the medial aspect of the patella with no evidence of bone reaction or sclerosis. It likely was inflicted postmortem by tomb thieves in antiquity.

Comments on mummification

The mummification style of the Elder Lady (Queen Tiye) is consistent with that commonly seen in the Eighteenth Dynasty. The queen's one crossed arm with clenched hand is often found on statues of royal women, though not on the few royal female mummies that are known.[38] The incision for mummification is not

Table 12. General CT findings for the mummy of the Younger Lady

Preservation status	Fair
Age	25–35 years
Gender	Female
Stature (vertex–heel)	158 cm

clear. The mummy of Tiye showed only very limited subcutaneous packing restricted to her lower neck, unlike other royal mummies of her time (her parents and husband), who had a more extensive process.[39] The hair's brown color, as well as the darkened skin of the face, could be a result of the materials used for mummification.

Manner and cause of death
The mummy offers no definite evidence for the manner or cause of death of Queen Tiye.

D. The mummy of the Younger Lady of KV35 (plates 29a–b)
Genealogy
Father: Amenhotep III
Mother: Tiye

Identification of the mummy
This mummy was found in tomb KV35 beside the older woman identified as Queen Tiye and a young boy. Like the other two mummies, the Younger Lady did not have a coffin or linen dockets to identify her. The mummy has been identified in a recent DNA study to be the mother of Tutankhamun, and a daughter of Amenhotep III and Queen Tiye[40] (see chapter 7).

CT findings for the Younger Lady of KV35
General CT findings
The CT study shows overall fair preservation of the mummy, despite a large defect in the anterior wall of the chest and disarticulated right upper limb, mutilations that likely were inflicted by tomb robbers in antiquity.

The morphological appearances of the skull and pelvis support the known gender of a female.

Judging from the condition of the epiphyseal union and closure of cranial sutures, the age at death was between twenty-five and thirty-five years.

The mummy's height measures 158 cm from vertex to heel. The length of the left humerus is 29.3 cm, left femur 40.5 cm, and left tibia 35.2 cm.

CT findings in different regions
Head (figs. 30a–b)
Reconstructed CT images of the head in multiple planes confirmed that the skull base was intact. A shrunken, desiccated brain and dura occupy the back of the skull cavity, with no evidence of intracranial embalming material.

The skull has an oval defect (38 mm x 30 mm) at the central part of the frontal bone in front of the coronal suture. The defect has sharp, beveled, festooned edges, with no CT evidence of attempted healing or sclerosis. This suggests that the defect was inflicted postmortem in several steps using a sharp instrument, like that used by the embalmers.

The left side of the lower face shows a large defect measuring 112 mm x 81 mm. The defect involves the left cheek, left maxillary sinus, and alveolar process, as well as part of the left mandible. The edges of the bony defect are sharp and show no evidence of sclerosis or attempted healing. Some bony fragments of the broken lateral wall of the left maxillary sinus are seen pushed within the antral cavity; however, most of the fragments

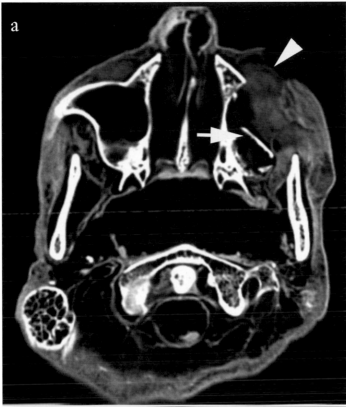

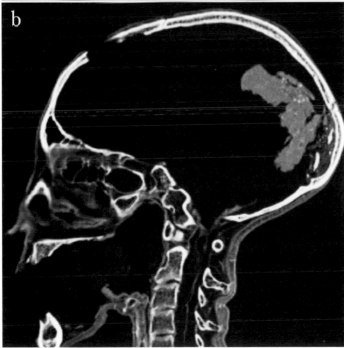

Figs. 30a–b: Axial CT of the head of the mummified Younger Lady of KV35 (a) at the level of the maxilla shows that the injury of the left side of the face involves the bones and soft tissues. The fractured lateral wall of the left maxillary sinus is seen pushed within the antral cavity (arrow). Embalming pack is placed on top of the facial gap (arrowhead).

Sagittal CT image of the head of the Younger Lady (b) shows an intact skull base with no evidence of bony removal or intracranial embalming materials. The sharp-edged defect in the frontal bone is also seen.

of the fractured bones are missing. The soft tissues adjacent to the facial defect are relatively thickened in comparison to the corresponding tissues on the right side. A rolled embalming pack of low CT density (likely formed of linen impregnated with resin) is seen placed on top of the facial gap, partly beneath the remaining skin (subcutaneous). This pack did not seem to be interrupted. A subcutaneous filling of heterogeneous CT density (likely formed of linen impregnated with resin) is also seen in the right side of the face at the level of cheek and mid-face.[41]

Both orbits contain packs of linen impregnated with resin at the periphery. The packs were placed in front of the dry eye globes. There is resin smearing the right nasal cavity.

The mouth cavity is filled with linen; no embalming materials were placed within the throat of the mummy. The right auricle is partly missing. The left auricle has two piercings in its lobe.

Teeth

The facial injury caused a fractured left alveolar plate and part of the left jaw, which resulted in multiple missing teeth; one tooth is seen within the oral cavity. The fracture involved most of the left alveolar plate just distal to the left first incisor, which is also missing. On the right alveolar plate, the sockets of the first incisor and the right canine are empty, and their teeth are missing. The rest of the teeth are present, including the non-erupted third molar.

The fracture of the mandible involved the midline and the adjacent part of the left mandible, which affected the right and left first incisors and the left canine. The sockets of the right second incisor, as well as the left first and second molars, are empty and their

teeth are missing. The first and second left upper molars are partly fractured. Both right and left upper third molars are non-erupted. The upper right canine, premolars, and first and second molars are present and show no attrition or occlusal surface irregularity.

Spine

The spine in the lumbar region shows a smooth lateral curve, with its convexity to the left (lumbar scoliosis). The upper limit of the curve is between the twelfth thoracic and first lumbar vertebrae, its lower limit between the fourth and fifth lumbar vertebrae, and its center between the second and third lumbar vertebrae. The scoliosis is mild; the angle of the curve, as measured with the Cobb method, is less than twenty degrees (16.6). There are no evident structural abnormalities of the vertebrae, such as fractures or congenital anomalies, and the curved spine could have been due to the position of the body during mummification.

Torso (chest and abdomen)

A large defect involves the anterior wall of the torso. The viscera had been removed by the embalmers, except the heart, which is seen in place. The embalming incision can be detected in the left inguinal region; the tissue gap is 56 mm and its depth is 135 mm. Similar findings were described by G.E. Smith.[42] The torso is filled with free linen fibers mildly smeared with resin, as well as linen packs treated with resin. A resin-treated linen pack is placed within the pelvis, plugging a large defect at the pelvic floor that could have been used for removing the viscera (perineal evisceration).

Upper limbs

The left upper limb extends beside the body with the hand placed over the left hip. There is a complete transverse fracture of the proximal shaft of the right humerus, with gaping ends and no evidence of callus formation or attempted healing. The disarticulated right upper limb is beside the body; the right hand is broken and completely separated at the wrist and lies loose at the foot level of the mummy.

Lower limbs

There are small fractures of the left iliac crest as well as the right inferior pubic ramus, without evidence of healing (likely postmortem). There is a defective area at the front (anterior cortex) of the distal shaft of the right tibia that extends 33.5 mm above the ankle joint. The metatarsal and phalangeal bones of both feet are broken and missing. There is a subcutaneous filling at the back of the right hip region (buttock).

Comments on mummification

CT findings indicating evisceration and stuffing of the torso with embalming materials are typical of the Eighteenth Dynasty mummification style. However, we noted the following (unusual) points in the mummification of this mummy:

1. Intact skull base without evidence of brain removal. Although this was detected in the mummies of so-called 'Thutmose I' and Thutmose II and III, all mummies dated to the later Eighteenth Dynasty show some sort of brain treatment. The frontal bone defect has sharp, beveled, festooned edges that could have been inflicted by the embalmers in several steps, using a sharp surgical instrument. However, there is no evidence of brain treatment to support this assumption.

2. The use of subcutaneous fillings and packs to remodel the injured left side of the face, the contralateral side of the face, and the right hip region.

Manner and cause of death

The CT study suggests that the injury of the left side of the face injury was likely inflicted before mummification took place, as the subcutaneous embalming packs and filling were not interrupted. In addition, the fractured fragments of the left maxillary bones were missing and were not found inside the gap. This may denote that the broken bony fragments were removed by the embalmers, who also partly cleaned the region of injury. There were no signs of healing at the edges of the broken bone, which implies that the injury must have happened perimortem, either shortly before death, or after death but before mummification. The few small fragments of bones seen within the maxillary antral sinus denote that the direction of trauma was 'pushing' rather than 'pulling.' Such injury was more likely inflicted by hitting the face with a heavy object rather than, for example, by pulling a stuck funerary mask from the mummy. An accident like a strong kick by an animal (such as a horse) may have also caused such an injury.

If we assume that the injury occurred perimortem during life, such acute facial trauma would have caused severe shock and bleeding that might have caused death.

The skull defect on the front of the skull and the defect in the anterior wall of the body might have been inflicted by the same accident that caused the facial injury, or alternatively could be postmortem, inflicted by tomb thieves, especially because the skull cavity contains fragments of the broken skull.

E. The skeleton from Tomb 55

This mummy was found in KV55, an uninscribed rock-cut tomb in the Valley of the Kings located near KV62, the tomb of Tutankhamun. The identification of this mummy is one of Egyptology's most enduring enigmas. The tomb, discovered by Edward Ayrton in 1907 in cooperation with Theodore Davis, has been convincingly interpreted as a cache of material from the Royal Tomb at Amarna. A number of Akhenaten's family members were apparently interred in this sepulcher, and the remains of their disturbed burials are thought to have been piously moved to Thebes and reburied by Tutankhamun.[43] The most important artifacts from KV55 are panels from a large gilded wooden shrine built to protect the sarcophagus of Queen Tiye, four exquisite canopic jars of Egyptian alabaster that had once been inscribed for Kiya, and a royal coffin of wood inlaid with gold and glass in a feathered style known as *rishi* (plates 30a–b).

It is this coffin, and the badly decayed mummy found inside, that has been the focus of Egyptological speculation. The lower three-quarters of the coffin's gilded mask were ripped away in antiquity, and the inlaid cartouches that once identified the coffin's owner were removed, leaving its final inhabitant faceless and nameless, a deliberate act of *damnatio memoriae*.

However, a recent study has suggested that the coffin was inscribed for Akhenaten himself.[44] This, plus the presence in the tomb of other artifacts bearing his name, has convinced a number of scholars that KV55 was intended primarily as a reburial of this mysterious king, brought to Thebes from his original tomb at Amarna. The biggest dilemma has always been the mummy itself, now reduced to a skeleton. The KV55 skeleton shares a blood group with Tutankhamun. A blood type matching that of the youth believed to be his son, a coffin bearing his name, and the simple answer is that the bones are Akhenaten's. However, most previous forensic studies have concluded that the skeleton is of a man who died at twenty-five or twenty-six years, plus or minus several years[45] (although one study did put the age at thirty-five[46]). Based on historical evidence, Akhenaten must have been well over thirty when he died. The majority of Egyptologists therefore identify the KV55 king as Smenkhkare, the enigmatic and ephemeral monarch, possibly Tutankhamun's older brother, who may have shared the throne with Akhenaten in his last years and then succeeded him.[47]

After the initial studies of Smith, Derry, and Harrison, further examination of the mummy was undertaken in 1988 by J.E. Harris and anthropologist Fawzia Hussein,[48] who concluded that the occupant of KV55 had died when he was thirty-five. The door was opened again for Akhenaten.

In 2000, the bones were studied again by Joyce Filer, an expert from the British Museum. Filer concurred with the earlier estimates of an age at death in the early twenties.[49]

CT findings in the KV55 skeleton (figs. 31a–b and 32)
The mummy is poorly preserved and is formed of separate remains of an incomplete skeleton with minimal soft tissues.

The CT study of the skeleton of the KV55 mummy indicates an adult man, 35–45 years old, with an estimated stature of 160 cm. There was no CT evidence of congenital anomalies or trauma. We were not able to

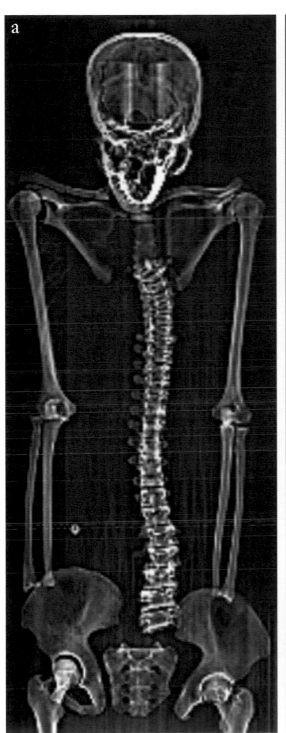

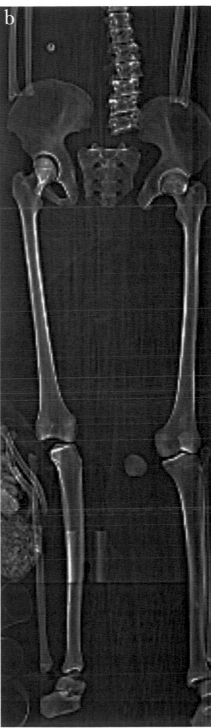

Figs. 31a–b: CT scout images of the upper (a) and lower (b) parts of the skeleton found in KV55.

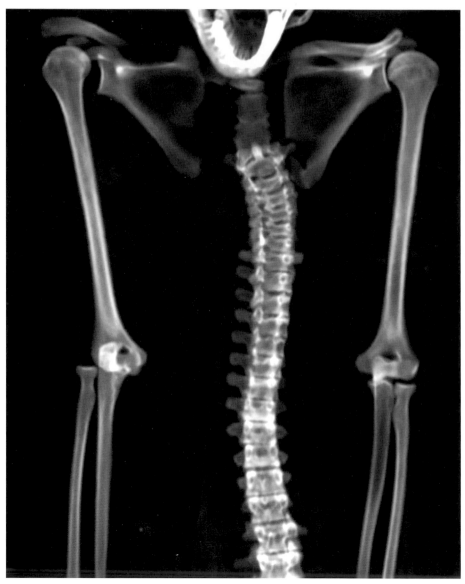

Fig. 32: Coronal CT image of the upper part of the skeleton found in KV55 shows the assembly of the separate bones of mandible, shoulder girdles, upper limbs, and spine.

suggest the cause or manner of death based on this incomplete skeleton. Although the mummy in KV55 was previously thought to be in his twenties when he died, our computed tomography investigations reveal that he lived to be much older, which would be consistent with an identification of the KV55 body as Akhenaten.[50]

Table 13. Inventory of the skeletal remains from KV55

Skull	Present, but displays multiple postmortem fractures involving the right occipital bone and right facial bones. The skull measures 189 mm in length, 153 mm in breadth, and 135 mm in height. The cranial sutures are detected.
Dental	All teeth are present. Non-erupted right upper third molar tooth and partially erupted right lower third molar tooth (wisdom tooth) (normal variant). Partially broken left lower incisors and left lower canine. Mild teeth attrition.
Pectoral girdle:	
Scapula	Both are present.
Clavicle	Right and left clavicles are present. Incomplete fracture at the posterior aspect of the middle of the right clavicle.
Upper limbs:	
Humerus	Right (317.6 mm in length) and left (313.4 mm in length). No fractures. Ossified.
Radius and ulna	On both forearms are present and intact. Right ulna measures 229 mm in length, right radius 236 mm, left ulna 229 mm, and left radius 234 mm.
Hands	Completely missing on both sides.
Spine:	
Cervical vertebrae	Present
Thoracic vertebrae	Present
Lumbar vertebrae	Present
Sacrum	Present
Coccyx	Missing
Pelvis and lower limbs:	
Hip bones	Present
Femur	Both femoral bones intact; the right measures 454.8 mm in length, and the left 455.8 mm. Right tibia measures 357.6 mm, right fibula 348.1 mm. Left tibia measures 360 mm, left fibula 348 mm.
Feet	Only talus and calcaneus bones are present; missing all other bones.
Loose bones beside the skeleton	3 vertebrae of unknown source were placed above the cervical spine. A few ribs are seen loose beside the skeleton.

5

The CT Scan of the Mummy of Tutankhamun: New Evidence on the Life and Death of the King

Historical Introduction

Tutankhamun[1] was born in approximately Year 11 of Akhenaten's reign[2] and was called Tutankhaten,[3] 'the living image of Aten.' He resided in Amarna, as suggested on relief blocks at al-Ashmunayn, which also indicates that perhaps Akhenaten was his father. When he acceded to the throne, he moved the religious capital back to Thebes, abandoning the religion of his father, changed his name to Tutankhamun, and married Ankhesenaten, a daughter of Akhenaten and Nefertiti, who also changed her name, to Ankhesenamun. A restoration decree was issued by Tutankhamun from Memphis, where he resided either in the palace of Thutmose I mentioned on the restoration stela or, because of his love for Memphis, in one built for himself. The decree indicates that there was a great deal of destruction and neglect of traditional religious monuments throughout the country during Akhenaten's reign, which the young king intended to reverse.

Thebes and Memphis[4] became the two central cities in the life of the king, and the young pharaoh was surrounded by influential courtiers, including the 'God's Father' and military officer Ay, and Horemheb, the army commander. The High Priest of Amun, Parennefer, whose tomb in Thebes (TT162) has many Amarna-style elements, may be linked to his reign. Other significant people were Maya, the treasurer of the king, who was buried in Memphis, and an officer in the army called Nakhtmin. The tomb of Sennedjem, found in the desert at Akhmim, contains cartouches of Tutankhamun; Sennedjem's title indicated that he was the tutor who instructed the king. The tomb of Maia, the king's wet nurse, was found at Saqqara by Alain Zivie. Tutankhamun is shown on reliefs within, at a young age, with his royal symbols while seated on her lap (fig. 33). Limestone blocks recently found at Memphis[5] show him smiting an enemy, as well as shooting an arrow, accompanied by his queen. John Ray discovered that these scenes on the blocks are from the tomb of Horemheb.[6] In addition, one of Tutankhamun's most important monuments at Memphis is a small rest house to the south of the Valley Temple of the Fourth Dynasty king Khafre (Chephren) at Giza, though there is no archaeological evidence of its plan.

Tutanhkamun died at the age of nineteen (plate 63a), and there are still many unanswered questions about the family of this young king.

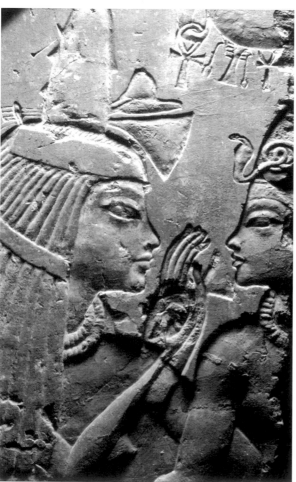

Fig. 33: Tutankhamun as a child, sitting on the lap of his wet nurse Maia. Tomb of Maia at Saqqara.

The Mummy of Tutankhamun

The mummy of Tutankhamun was studied by the Egyptian Mummy Project four times. The first time was in 2005, and marked the first occasion that a royal mummy was CT scanned.[7] The scanner, donated by Siemens, Ltd. and the National Geographic Society, is a portable unit mounted on a trailer, and it traveled to Luxor in the company of Hisham el-Leithy, one of the team members. The scanning of the mummy took place on January 5, 2005, outside the tomb. The second examination was done in conjunction with the conservation of the mummy, before it was moved to an exhibition case for its protection. The evidence was examined again during the study of the family of the king, and on a fourth occasion DNA samples were taken from the mummy.[8]

Previous studies

The mummy of Tutankhamun was first studied by Howard Carter, Douglas Derry from the Faculty of Medicine at Cairo University, and Saleh Bey Hamdy from the Faculty of Medicine at Alexandria University on November 11, 1925, in the Valley of the Kings.

Carter had opened the innermost coffin on October 28, 1925, and discovered that the embalmers had poured resins and oils onto the coffins and the gold mask that protected the king's head. As a result, the inner two coffins were stuck together, the body was stuck to the base of the innermost coffin, and the mask was firmly glued to the head and chest. After trying in vain to melt the

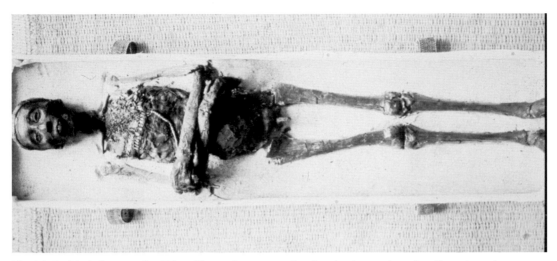

Fig. 34: Archival photograph of Tutankhamun's mummy, showing the destruction after Carter's work.

unguents by leaving the assemblage in the hot Egyptian sun for several hours a day, Carter and his colleagues decided to unwrap the mummy while it was still in its coffin.[9] Using the nearby tomb of Seti II, KV15, as a workshop, they freed the head by severing it from the body, and then used heated knives to remove the mask. In the process of unwrapping and studying the mummy, they also detached the arms and legs, and broke the mummy into a number of separate pieces—a fact that Carter did not mention in his publication,[10] though it can be seen clearly in the original excavation photographs (fig. 34).[11] The full results of the analysis of the body were not made available until F. Filce Leek published them in 1972, using Carter's diary and Derry's unpublished manuscript.[12]

In his initial study of the mummy,[13] Derry inferred that the king had been about 1.67 m tall (5'6") and lightly built, and deduced, based on the union of the epiphyses, that the king died between the ages of seventeen and nineteen, with eighteen being the most likely. He also noted a break in the left leg, but could

reach no conclusions about the possible cause of the king's premature death. Carter's team brought the mummy back to the tomb in October 1926.

In 1968, R.G. Harrison, professor of anatomy at the University of Liverpool, undertook the first x-ray analysis of the mummy inside the tomb (fig. 35), which confirmed that it had been broken into pieces.[14] The x-rays revealed that some of the king's ribs were missing. In addition, a photograph of the mummy left by Carter shows the head covered with linen and a gold band around the head. The band had completely disappeared by the time that Harrison x-rayed the mummy. Harrison also discovered dislodged bone fragments within the king's skull,[15] which some have subsequently taken as possible evidence of murder by a blow to the head.[16]

Following his investigation, Harrison estimated that the king died at age eighteen, more specifically, and analysis of the teeth suggested an age early in the range of eighteen to twenty-two years.[17]

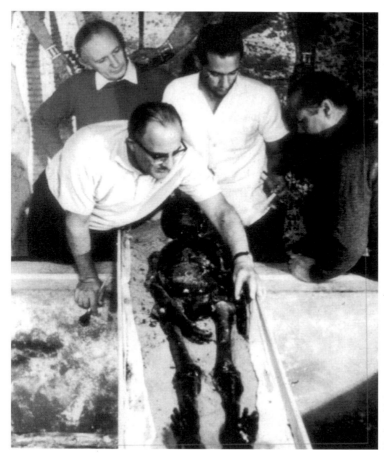

Fig. 35: The team accompanied by Ibrahim al-Nawawi during the 1968 reexamination of the mummy of Tutankhamun.

In 1978, James Harris from the University of Michigan also performed an x-ray examination of the skull inside the tomb. He stated that both eye sockets had collapsed, so that the lids and lashes were now gone, and the right ear was missing.[18] Unfortunately, Harris never published his observations.

CT Scanning of the Mummy

Although both the original examination and the subsequent x-rays revealed much about the life of the king, they also left many questions open and have provided fuel for much speculation. The current investigation was designed to confirm or refute the conclusions of the previous examinations, and to look for additional details that earlier investigators might have missed. In this it was extremely successful.[19]

We began our investigation on the evening of January 5, 2005, though we were faced with bad weather in the form of a driving rainstorm that occurred in the valley. The trailer housing the CT scanner was situated in front of the tomb of Tutankhamun. Dr. Hany Abdel-Rahman operated the machine.

We removed the lid of the sarcophagus and found that the mummy was lying on a wooden tray placed in sand (plate 31). The Egyptian team carefully moved the mummy out of the tomb and positioned it under the CT scanner inside the trailer (plate 32). The scanning was delayed by a technical glitch (sand in the cooling system) that took about an hour to fix. CT scanners are able to scan the whole body in a very short time, and their ability to distinguish various types of soft tissues and bone and differentiate between diseases is far superior to conventional x-rays. The body does not need to be moved repeatedly as it does for x-rays, which meant that there was less chance for damage to the mummy during the process. The scanning of Tutankhamun's mummy was completed in half an hour. More than 1,700 images were generated, which the team examined over the course of the next two months.

When the mummy was returned to the tomb, a card was discovered in the sarcophagus that had originally been placed there by Howard Carter, recording the dates that he examined the mummy. This had been added to by Harrison, then Harris, and we added this most recent study, naming Zahi Hawass and the team.

On March 4–5, 2005, the group of scholars convened to discuss the results. The conclusions follow, and the scientists were in agreement on almost all points.[20]

CT findings for the mummy of Tutankhamun
General CT findings
Preservation
In general, the remains of the king were in a poor state of preservation. The body is in a number of pieces, and many parts present at the original examination in 1925 are now missing, although numerous fragments remain loose in the sand tray on which the mummy rests. In fact, CT scanning revealed the presence of parts of the ribs, clavicles, fingers, toes, and possibly the penis buried in the sand of the wooden box into which Carter's team placed the dismembered mummy. The mummy had been decapitated at vertebral level thoracic one by Carter and his team. The extremities were disarticulated, including elbow, wrist, and knee joints, and there was a complete separation of the body at vertebral level lumbar three. The arms were no longer crossed at the chest as they had been originally, and now lay at his sides (plates 33a–b).[21]

Some bones were completely missing (finger phalanges, sternum, parts of the clavicle, both scapulae, and pelvic bones).

The skeleton was slender in appearance, and the soft tissues were shrunken in varying degrees. Variations of the anatomy included bilateral lambdoid sutural bones, an incomplete cleft palate, and a left os tibiale externum. Changes that appeared to be postmortem in nature were cracks in the skin and adjacent soft tissues, as well as the presence of small dots of high density (ca. 1000 HU) in several places, especially in muscle areas, which may be a result of the embalming process. There was a mild right-convex scoliosis (see below). There were many traumatic lesions, some clearly caused by mummification, including the destruction of the nasal septum, ethmoid cells, and cribriform plate, during transnasal removal of the brain.

Other changes clearly resulted from modern unwrapping of the mummy. Much of the front chest wall, including the sternum and large parts of the ribs, front and back, are missing. The ends of the fragmented ribs were clearly cut by a sharp instrument at different places, which could not have been the result of an intra vitam (during life) trauma. These chest lesions were most likely caused by Carter's use of chisels to extract the mummy from its inner coffin and mask.[22] Other apparently modern fractures, based on their location and appearance (sharp cuts at most dorsal exposed body parts) were seen in the lumbar back region with absence of soft tissue (erector spinal muscle area), and the first four lumbar vertebral arches.

Stature

The overall height of the king was estimated at 167 cm (five and a half feet), based on the measurements of his tibia (lower leg), the only intact major long bones. He was slightly built (gracile).

Age at death

Tutankhamun was about nineteen years old when he died, based on the following observations and using modern developmental tables.[23]

The fusion of the epiphyseal plates matches the development of a young man of eighteen to twenty years. The cranial sutures of the skull could be seen, the sagittal suture in particular. The epiphyseal plates were not fused at the distal right femur, or the proximal humeral and femoral ends on both sides, but were united at both proximal and distal tibial ends on both sides.

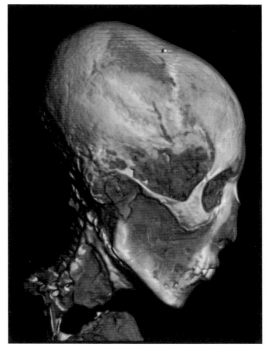

Fig. 36: Three-dimensional reconstructed CT image of the skull of Tutankhamun in right profile projection.

Three wisdom teeth were partially erupted, with minor malalignment. The fourth (left upper) was impacted and unerupted, and there is a slight thinning of the sinus cavity above. This was not life-threatening, and there are no signs of infection.

CT Findings in different regions
Head

Tutankhamun has a brachycephalic skull (ca. 190 mm x 160 mm, total circumference ca. 580 mm, and cranial index 84) (fig. 36).[24]

The nasal septa were destroyed by the embalmers when the brain was extracted through the nose.

The king had a small cleft in his hard palate (the bony roof of his mouth), not associated with an external expression such as a harelip or other facial deformation.

Table 14. General CT findings for the mummy of Tutankhamun

Preservation Status	Poor
Age	About 19 years (18–20 years)
Gender	Male
Stature (from tibia)	167 cm

Teeth (figs. 37a–b)

The general condition of the teeth was excellent, with no caries, periodontal abcesses, or abrasion. The lower teeth are slightly misaligned. There was a mild prognathism (projection forward of the jaw). Tutankhamun has large front incisors and the overbite characteristic of other kings from his family (the Thutmosid line).[25]

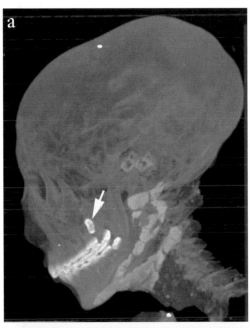

Torso

There is a slight bend in the spine, producing minimal right-convex scoliosis, with its apex at the twelfth vertebral level, without vertebral deformations or rotation, with attendant mild tilting of the pelvis towards the left, as far as could be determined in its present fragmented state. The scientists agreed that it is not a pathological scoliosis, since there is no rotation and no associated deformation of the vertebrae. This bend most likely reflects the position of the body during embalming or resulted from the severing of the spine by Carter and his team.

The sternum and a large percentage of the front ribs are now missing, evidently along with much of the front chest wall (fig. 38). The ends of the missing ribs have clearly been cleanly cut with a sharp instrument. However, photographs of Carter's work clearly show a beaded collar and string of beads placed upon the breast, before the unwrapping was complete. It is most likely that the damage was caused by the removal of these objects. Carter does not mention this in his notes, nor does he report missing ribs or sternum. Archaeological investigation will continue in an effort to resolve this issue.[26]

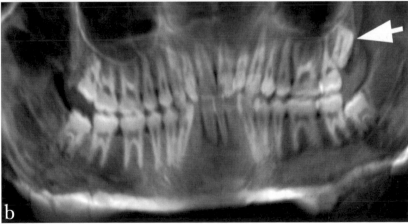

Figs. 37a–b: Three-dimensional reconstruction of the head of Tutankhamun using MIP in the lateral view (a) shows the impacted, nonerupted upper wisdom tooth (arrow).

Curved multiplanar reconstructed CT image along the dental arcades of Tutankhamun (b) shows the nonerupted, impacted left third molar (wisdom tooth) (arrow) as well as noneruption of the other three wisdom teeth.

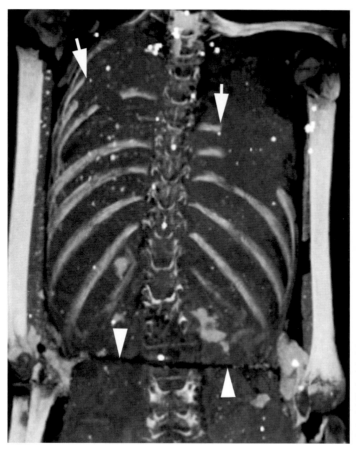

Fig. 38: Three-dimensional reconstruction of the torso of Tutankhamun using MIP in frontal view shows multiple missing ribs with sharply cut edges (arrows). Note also the severed lower trunk (arrowheads), which was likely responsible for the mildly bent spine (scoliosis).

The phallus of the king was intact during Carter's exhumation of the body, but was reported missing during the 1968 examination. The team has tentatively located it loose in the sand surrounding the mummy.

Lower limbs

The team noted a fracture of the left lower femur at the level of the epiphyseal plate. In contrast to the multiple traumatic lesions caused by embalming or Carter's modern unwrapping, the left femur shows a fracture line at the medial epiphyseal region with mild ventral dislocation from the axis of the femur. Reactive physiologic changes, in vivo, were present, including irregular bony fragments with ragged edges on the lateral and medial epicondyles, rather than the sharp edges found in modern damage. Along the fracture line (width ca. 2–5 mm), a clearly distinct spotted increased density of the spongiosa is visible. This type of fracture of the femur corresponds to the clinically well-known multi-fragmentary intra-articular distal femur fracture (type 33 C3 according to AO classification[27]) found in individuals with still unfused epiphyses, such as the king, a young man in his late teens (fig. 39). Furthermore, within the space of the medial femoral fracture and in the subcutaneous tissues of the

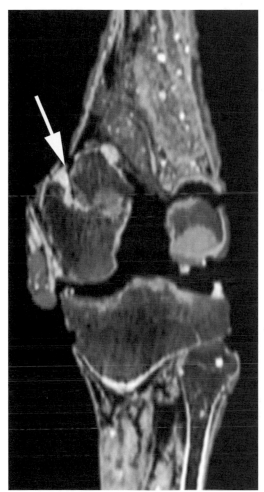

Fig. 39: Two-dimensional reconstructed CT image of the left knee in coronal plane shows a fracture of the inner side of the lower part of the thigh bone, with the dense embalming material covering its edges (arrow), suggesting its occurrence shortly before death.

associated skin would still have been open, the fracture would have taken place shortly before death, a matter of days at most. In addition, Carter's team had noted that the patella of this leg was intact but loose[28] (and is now completely separated and enclosed within the left hand), which may indicate further ancient damage to this part of the body. The members of our team who subscribe to this theory also noted a fracture of the right patella and right lower leg. These team members maintain that the king may have suffered an accident that badly broke his leg and left an open wound. The fracture would not have been fatal, but could have triggered lethal cascades, such as bleeding, pulmonary or fat embolism, or infection. However, they also indicated that this fracture could have been caused by the embalmers, though this was less likely, or that it was caused by Carter's actions.

At the outset, part of the team believed that the above scenario was absolutely incorrect. They suggested that the leg fracture mentioned above could only have been done by Carter's team during the removal of the mummy from the coffin. They argued that if such a fracture had taken place during the king's life, the CT scans would have produced evidence of hemorrhage or hematoma. They maintained that the embalming material was pushed into the fracture by Carter's team. However, in the final analysis, this interpretation was rejected, and the traumatic fracture was seen as the correct diagnosis.

Feet

Although the CT scanning was done in 2005, a re-examination of the images was carried out in 2009 by Ashraf Selim, Sahar Saleem, and Paul Gostner to investigate the king's feet in order to ascertain further details. The scientists

popliteal fossa (back of knee), two different embalming-like substances of unknown chemical components had infiltrated, suggesting an associated open wound. There is no apparent evidence that healing took place, though it is possible that any such healing would be masked by the embalming material. Since the

analyzed the images of Tutankhamun's feet separately and blinded from each other's work. The scientists were unanimous on most of the points, and the final decision was rendered by consensus.

The CT examination revealed multiple bony fractures that were likely inflicted after the king's death, possibly by Carter's team. One notable fracture occurred at the outer side of the right ankle (lateral malleolus), whose location and appearance is a well-recognized injury caused by forcible twisting of the ankle. This could have been caused before death, though the lack of associated healing or embalming material within makes it impossible to rule out postmortem damage.

Tutankhamun had a flat arch of his right foot (pes planus). The CT image also revealed a left club foot deformity. The foot was moderately turned downward and inward in a manner that simulated the position of a horse's foot (talipes equinovarus). The CT observations of the king's feet (plates 34a–b) could also be detected in a recent inspection of the mummy itself. The toes of the left foot were also widely separated. Both of these conditions are usually present from birth (congenital), and were probably not due to the embalming process. The embalmers actually treated the feet quite carefully, wrapping each toe individually in linen and encasing them in gold toe stalls (fig. 40), as can be seen in early photographs taken at the time of the discovery. With such a deformity in his left foot, the king would have walked on his ankle or on the side of his foot.

In addition to the club foot, the CT images of the left foot showed that the middle bone of the second toe was missing, so that the toe appears shorter (oligodactyly). This supports the conclusion that the left-foot deformities of the king were congenital.

Moreover, the heads of the second and third midfoot bones (metatarsals) showed abnormal mixed high and low densities within that correspond to the diagnosis of Freiberg's Disease of the midfoot bones (usually the second and third metatarsals) that affects adolescents. The etiology of Freiberg's Disease is not clear. It could be attributed to the insult (injury, irritation, or trauma) of the midfoot bones during their growth (epiphyseal maturation). The insult could have been caused by one acute injury, small repetitive micro-injuries, or insult of the blood supply. The deformity may be predisposed by genetic variables, as it has been reported also in twins. The modern treatment of Freiberg's Disease is removal of the defective bone through surgery or repair using a bone graft. In the absence of this treatment, King Tutankhamun would have suffered from painful, swollen joints (second and third metatarso-phalangeal), and limited motion.

In conclusion, Tutankhamun had a painful foot, with multiple deformities in his left foot. The medial longitudinal arch of this foot was slightly higher than normal (Rocher angle 120°). Archaeological evidence also documents the foot problems of the king. Howard Carter found 130 walking sticks in his tomb.[29] One of these sticks has an inscription that reads "a reed which His Majesty cut with his own hand."[30] In addition, on a painted plaque or relief from Amarna, now in Berlin,[31] the king leans on a staff, and he is shown holding a staff while accepting flowers from Ankhesenamun on an ivory plaque from a box lid found in his tomb (plate 35). However, the staff can also be viewed as a symbol of authority over others that occurred from the Old Kingdom on. Akhenaten is portrayed holding a stick on *talatat* from the Ninth Pylon at Karnak.[32] Reliefs of Amenhotep III from the area of the

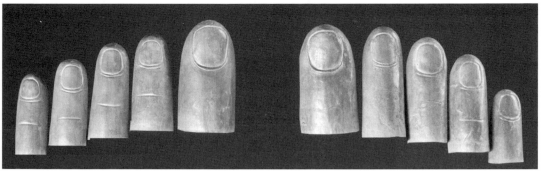

Fig. 40: Gold stalls found on the feet of Tutankhamun. Egyptian Museum, Cairo.

Fourth Pylon at Karnak depict the king holding staves, and royalty and high nobility are shown with staves in their tomb reliefs.

Further evidence for Tutankhamun's affliction, however, is seen in portrayals of the king seated while engaged in activities for which one usually would stand, such as hunting.[33] In one limestone relief found in the area of Memphis, from the tomb of Horemheb at Saqqara, he is seated and shoots an arrow, with his queen beside him (fig. 41).[34] Scenes of non-royal people seated while catching birds or fish exist, such as in the Middle Kingdom tomb of Khnumhotep[35] and the Eighteenth Dynasty tomb of Kenamun, TT93.[36] The context of these scenes, however, is very different from

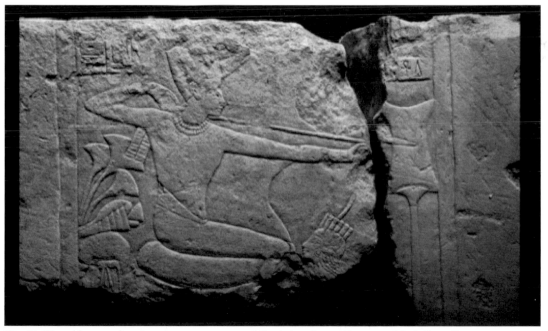

Fig. 41: Tutankhamun shooting arrows at a target while sitting. Loose limestone block from Saqqara.

those of Tutankhamun, for which there is no known royal parallel.[37] Some scholars maintain that this royal scene does not indicate weakness, but the king's dignity and status as a god, but the physical evidence from Tutankhamun's mummy suggests a different interpretation.

It seems possible that the boy king had these medical conditions due to the brother–sister marriage of his father, Akhenaten (see chapter 7, "Investigations into King Tutankhamun's Family"). Such inbreeding carries an increased risk of congenital disorders in children of the union.

Conclusions
Embalming of the head: principal route
The scientists agreed that various types of liquids were introduced into the cranial cavity several times through the nose, based on the differing densities of the material and the way the now-solidified liquids appear. At first, the body lay on its back, and the embalming fluid pooled along the back of the skull. Later in the process, the head was tipped back, and the liquid pooled in the top of the skull.

Possible second route for embalming of the head
Part of the team saw evidence for a second

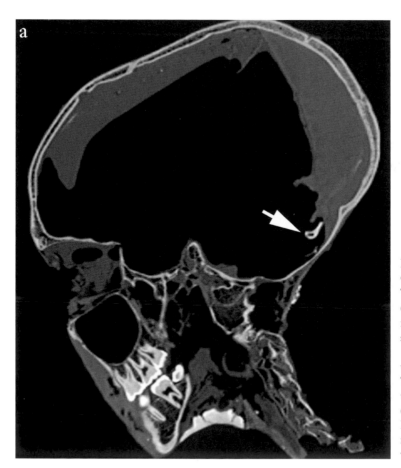

Figs. 42a–b: Reconstructed CT image of the skull of Tutankhamun in sagittal plane (a) shows a free bony fragment inside and at the back of the skull (arrow).

Reconstructed CT image, using MIP, of the skull of Tutankhamun (b) identified two free bone fragments (arrows). These fragments are likely detached from the foramen magnum and first cervical vertebra (atlas).

route through which embalming liquid was introduced into the lower cranial cavity and neck. This would have been through the back of the upper neck. In this area, there are two layers of solidified material of different density from that seen above in this area.

According to the report, an extensive irregular defect was seen in the soft tissues and adjacent bones at the left occipito-cervical region, including the left posterior border of the foramen magnum and adjacent occipital bone (defect ca. 20 x 6 mm) and the posterior arch of the atlas. The soft-tissue lesion extends on the left side of the neck anterior to the mandibular angle with partial destruction of the masseter muscle area. The vast majority of the surface lesion is covered by a high-density substance (ca. 2000 HU). Two free bone fragments were found, one consisting of cortical and spongiotic bone of clasp-like shape (ca. 21 mm x 7 mm x 6 mm) in the right posterior cranial fossa and the other (ca. 11 mm x 3 mm x 3 mm) in the left parietal region (figs. 42a–b). These fragments are clearly the detached part of the foramen magnum border and the posterior arch of the atlas, respectively. They are obviously loose, as they are currently at different locations

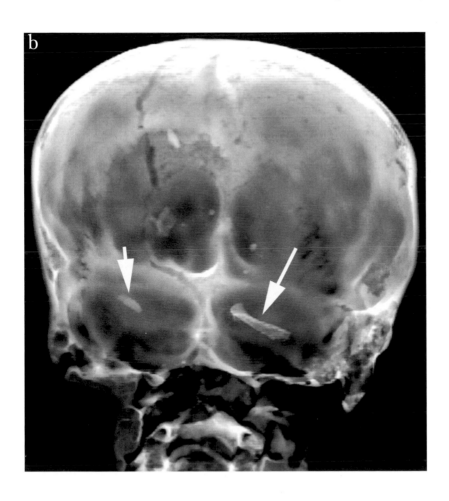

than were shown by x-rays in 1968 and 1978.[38] (These x-rays have never been fully published.) Therefore, the fragments are postmortem, and a penetrating intra vitam skull bone lesion can now be completely ruled out. There is no associated thinning of the skull bone or calcified hematoma as possible evidence for major intra vitam cranial trauma. Since the bony pieces were not adherent to the intracranial embalming liquids, it is believed that these fragments were either caused by the modern unwrapping or, less likely, were remnants of a second attempt at embalming through the foramen magnum. The remainder of the team saw no evidence for an embalming route through the back of the neck. They believe, instead, that the embalming liquid in this area was also introduced through the nose or trickled down from the cranial cavity, and that the vertebra and foramen magnum were definitely damaged by Carter's team while removing the head from the mask, and could not have been damaged by the embalmers.

A trans–foramen magnum embalming approach, including removal of the atlas bone, has been continually described as being performed for the founder of the Eighteenth Dynasty, King Ahmose.[39] This approach in Ahmose would have to be confirmed by a CT scan as well.

The use of both transnasal and trans–foramen magnum embalming approaches in the same individual has never been described before. More royal mummies would need to be CT scanned to see whether or not this was a common practice.

The 'murder' theory

The entire team agreed that there was no evidence in the skull that would suggest Tutankhamun was murdered.[40] There is no area in the back of the skull that indicates a partially healed blow. There are two bone fragments loose in the skull, but these cannot possibly have been from an injury during his lifetime, as they would have adhered to the embalming fluid. The scientific team has matched these pieces to the fractured cervical vertebra and foramen magnum, and concluded that these were broken either during mummification or by Carter's team.

Sahar Saleem studied in detail the embalming approach used on the remains of Tutankhamun, including evisceration incisions, the presence of the heart and other viscera, and attempts at beautification. These studies will be addressed below; see chapter 11, "CT Findings on the Mummification Process of Royal Ancient Egyptians."

Malaria

The skin of the left cheek and neck of the mummy showed patchy changes, possibly indicating an 'Aleppo boil,' plague spot, or inflamed mosquito bite. Blood tests indicated that the king had multiple malaria infections, as two alleles of the pathogen causing malaria (*Plasmodium falciparum*) were extracted.[41]

Some modern dietary treatments for malaria prescribe a substantial quantity of fresh fruit to bring the fever down, and specify that patients should stay away from alcohol and meat.[42] Although a lot of fruit was found in Tutankhamun's tomb, and there is a lack of beer, there were wine and meat, which would not help recovery. The food in the tomb cannot, therefore, be firmly linked to any medical treatment that the king may have received. Also, others simply state that there are no dietary restrictions for those suffering from malaria. In addition, the food provisions placed in other royal tombs of the New Kingdom are unknown, and those found in Tutankhamun's tomb may have been standard. Since there is no evidence for the treatment of malaria in the ancient texts, we cannot discern what measures the ancient Egyptians would have taken to aid the young king. There can thus be no firm link between the food found in the tomb and the treatment of malaria.[43]

Did malaria kill the king? Perhaps. The disease can trigger a fatal immune response in the body, cause circulatory shock, and in its most dangerous expression, infect the brain, leading to hemorrhaging, convulsions, coma, and death. As other scientists asserted, however, malaria was probably common in the region at the time, and Tutankhamun may have acquired some partial immunity to the disease. On the other hand, it may well have weakened his immune system, leaving him more at risk to developing infections such as might have followed the fracture of his leg.

Tutankhamun's health was compromised from the moment he was conceived. His mother and father were full brother and sister,

as described in chapter 7. Pharaonic Egypt was not the only society in history to institutionalize royal incest, which has political advantages, but there is a dangerous consequence. Matings between siblings are more likely to burden progeny with twin copies of deleterious genes, leaving them vulnerable to a variety of genetic defects. Tutankhamun's deformed foot, which he dragged behind him all his life, may have been one such flaw. We know he also had a cleft palate, another congenital defect. Perhaps he battled others, until a severe bout of malaria or complications from a broken leg added one strain too many to a body no longer able to bear the burden.[44]

In conclusion, it is possible that Tutankhamun had an accident a few hours before his death, based on the result of the CT scanning in 2005. It could have been the result of a chariot accident while hunting in Memphis. As mentioned above, he resided in a palace there and also had a rest house south of the Valley Temple of Khafre. A leg fracture possibly complicated by infection resulted in a life-threatening situation, especially in the presence of malaria.

A New Theory about the 'Burned' Mummy of Tutankhamun

Recently, a new theory about the mummy of Tutankhamun has emerged, proposed by Chris Naughton, director of the Egypt Exploration Society, and Robert Connolly, an anthropologist from University of Liverpool, working in conjunction with forensic anthropologist Matthew Ponting and scientists at the Cranfield Forensic Institute. Using a tissue sample obtained in 1968 and a 'virtual autopsy,' they claim that the mummy was burned while sealed in its coffin, had extensive damage on one side, and was missing its heart. They further theorized that a chariot accident could explain the shattering of the ribs and pelvis.

It is our belief that this theory is unlikely to be true, for many reasons:

1. *Tissue sample*: The authenticity of the tissue sample is unknown and it cannot be proved to have belonged to Tutankhamun.

2. *Damage to the mummy during unwrapping by Howard Carter and his team*: With the assumption that the tissue really belongs to the royal mummy of Tutankhamun, the well-known, brutally invasive methods that Howard Carter and Douglas Derry used during the original examination of the mummy in November 1925 must be taken into consideration. It was difficult for them to remove the body from the inner coffin as they were adhered to each other by resin, so Carter and his team removed the mummy in pieces. They cut the neck to separate the head from the body, used hot knives to extract the skull from the mask and front of the chest, separated the pelvis from the trunk, and detached the arms and legs. Such documented damage of the mummy during its unwrapping should be considered before claiming stories about injuries that might have happened to the king or caused his death. The tissue sample could have been obtained from a section that had been burned by Carter's knives.

3. *Chemical reaction of mummification*: The report claims that a chemical reaction between embalming oils and linen in the presence of oxygen burned the mummy inside the coffin, with a temperature of 200 degrees Celsius.

However, this was based on some mummies with poor mummification that were reported to suffer from this phenomenon due to improper drying and exposure to wet hot resin that scorched the mummy without causing it to go up in flames.

Although poor mummification could also theoretically happen due to an abusive excess of material as an expression of piety, we attest excellent mummification procedures in the royal mummies. During our forensic examinations, which included tissue sampling of dozens of the royal mummies dating to the same period as that of Tutankhamun, we did not report any burning effects or charring.

4. *Missing heart*: The claim was made that a fatal accident damaged the chest and accounts for the missing heart in the mummy of Tutankhamun. Our CT examination showed clearly that much of the front of the chest wall, including the sternum, and large parts of the ribs are missing. The ends of the fragments were clearly cut by a sharp instrument at different sites. This could not have been the result of a trauma during the life of the king (intra vitam). In fact, parts of the missing bones of the ribs and clavicles were buried within the sand beneath the mummy, inside the wooden box into which Carter's team placed the dismantled mummy. In our CT examination, we noted no evidence of heart tissue, and it is apparently missing in other royal mummies, such as Yuya, Amenhotep III, and Merenptah. A missing heart thus cannot be taken as evidence for intra vitam trauma.

5. *Virtual autopsy*: The results of the thorough study of the CT images, done by our Egyptian scientists and approved by international experts, indicated clearly an injury at the lower left femur of the mummy and put forth the possibility of a chariot accident. We announced this and published it in several studies since 2010, so this report does not provide any new data.

6. *Recent examinations of the mummy by Zahi Hawass*: The mummy has been examined three times in recent years, and there was no visual indication that the body had been burned.

There is also a serious ethical issue here. By claiming that he obtained a tissue sample from the royal mummy, Robert Connolly breached the ethical code, as his job was only to x-ray the mummy in 1968. The sample was thus obtained illegally.

For all of the above reasons, we can conclude it is unlikely that the body was burned by the mummification process.

S.N.S. and Z.H.

6

The Two Fetuses Found
in the Tomb of Tutankhamun

Historical Introduction

In 1922, Howard Carter found two miniature mummies inside an undecorated wooden box in the Treasury of King Tutankhamun's tomb (fig. 43).[1] Nestled within the box were two miniature anthropoid coffins placed side by side in opposing directions. Both coffins were covered in a layer of black resin and decorated with gold bands, which simply named each deceased fetus as "the Osiris." The lids were attached to the coffin bases with eight flat wooden tenons. Around the coffins were bands of linen with clay seal impressions of a jackal and nine captives, referring to the "nine bows" or enemies of Egypt. Bands were also wrapped around the mummy bundles beneath the chin and around the waist and ankles. A second coffin, which was covered in gold foil, was placed inside each outer coffin. Within these gilded second coffins were the mummified fetuses. The wooden box was designated by Carter as number 317,

and the two coffins and their respective mummies were recorded as 317a (the smaller mummy, plate 36a) and 317b (the larger one, plate 36b).[2]

In 1925, Howard Carter removed the bandages of mummy 317a, and in 1932 both fetuses were autopsied by Douglas Derry. In this examination,[3] Derry described the mummies as female fetuses at five and seven months of gestation. At that time, mummy 317a was almost perfectly preserved, though it had no eyebrows or eyelashes. It measured 25.75 cm in height, and the arms were placed on the front of the thighs. Part of its umbilical cord (21 mm) was still attached to the mummified fetus. Derry did not report any abdominal incisions, which raised the possibility that it was naturally mummified. The larger fetus, 317b, was less well preserved. It measured 36.1 cm in length, and the arms were extended and placed beside the thighs. The eyes were open, and eyebrows and eye-

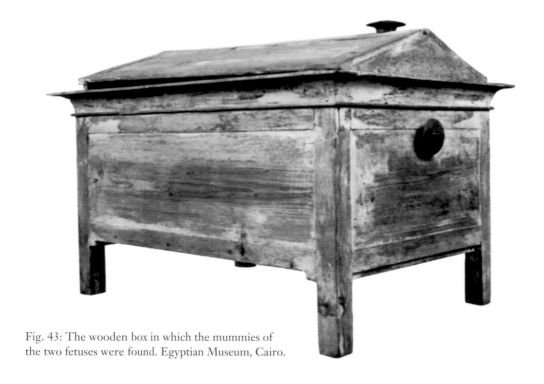

Fig. 43: The wooden box in which the mummies of the two fetuses were found. Egyptian Museum, Cairo.

lashes were preserved. There was downy hair on the scalp. Derry reported that this fetus had been artificially mummified, due to the presence of a small left inguinal embalming incision, measuring 1.8 cm, as well as linen packs inserted through the nose into the skull.[4] The two mummies were placed in the Faculty of Medicine at Cairo University for safekeeping, and they have remained there since Derry's examination.

Previous Plain X-Ray Study of Mummy 317b
In 1978, Ronald Harrison and colleagues examined the 317b mummy by x-ray. They theorized that the mummy was thirty-five weeks' gestation to full term at the time of mummification and had multiple congenital anomalies of Sprengel's deformity, spinal dysraphism, and scoliosis.[5] In 2008, Catherine Hellier and Robert Connolly reassessed the

x-ray of the mummy and suggested a younger age of thirty weeks' gestation.[6]

Results of the CT Scan of the Two Fetuses
Ahmed Sameh Farid, the head of Kasr Al-Ainy Hospital and the dean of the Faculty of Medicine at Cairo University at that time, was contacted about the possibility of studying the two fetuses. He gave his approval, supported the project, and was instrumental in the establishment of a DNA lab at Kasr Al-Ainy (see chapter 7, "Investigations into King Tutankhamun's Family"). Fawzi Gaballa, professor of anatomy at Kasr Al-Ainy, was in charge of the fetuses and worked with us closely. It was discovered that they were in very fragile condition. It was not possible to move them for scanning at the Egyptian Museum, so it was necessary to scan them at the Faculty of Medicine.[7]

Special technical points in the CT examination of the two mummies (317a and 317b)

CT scanning was done on July 27, 2008, using MDCT at the radiology department of Cairo University supervised by Ashraf Selim and Sahar Saleem. Inside the gantry of the CT machine, each mummy was placed separately in an open wooden box. To maximize the results of the study, the CT and image analysis were tailored to suit the examination of small, poorly preserved ancient human remains.

The settings were adjusted so as not to exceed the thermal capability of the x-ray tube, to 120 kilovolt (kVp) and 140 milliamperes (MA). Antero-posterior and latero-lateral scout images were chosen to include the whole mummy. The minimal scanning thickness permitted by the CT (0.625 mm) was chosen. A total of 495 CT images were taken of mummy 317a and 701 images of 317b. On a separate workstation, Sahar Saleem handled the reconstruction of the images, image analysis, and the forensic research studies. Image reconstruction included MPR, curved images along dental arcades (orthopantomographic-like), advanced 3D reconstruction, and manual tracing and virtual removal of linen tissues and other embalming materials. Three-dimensional reconstruction was accomplished using preset reconstruction algorithms for soft tissues with varying window-width parameters using volume-rendering techniques. Measurements of bony lengths and densities of soft-tissue structures, linen, and embalming materials were precisely obtained electronically; each measurement was precisely taken once.[8]

CT findings in mummy 317a

At the time of CT study, the mummy was in very poor condition. The 2D and 3D reconstructed CT images showed such extensive soft-tissue and bony damage that it was not possible to measure the stature of the mummy on CT images (plate 37). Instead, the body stature was extrapolated from the left humerus, which was reasonably preserved, to be 29.9 cm. We used the following equation: Stature (cm) = 7.92 × (humeral length (cm) − 0.32) + 1.8.[9]

The age of the fetus (gestational age) at the time of mummification was inferred from the humeral bone length to be 24.6 weeks (5–6 months) by using fetal age (weeks) SD 2.33 = 0.4585 x humerus length (mm) + 8.6563.[10]

The morphology of the external genitalia can be used in assignment of fetal sex starting from twelve weeks and is normally fully developed at twenty weeks of gestation.[11] At the estimated age of mummy 317a of 24 weeks' gestation, the external morphology of genitalia can determine the sex clearly. However, we could not assign the gender of the mummy from the CT images due to its poor condition. We depended on the forensic examination done in 1932 by Douglas Derry, who indicated the mummy to be a female.[12] At that time, the mummy was almost perfectly preserved, which enabled Derry to describe the mummy's anatomy in detail. Derry was a professor of anatomy at Cairo University who had experience in performing autopsies on several mummies; thus we think that his testimony of the sex of fetus 317a can be relied upon.[13]

The skull was severely damaged, but we could detect contents of mixed high and low CT densities within. These in all probability represented atrophic brain tissue with possible embalming material (fig. 44). Based on physical examination of mummy 317a in 1932, Douglas Derry did not notice any abdominal incisions, and thus he assumed that it was mummified naturally. Despite the

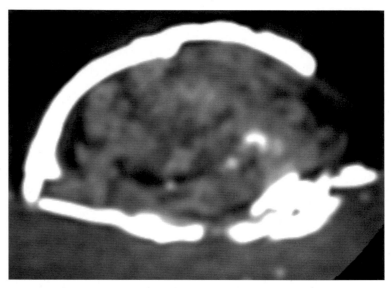

Fig. 44: Transverse CT section through the skull of mummy of fetus 317a shows multiple postmortem skull fractures that hampered detection of a transcranial route of mummification. However, the skull contains substances of mixed high and intermediate CT densities that may represent atrophic brain residue and/or embalming materials.

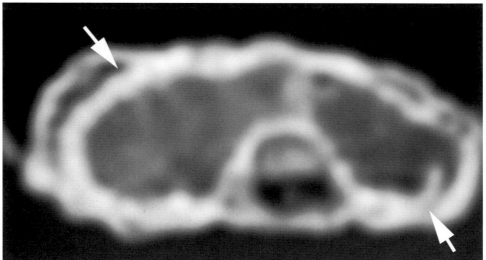

Fig. 45: Transverse CT section through the torso of mummy 317a shows low-density structures with dense periphery (arrows) within the torso cavity, probably representing linen packs coated with resin.

marked deterioration of the condition of the mummy since Derry's report, we suggest that the mummy may have been subjected to artificial mummification. CT images of the body cavity show elaborate structures of mixed CT densities that most likely represent visceral packs (fig. 45). However, detection of such embalming routes as skull defects or abdominal incisions was not possible because of the poor condition of the mummy. The CT images could not detect gross skeletal deformities or an evident cause of death.[14]

CT findings in mummy 317b

CT images confirmed the poor condition of the mummy that was apparent from physical inspection. However, the preservation of this mummy was better than the other; this permitted more thorough CT study. Full-body 2D and 3D reconstructed CT images revealed multiple fractures in the skull, neck, shoulders, and feet (plates 38a–b). The presence of multiple skeletal and craniofacial fractures hampered direct vertex-to-heel measurement. Body stature extrapolated from humeral length was 45 cm.

The mummy was likely subjected to artificial mummification, as supported in CT images by the presence of a left inguinal incision that extended for 18 mm with a maximum depth of 13 mm, and opened lips of 5–11 mm (fig. 47). In addition, CT images identified multiple convoluted structures in the body cavity of mixed high and low CT densities; these probably represent visceral packs (fig. 46). The mummification seems to be of high quality, as there was evidence of subcutaneous high-density fillings in the lower limbs, which were probably used to

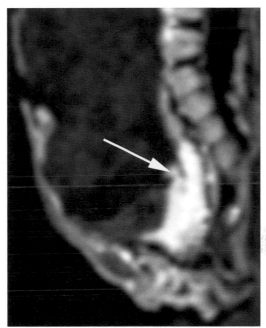

Fig. 46: Sagittal CT image of the lower torso of fetus 317b shows dense structure, likely an embalming pack (arrow).

restore the contour of the mummy's legs. As a result, the left thigh was noticeably larger than the right (fig. 48).

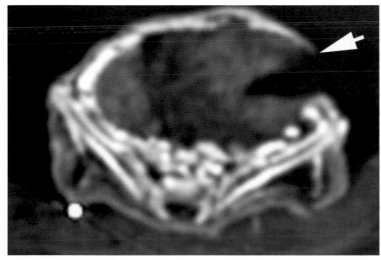

Fig. 47: Axial CT of the torso of mummified fetus 317b shows the embalming incision at the left inguinal region (arrow).

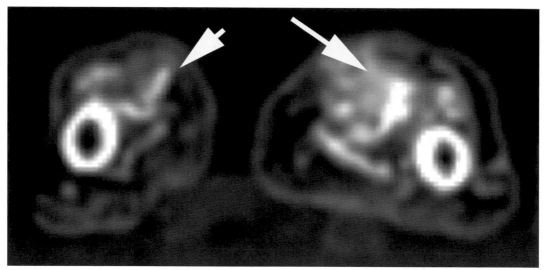

Fig. 48: Axial CT image of both thighs of mummy 317b shows structures with mixed density within the soft tissues of both thighs (arrows), probably subcutaneous packs placed by the embalmers to restore the contours of the limbs. Note the asymmetry of size of the packs that resulted in larger left thigh (long arrow).

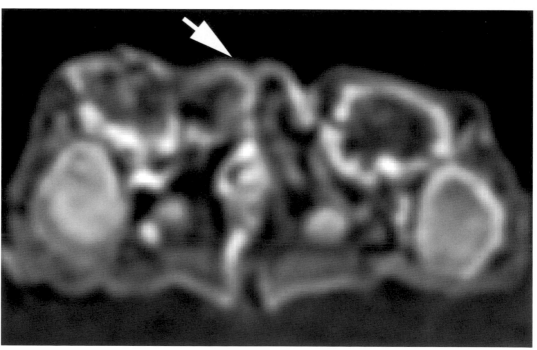

Fig. 49: Axial CT image of the lower pelvic region of mummy 317b shows the female morphology of the external genitalia (arrow).

The morphology of the fetus's external genitalia was consistent with that of a female (fig. 49), as well as the morphological appearance of the hip bone (os coxae), with a wide sub-pubic angle of 118 degrees and an ischio-pubic ratio of less than 1.

We employed different radiographic methods using CT findings to estimate the gestational age of the mummy, which was nine months (36.78 weeks SD 1.91) (details below).

Ossification centers

At the knees, the distal femoral epiphysis (DFE) and proximal tibial epiphysis (PTE) are present bilaterally, being slightly more developed on the left side. Right knee: DFE diameter is 4 mm and PTE diameter is 1.6 mm. Left knee: DFE diameter is 4.1 mm and PTE diameter is 1.7 mm (fig. 50).

Two ossification centers at the talus and calcaneus bones are present on both sides. The cuboid ossification center was not visualized. The talus ossification center is present on both sides, with concavity at the upper and plantar surfaces. The superior pubic ramus is ossified, with a dumb-bell-shaped appearance. The ischial ramus is ossified, with a concave anterior surface. The sternum is ossified. The inferior radial metaphysis and inferior tibial metaphysis are flat.

Teeth mineralization

We detected on the orthopantomographic-like reconstructed CT images the ossified crowns of maxillary and mandibular teeth: the central and lateral incisors, canines, and first and second molars on both right and left sides (figs. 51a–b).

We used Stempflé's Score 1 formula[15] and Olsen's method[16] to estimate the fetal age of the mummy at death based on ossification

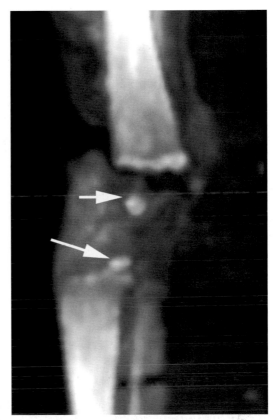

Fig. 50: Sagittal CT image of the knee of mummy 317b. The arrows point to the ossified centers at the knee: short arrow points to distal femoral epiphysis and the longer arrow to the proximal tibial epiphysis. These findings helped in estimating the age of the fetus to be around nine months of gestation.

centers, teeth mineralization, and bone morphology. The mean gestational age of the mummy is estimated to be 36.78 weeks (SD 1.91) by considering the results of the different methods we used for age estimation.[17]

Postmortem fractures and soft-tissue injuries

Reconstructed CT images in this study showed multiple comminuted fractures involving the cranial vault and skull base (fig. 52). This resulted in a false impression of an

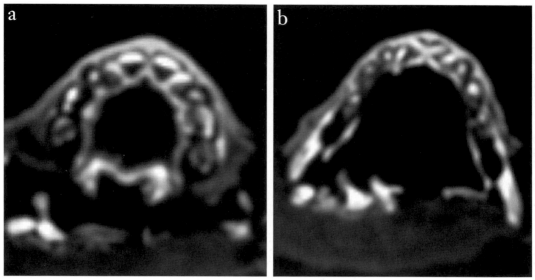

Figs. 51a–b: Axial CT images of the maxilla (a) and the mandible (b) of the mummy of fetus 317b show ossification of multiple crowns.

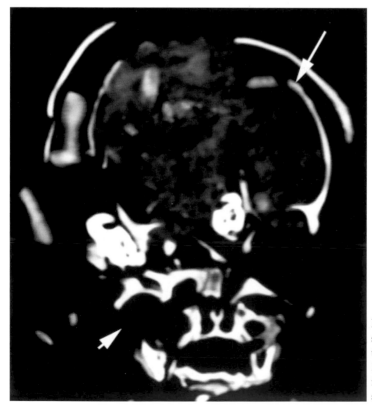

Fig. 52: Coronal two-dimensional CT reconstructed image of the skull of mummified fetus 317b shows multiple comminuted fractures in the face (short arrow) and the skull (long arrow).

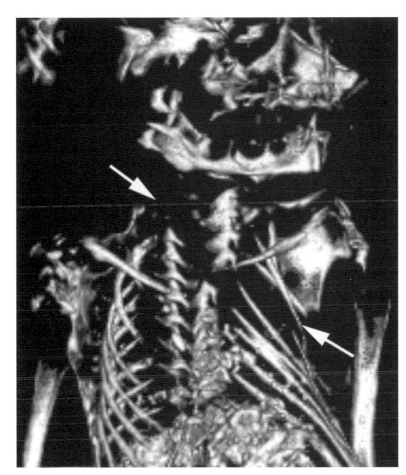

Fig. 53: Coronal oblique three-dimensional CT reconstructed image of mummified fetus 317b shows an oblique postmortem fracture (arrows) that involved the laminae of the upper thoracic vertebrae, and resulted in complete separation and upward displacement of the left shoulder.

abnormally enlarged skull. There were comminuted postmortem fractures of the cervical vertebrae from C1 to C7. An oblique fracture crosses the upper four dorsal vertebrae, disrupting the vertebral rings and widely separating the laminae of the dorsal spine from D1 to D4. There is no evidence of the anomalous defects in the preserved skeleton and vertebrae that were falsely suggested by the 1978 study. The left shoulder region was completely separated from the rest of the fetal body; consequently, the left scapula was displaced upward and the left clavicle was dislocated (fig. 53). However, both scapulae and clavicles have normal comparable dimensions, which ruled out the previous erroneous suggestion of a small-sized left scapula or long left clavicle in the plain x-ray study by Harrison and colleagues.[18]

Comparison between Findings of the CT Study and the Previous Plain X-Ray Studies

Harrison's 1978 study theorized that the mummy 317b was thirty-five weeks' gestation to full term at time of mummification. A restudy of the plain x-ray examination by

Hellier and Connolly in 2008 suggested a younger age of thirty weeks' gestation. CT enabled detection of tooth mineralization and multiple ossifying centers that were missed by plain x-rays. These findings helped the CT to estimate the age of the mummified fetuses more precisely than the plain x-rays and suggested a higher gestational age, around thirty-seven weeks.

Plain x-ray study also suggested the presence of multiple congenital anomalies,[19] because the mummy seemingly displayed signs of Sprengel's deformity (a raised left scapula and long left clavicle) and opened vertebral laminae. The CT study ruled out the presence of these congenital anomalies and clarified that the changes were due to postmortem trauma and fractures.

This study sets a precedent for the use of CT and forensic image analysis in the study of ancient mummified fetuses.[20] The study also documents the elaborate burial rites and mummification process provided for the fetuses that were similar to those provided for royal adults in their time. The study results reflect that fetuses in ancient Egypt were considered as entities with cultural, social, and biological significance.[21]

7

Investigations into
King Tutankhamun's Family

Historical Introduction

There are many unknowns surrounding the family of Tutankhamun. First, his parentage has always been in dispute, and some of the familial relationships between individuals who were presumably his close relatives are uncertain from the archaeological record. Second, there are a number of unidentified mummies thought to belong to members of the late Eighteenth Dynasty royal family. Our study uses a combination of Egyptology and forensic science to shed light on the identities of previously nameless royal remains, and to draw links between the historical players of the Amarna Period and its aftermath. The Egyptian team concentrated on this study of the late Eighteenth Dynasty, in particular the kings who reigned from Amenhotep III to Tutankhamun.

Between the reigns of Akhenaten and Tutankhamun appeared the kings' names of Neferneferuaten and Smenkhkare. Neferneferuaten seems to have been a female king whose reign overlapped entirely or almost entirely with that of Akhenaten. Smenkhkare seems to have been a male king who ruled for less than a year, perhaps partly or entirely as a coregent of Akhenaten.[1] Already during the reigns of the two ephemeral successors of Akhenaten, the return to orthodoxy seems to have begun.[2]

It has been suggested that Ankh(et)kheperure Neferneferuaten ruled briefly with Akhenaten late in his reign and possibly survived the old king for several years, perhaps serving as Tutankhaten's regent at the outset of his reign.[3] Many scholars believe that this king was actually Akhenaten's queen, Nefertiti.[4] Smenkhkare, who was apparently married to the eldest Amarna princess, Meritaten, ruled either between Akhenaten and Tutankhaten or for several years beginning in the middle of Akhenaten's reign.[5] Some scholars believe that Smenkhkare was actually Nefertiti in yet another guise,[6] and

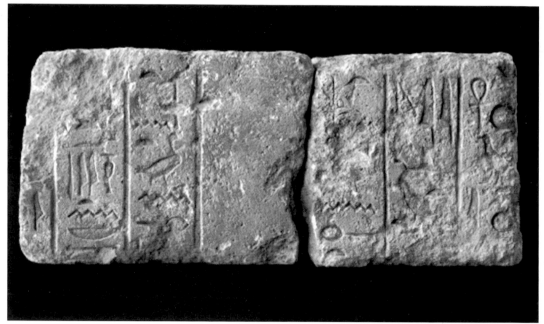

Fig. 54: An inscribed block from Hermopolis; the name of Tutankhaten (later Tutankhamun) is mentioned after the title "king's son." The name of the princess Ankhesenpaaten (later Ankhesenamun) also appears.

still others propose that he was male and the son of either Akhenaten or Amenhotep III.[7]

Shortly after Tutankhaten ascended the throne, he changed his name to Tutankhamun. The city of Akhetaten seems to have been abandoned within a few years of his accession. Tutankhamun's reign saw extensive restoration of the monuments of the orthodox gods of Egypt, and he died while still in his late teens (plate 39) and was succeeded by the elderly Ay.[8]

Tutankhamun's royal origins can be seen on a block from Amarna, reused at Hermopolis (fig. 54). Tutankhamun is identified as "King's Son of his body, whom he loves, Tutankhaten."[9] This block can confirm that Tutankhaten lived in Amarna and that he was a direct descendant of a king.[10] Amenhotep III has been proposed as

the father of Tutankhamun.[11] The evidence for this comes through additions to the temples of Luxor and Soleb made by Tutankhamun, suggesting a connection to Amenhotep III, under whose reign these temples were originally built. Tutankhamun describes himself as "renewing the monuments of his father," Amenhotep III.[12] However, this inscription does not necessarily mean that Amenhotep III was the biological father of Tutankhamun. The term 'son' can refer to a grandson, great-grandson, or even a son-in-law.[13]

Since Tutankhamun reigned for about nine years and died at approximately age nineteen, he must have been born between the seventh and eleventh years of Akhenaten's reign, depending on the length of time that passed between the latter's death and Tutankhamun's accession.[14] He could only have been the literal son of Amenhotep III if the coregency of Amenhotep III and Akhenaten was long.

Many other scholars have suggested that Akhenaten is the father of Tutankhamun.[15] Tutankhamun is identified on an astronomical instrument in the Oriental Institute, Chicago, as "the great-grandson of Thutmose IV,"[16] or one generation younger than Akhenaten. Archaeological evidence supports the identification of the mummy found in tomb KV55 in the Valley of the Kings with Akhenaten, and establishes a connection between this mummy and Tutankhamun. It has been suggested, in fact, that the coffin and its remains, along with the canopic jars found in the tomb, belonged to Akhenaten, based on the fact that the 'magic bricks' found in the corners of the tomb were inscribed for him.[17] These objects may indicate that Akhenaten was moved to KV55 by Tutankhamun, as seals with the young king's name were also found in the tomb, a further link between the two.[18] This connection is strengthened by the location of KV55 very close to the tomb of Tutankhamun, though this is not direct evidence that Tutankhamun was the son of Akhenaten. He could simply have been performing his duties as a member of the extended family.

Another connection to Akhenaten is provided in Room Alpha of the Royal Tomb at Amarna (fig. 55).[19] In a scene adjacent to one depicting a deceased woman, a female figure appears holding a baby under a flabellum, a symbol of royalty. The woman with the baby has just left the chamber of the deceased woman, who has apparently died in childbirth. It has been proposed that the child is Tutankhamun,[20] although this is by no means certain and has been disputed.[21]

Smenkhkare has been named by some as the father of Tutankhamun.[22] This suggestion seems to be based on the identification of the KV55 mummy as Smenkhkare,[23] combined

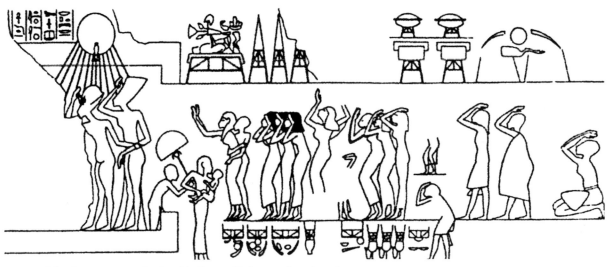

Fig. 55: The funerary scene depicted in Room Alpha, royal tomb at Amarna.

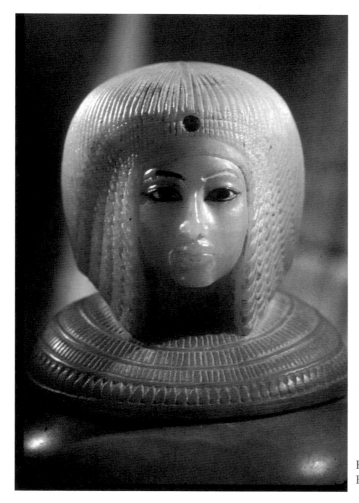

Fig. 56: Canopic jar lid of Kiya.
Egyptian Museum, Cairo.

with physical evidence tying the KV55 mummy to Tutankhamun.[24]

The identification of the mother of Tutankhamun is also a conundrum. It has been suggested that Queen Tiye could be his mother.[25] At the outset of the present study, Tiye's remains were unidentified, although the mummy known as the Elder Lady in KV35 had been suggested as belonging to her.[26] The lock of hair discovered in the tomb of Tutankhamun, which tests had found iden-

tical to the hair of the Elder Lady,[27] seemed to indicate a family relationship, but not necessarily maternity.

Others suggest that Kiya (fig. 56) could be the mother of Tutankhamun.[28] Kiya was a secondary queen of Akhenaten, and it has been theorized that she died delivering Tutankhamun, as depicted in Amarna's Royal Tomb.[29]

Still other scholars have proposed that Queen Nefertiti could be the mother of

Tutankhamun.[30] Another possibility is a princess,[31] possibly Tadukhepa, who was married to both Amenhotep III and Akhenaten, and has been identified by some as Kiya.[32]

Other princesses, such as one of Akhenaten's daughters (Meketaten or Meritaten), are further candidates,[33] or perhaps Beketaten, the youngest daughter of Amenhotep III and Queen Tiye.[34]

One of Akhenaten's sisters, perhaps Sitamun, who was the daughter and royal wife of Amenhotep III, has also been suggested. This scenario posits Amenhotep III as the father.

Finally, the identities of Tutankhamun's wife and children are known. His wife was Ankhesenamun (plate 40), the daughter of Akhenaten and Nefertiti. It has been suggested by Howard Carter[35] that the two fetuses found in the tomb of Tutankhamun were stillborn daughters of this king and his wife (see chapter 6, "The Two Fetuses Found in the Tomb of Tutankhamun").[36]

As we can see from the above discussion, it will be necessary to elucidate the issue concerning the family of Tutankhamun using modern technology.

The Parentage and Family of Tutankhamun: The DNA Evidence

Nine mummies possibly or definitely closely related in some way to Tutankhamun will be considered here. Of these, the identification of four mummies was certain, while the identities of the other five were previously undetermined or only tentatively established.[37]

The four identified mummies

Tutankhamun

The identity of this mummy is secure, as it was found intact inside his coffins.

Yuya

The body of Yuya, the father of Queen Tiye and thus the grandfather of Akhenaten, was found inside his clearly labeled nest of coffins in the tomb that he shared with his wife in the Valley of the Kings, KV46.[38]

Thuya

The mummy of Thuya, wife of Yuya, was also found in a nest of coffins in KV46.

Amenhotep III

This king was originally buried in his tomb in the western branch of the Valley of the Kings, WV22 (plate 41), but was moved in antiquity to a side room in KV35, the tomb of Amenhotep II, where he was found in 1898.[39]

The mummy of Amenhotep III is in poor condition. Though his name was inscribed on his coffin, there has always been some doubt about the mummy's identity because of the style of mummification. The limbs were stuffed with resin, a practice previously unknown in Eighteenth Dynasty mummies at the time of the study. The current study was important to securely establish the identity of this mummy.

The tentatively identified or unidentified mummies

The Elder Lady

This mummy was found next to the mummy known as the Younger Lady in KV35. She was well mummified and even in death is lovely, with a regal expression and long, curly, reddish hair falling across her shoulders. (For CT results, see chapter 4, "CT Examination of Selected Mid- to Late Eighteenth Dynasty Mummies.")

The style of mummification, the treatment of the mummies by the tomb robbers, and the lack of bandages and coffins seem to indicate that this mummy, the Younger Lady, and the Young Boy found together in KV35 were somehow associated with one another.[40] She was tentatively identified as Queen Tiye, based on the analysis of the lock of hair found in Tutankhamun's tomb, and the mummy was added to our study in the hope of confirming her identity.

The KV55 mummy

As is apparent from the previous studies on the KV55 mummy, its identity has never been confirmed. It was therefore imperative that it be included in our recent project. (For CT results, see chapter 4.)

The Younger Lady

This female mummy, found alongside the Elder Lady, was also included in the study. (For the CT results, see chapter 4.)

The two fetuses (possibly daughters of Tutankhamun)

The two fetuses (a and b) that were buried in their own small nest of coffins in the treasury room of Tutankhamun's tomb were added to the study. (For CT results, see chapter 6, "The Two Fetuses Found in the Tomb of Tutankhamun.")

Results of the Research

Through our recent study,[41] we were able to answer many of the hotly debated questions raised by Egyptologists: who were the parents of King Tutankhamun, and who are the unidentified mummies in KV35?

In this study, DNA played an important role. The project utilized two labs that were dedicated solely to DNA research on the mummies. They are located far from each other in Cairo and had separate, well-qualified Egyptian teams at work in full cooperation with two European experts, Carsten Pusch of the University of Tübingen, and Albert Zink of the EURAC Institute for Mummies and The Iceman, Bolzano, Italy.

Isolating the DNA of a mummy that is more than three thousand years old requires exceptional skill, patience, and a certain amount of luck. To obtain at least one workable sample, the geneticists extracted tissue from several different locations in each mummy, always from deep within the bone, where there was no chance the sample would be contaminated by the DNA of previous archaeologists or of the ancient Egyptians who performed the mummification. Extreme care was taken to eliminate any contamination by the researchers themselves. After the sample was extracted, the DNA had to be separated from superfluous substances, including those that the ancients had used to preserve the bodies. The purification steps varied from sample to sample, each step capable of destroying the material.

The crux of the study was Tutankhamun himself. If the extraction and isolation were successful, his DNA would be captured in a clear liquid solution, ready for analysis. To our dismay, however, the initial solutions were a murky black. Two more months of effort were required to figure out how to remove the contaminant, which was an unknown product of the mummification process, and obtain a sample ready for amplifying and sequencing using standard techniques.

Our chief 'informant' was the mystery mummy in KV55. The main issue was that previous studies concluded that he died at the age of twenty-five, too young to be Akhenaten. He had thus been identified as Smenkhkare.

Once the DNA team under Dr. Gad had isolated DNA from the mummies, it was a fairly simple matter to compare the Y-chromosomes of Amenhotep III, KV55, and Tutankhamun and see that they were indeed related. (Related males share the same pattern of DNA in their Y-chromosomes, since this part of a male's genome is inherited directly from his father.) But the clarification of their precise relationship to one another required a more sophisticated analysis known as genetic fingerprinting. Along the chromosomes in our genomes there are specific known regions where the pattern of DNA letters—the A's, T's, G's, and C's that make up our genetic code—varies greatly between one person and another. These variations amount to different numbers of repeated sequences of the same few letters. When one person might have a sequence ten times, for instance, another unrelated person might have the same sequence stuttered fifteen times, a third person twenty, and so on. A match between just ten of these highly variable regions is enough for police investigators, such as the FBI, to determine that the DNA left at a crime scene and that of a suspect is the same.

The same standards of reliability apply whether solving a crime or reuniting the members of a family separated 3,300 years ago. By comparing the mummies' genetic fingerprints, our team was able to establish with a probability of better than 99.99 percent that Amenhotep III was the father of the individual in KV55, who was in turn the father of Tutankhamun. Except for the alleged young age of the body, most other evidence pointed to the mummy also being Akhenaten. However, our CT scans did not rule out the possibility that the mummy found in KV55 could have reached forty at death. We thus suggest that the body found in KV55, the father of Tutankhamun, is most likely Akhenaten—he is displayed with this identification at the Egyptian Museum. But since we know so little about Smenkhkare, he cannot be completely ruled out.

Our search for the women in Tutankhamun's life focused on the two anonymous mummies found in KV35, the Elder Lady and the Younger Lady (plate 42). We already had a clue about the identity of the Elder Lady as Queen Tiye, due to the lock of hair found in Tutankhamun's tomb. The DNA results bore this out: this mummy is the daughter of Yuya and Thuya, whom we knew historically to be Tiye's parents.[42]

As would then be expected, the combination of Tiye's DNA with that of her husband, Amenhotep III, matched up perfectly with that of their own son, Akhenaten. More of a surprise was that Amenhotep III and Tiye also proved to be the parents of the Younger Lady, found lying beside Tiye in the alcove of the tomb. And, most revealing of all, her DNA matched that of Tutankhamun himself. Akhenaten had married his own sister, and their son was Tutankhamun (plate 43).

With this discovery, we now know that it is unlikely that either of Akhenaten's known wives, Nefertiti and Kiya, was Tutankhamun's mother, since there is no evidence from the historical record that either was Akhenaten's sister. Just which of Akhenaten's many sisters is the Younger Lady will probably never be known—he seems to have had almost forty, including five probable full sisters. To this author, knowing her name is less important than the blood relationship with her husband. In this case, it planted the seed of their son's early death.

The results of the research were sent to a peer-reviewed journal,[43] and a press conference was held at the Egyptian Museum on February 17, 2010, to announce these discoveries. The results of our DNA analysis provide convincing evidence that genetics can provide a powerful new tool for understanding Egyptian history, especially when combined with radiological studies of the mummies and insights gained from the archaeological record.

Marfan's Disease and the Family of Tutankhamun

Because Akhenaten was portrayed in ancient reliefs with an elongated head, narrow face, and long limbs (plate 44), some scholars have postulated that an ailment, Marfan's Disease, afflicted the king and his son Tutankhamun.

Marfan's Disease is a genetic condition that is caused by a fault in a gene on chromosome fifteen, which controls the production of fibrillin, a fiber in connective tissue throughout the body.[44] This tissue connects, supports, and controls the elasticity of the body's organs. The weakened connective tissue found in those with Marfan's Disease can lead to problems in many parts of the body, including bones, eyes, heart, aorta, lungs, skin, and dura.[45]

People suffering from Marfan's Disease tend to share certain physical traits that usually occur together as a group (syndrome). Skeletal abnormalities that have been noticed in Marfan's patients are a long face, elongated skull, wide pelvis, unusually tall stature, and unusually long arms, fingers, and toes (described as spider legs or arachnodactyly).

There are two types of diagnostic criteria for Marfan's: major and minor. The major diagnostic criteria carry high diagnostic precision

because they are infrequent in other conditions, while the minor criteria are common in Marfan's as well as in other diseases. Major diagnostic criteria of Marfan's Disease include disproportionate body with reduced ratio of the upper to lower body segments or increased armspan-to-height ratio.[46] Severe chest deformity (depressed sternum), severe bending of the back (scoliosis >20 degrees), and flat feet are also important major criteria for the diagnosis of Marfan's Disease. Minor criteria include elongated skull (dolichocephaly), narrow face (hypoplasia of cheek bones), high arched palate, and crowding of teeth.[47]

The question: Is it possible to confidently diagnose Marfan's Disease in a mummified body?

At least three different organ systems must be involved before a diagnosis of Marfan's is made; two of the systems must have major criteria.[48] However, among the different organ systems that might be involved in Marfan's Disease, only one system (the bones) can be assessed in a mummified body. The other body systems that involve the soft tissues cannot be reliably examined, owing to the alteration of these tissues during the embalming process. Embalming procedures include removal of some of these organs (lungs) and desiccation of others (heart, aorta, and skin).

There are even more difficulties in assessing the bones of a mummy for the presence of Marfan's Disease, as some criteria include clinical signs (such as the wrist and thumb signs).[49] In addition, a mummy has to be complete and well preserved in order to obtain the measurements needed for body ratios, hand indices, and craniofacial measurements. Table 15 includes the applicability of the criteria for diagnosing Marfan's Disease in a mummy. The table shows the limited applicability of the known criteria needed for diagnosing Marfan's Disease in a mummy, as well as the pitfalls of false positive findings.

Thousands of CT images of the KV55 mummy (Akhenaten), as well as the mummies of other family members, were examined to refute or confirm the presence of Marfan's Disease as a familial congenital abnormality. The CT images were studied by Ashraf Selim and Sahar Saleem, who for scientific reasons worked separately, blinded from each other's work.

Analysis of CT images of the full body and precise measurements were attempted for each of the studied mummies. The shape of the head and face was described and objectively determined by obtaining accurate CT measurements (such as skull indices[50]) whenever possible. However, the limited preservation of some of the mummies hindered proper assessment for some findings or obtaining body measurements. These difficulties were encountered in the skeletonized mummy of KV55, which is formed mostly of separate bones, as well as in other mummies with detached or missing body parts, such as Amenhotep III, Thutmose III, and Seti I.

Some features of Marfan's Disease were claimed to be in the mummy of Akhenaten, as well as in some of his family or dynasty. However, we found that these were either doubtful findings or of low diagnostic precision for Marfan's Disease. These features included a mildly elongated skull (dolichocephaly), which was objectively diagnosed by obtaining measurements (cephalic index of 75 or less). With the exception of Yuya (cephalic index 70.3), none of the other mummies of Tutankhamun's lineage have dolichocephaly. Neither Akhenaten (cephalic index 81), nor Tutankhamun (cephalic index 84.2) have this skull shape. Mummies early in the Eighteenth Dynasty (so-called 'Thutmose I' and Thutmose II) have mildly elongated skulls, which are likely exaggerations of family traits, rather than abnormalities related to congenital ailments. Other features, such as spine deformity (scoliosis), were significant only in the mummy of Thuya (with angle > 20°). Although reported in some other mummies, scoliosis was either mild or related rather to the presence of postmortem spine fractures or the position of the body during mummification.[51]

To conclude, confident diagnosis of Marfan's Disease in a mummy cannot depend solely upon CT examination of the bones. We could not find significant changes in the mummies of Akhenaten or his lineage to suspect the diagnosis of Marfan's Disease. The strange (androgynous) depiction of Akhenaten in art does not seem to be his reality; it could be a stylistic reflection of his identification with the god Aten, who in one hymn was described as both male and female, and thus the source of all life.

Table 15. Potential applicability of the diagnostic criteria of Marfan's Disease in a complete, well-preserved ancient Egyptian New Kingdom mummy, using CT examination

Body system	Diagnostic criteria*	Potential applicability of the criterion in a complete, well-preserved mummy
Skeleton	**Major criteria**	
	Severe chest deformity: Pectus carinatum; pectus excavatum	Possible. Pitfall: may be mistaken for collapsed thoracic cavity as the result of evisceration and inadequate packing
	Body ratios: Reduced upper to lower segment ratio (0.85 vs normally 0.93) or armspan to height ratio (>1.05)	Possible. Pitfall: dry, reduced-height discs may cause reduction of the measurements of the upper body segment
	Clinical signs: Wrist sign and thumb sign (see note 49)	No
	Severe scoliosis (>20 degrees)	Possible. Pitfall: Mild scoliosis can possibly be caused by the position of the mummy during mummification, especially in absence of vertebral deformities
	Extension of elbows<170	No
	Pes planus (flat foot)	Possible
	Protrusion acetabuli	Possible
	Minor criteria	
	Highly arched palate with crowding of teeth	Possible
	Facial appearance: slender face, prominent glabella, retrognathia	Possible
Other findings (non-pathognomonic) not included in the criteria of diagnosis		
	Dolichocephaly	Possible
	Increased skull height	Possible
	Thick skull at lambdoid	Possible
	Prominent frontal sinus	Possible
	Metacarpal index	Possible

* Data under "Diagnostic criteria" are from De Paepe et al., "Revised Criteria for the Marfan Syndrome."

2. Eye	Major criterion	
	Ectopic lens	No
	Minor criteria	
	Flat cornea	No
	Longer globe	No
	Miosis (hypoplastic iris/ciliary)	No
3. Cardiovascular	**Major criteria**	
	Dilated ascending aorta	No
	Dissection of ascending aorta	No
	Minor criteria	
	Mitral valve prolapse	No
	Pulmonary artery dilatation	No
	Mitral annulus calcification	Possible. Pitfall: localization of mitral annulus in desiccated heart may not be possible
	Dilatation/dissection of descending thoracic/abdominal aorta	No
4. Lungs	**Minor criteria**	
	Spontaneous pneumothorax	No
	Apical blebs	No
5. Skin	**Minor criteria**	
	Stretch mark	No
	Recurrent hernias	No
6. Dura	**Major criterion**	
	Lumbosacral dural ectasia	Possible only if it caused scalloping of vertebrae

8

The Search for the Mummy
of Queen Nefertiti

Historical Introduction

Nefertiti (fig. 57) is one of the most famous queens of ancient Egypt. She was Akhenaten's main wife and lived with him at the new capital known as Akhetaten, 'Horizon of the Aten,' today Amarna. In spite of her fame, there are many questions about her that remain unanswered, such as the date of her death; new evidence suggests that she lived into Year 16 of Akhenaten's reign (see chapter 4, note 15). Was she in disagreement with her husband at the end? Did Queen Tiye play any role in opposition to her? Or perhaps Nefertiti became coregent with Akhenaten? Did she rule after his death? Nefertiti's mummy has never been found, and there is no evidence as to the circumstances of her death or the location of her tomb.

Some scholars have suggested that she was of foreign origin,[1] the daughter of the king of Mitanni, but most believe that she was Egyptian, perhaps the daughter of King Ay.

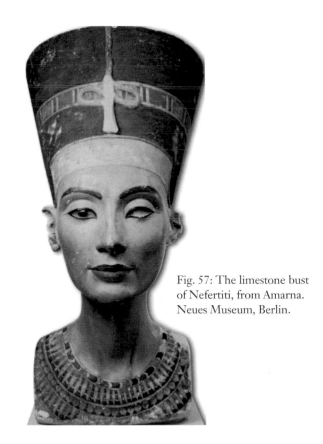

Fig. 57: The limestone bust of Nefertiti, from Amarna. Neues Museum, Berlin.

She played an important role in supporting her husband and his new religion, and was shown accompanying him in the worship of Aten. In Year 5 of Akhenaten's reign, she changed her name to Neferneferuaten Nefertiti, which means "The Aten is radiant of radiance."

The tomb of Meryre II at Amarna is one source of information about the political situation in the city. A scene in this tomb[2] shows a procession and ceremony dated to the second month of Year 12 of Akhenaten's reign. This scene shows the royal family, at that time composed of Akhenaten, Nefertiti, and their six daughters, and is the latest known securely dated appearance of the seven women.[3] Nefertiti and Akhenaten are seated next to each other so that their figures are superimposed (one is drawn on top of the other, and they share most of their outlines.) Nicholas Reeves interprets this to mean that at the time the scenes were carved, Nefertiti was beginning to be considered Akhenaten's coruler.[4] She may have changed her name once again, to "Ankh(et)kheperure Neferneferuaten," due to her elevation to this position.[5] From the beginning, her name was written inside two cartouches parallel to each other, similar to the two names of each king.

Elsewhere, Nefertiti was depicted sitting beside Akhenaten wearing the kingly double crown.[6] She was also shown smiting an enemy, on a block in the Museum of Fine Arts, Boston[7] and another *talatat* block found at Karnak.[8] The scene of smiting an enemy is a part of the iconography of kingship, reflecting one of the king's duties to destroy the enemies of Egypt. It is not a part of the queenly artistic program. This suggests that Nefertiti actually ruled. This could have taken place at the end of Akhenaten's reign when she took the name

Ankh(et)kheperure Neferneferuaten. This theory, however, may disregard the existence of a brother or half-brother of Tutankhaten.

There exists a letter sent by an Egyptian queen to Suppiluliumas, king of the Hittites, asking him to send one of his sons to marry her. The letter states:

> My husband died. A son I have not. But to you, they say, the sons are many. If you were to give me a son of yours, he would become my husband. Never shall I pick out a servant of mine and make him my husband! . . . I am afraid![9]

Some scholars believe that this letter was sent by Nefertiti; others have suggested the more likely scenario that it was sent by Ankhesenamun, wife of Tutankhamun. However, the reign of Akhenaten and Nefertiti is a mysterious period, and the excavations in Amarna by Barry Kemp may still reveal important clues about the queen's role.

The Mummy of Nefertiti: Recent Theories

Regarding the mummy of Nefertiti, two recent theories have emerged: the first, when tomb KV63 was found in the Valley of the Kings, and the second, when Joann Fletcher, an Egyptologist from England, announced that the mummy of the Younger Lady from KV35 was the mummy of Nefertiti.

The discovery of Tomb KV63[10] (plate 46) by Otto Schaden and a team from the University of Memphis was announced on February 5, 2006. Found within the tomb were seven wooden coffins (plate 45), including one for a child and one for an infant, and twenty-eight storage jars. There was much speculation about the identification of the tomb owner and the possibility that the queens of the Eighteenth Dynasty could be found within, especially Nefertiti as the possible mother of Tutankhamun. Others conjectured that the tomb could contain remains of the six daughters of Akhenaten and Nefertiti.

When opened, however, the coffins and jars were found to contain refuse from the embalming process, as well as a pink anthropoid coffinette and several pillows inside the child's coffin (plate 47). A seal impression found in a storage jar contained part of a cartouche that can be restored as the name of Tutankhamun or Ay. In addition, the ceramics found there are similar to those of the late Eighteenth Dynasty. It has been suggested that the tomb was a cache for material used by embalmers. Though no royal remains were found in the tomb, Earl Ertman of University of Akron, who was a member of the KV63 expedition, studied the coffins found there, and suggested that the eyes on three of the coffins were reminiscent of the eyes of Queen Nefertiti[11] on the famous bust as well as other representations, linking her to the tomb.

The second theory, equating the mummy of the Younger Lady with Nefertiti, was announced on June 9, 2003 by Joann Fletcher. The Supreme Council of Antiquities had given York University permission in 2003 to do an x-ray study of the two female mummies found in the side room of the burial chamber in KV35. Joann Fletcher was a member of the expedition. In contravention to the SCA rules put in place in the interest of science, that an expedition must report its findings to the SCA, which reviews it and makes an initial announcement of any discovery, the York University team announced their findings in a Discovery Channel press release.

The mummy of the Younger Lady (see chapter 4, "CT Examination of Selected Mid- to Late Eighteenth Dynasty Mummies," and chapter 7, "Investigations into King Tutankhamun's Family") had been badly damaged, and its right arm had been ripped off. Fletcher concluded that a bent arm with a clenched fist found nearby in KV35 belonged with the mummy, rather than a straight arm also discovered close to the mummy.[12] This might support an argument that the mummy is royal, as queens often have one arm (though usually the left) bent and the other straight. (In fact, this arm position is also seen in nonroyal women.) The Egyptian Mummy Project examined both arms by CT scan. Ashraf Selim concluded that the bent arm's bone was different in consistency from the attached left arm and that it was too long to belong to this mummy. The straight arm, however, was similar to the left arm in consistency and therefore most likely belonged to the Younger Lady. The Egyptian Mummy Project has concluded, based on the density of the bones as well as the relative lengths of the arms, that it is the straight arm that belongs with the mummy, not the bent one. The CT report indicates that both arms are extended beside the body and that the right arm has two breaks, one in the upper arm and one at the wrist. The right hand is completely separated from the limb. Ashraf Selim does not mention the broken "bent" forearm in his report, but he stated in a scientific discussion in 2008 that it definitely does not belong to that mummy.

Another point raised by Fletcher is that the lower portion of the Younger Lady's face is badly damaged, with a large gash in the right check. This at first was taken as evidence, caused by tomb robbers, of the malice felt towards Nefertiti, an extreme form of *damnatio memoriae* appropriate for someone as controversial as Akhenaten's Great Wife. A member of Fletcher's scientific team later noted that this wound was possibly premortem, though this was uncertain.[13] Ashraf Selim, however, is certain that the gash on the check was a premortem wound and was so violent as not to be accidental. He argues that if the mummy's face had indeed been smashed after embalming, one would expect to see bits of dried bone and flesh within the wounds; the CT scanning performed by the Egyptian Mummy Project revealed very few pieces of the relevant broken bones within the sinus cavity, suggesting that the damage to the mummy's face occurred before embalming, most likely even before death. Indeed, it probably was the cause of death.[14]

The age range of the mummy suggested by CT scan is between twenty-five and thirty-five years. This would fit any number of important New Kingdom females.

Other points made in support of the identification of the Younger Lady as Nefertiti can be refuted without reference to the CT scans. This includes a wig of the type worn by Nefertiti found in the tomb,[15] as well as the fact that the mummy has a double-pierced ear,[16] both of which attributes are seen in nonroyal women of the New Kingdom, so they do not prove that this is Nefertiti. In summary, there is no convincing reason to identify the Younger Lady as Nefertiti.

In the face of this scientific and Egyptological evidence, this author (Z.H.) rejected the theory that equated the Younger Lady of KV35 with Nefertiti, and the Permanent Committee of the SCA formally denounced it.

In 2007, with the advent of the Egyptian Mummy Project's attempt to identify the family of Tutankhamun through DNA analysis, we

discovered that the Younger Lady is the daughter of Amenhotep III and Queen Tiye, that she married her brother Akhenaten, and that Tutankhamun was her son (see chapter 7). In this case, there is no way that the Younger Lady could be Nefertiti, because we know that Nefertiti was not the daughter of Amenhotep III and Tiye.[17] Also, if she was Nefertiti, we would expect that Tutankhamun would have been portrayed with her on reliefs at Amarna, especially with the emphasis on family characteristic of Amarna art. On the contrary, we see Nefertiti always accompanied by her six daughters, never Tutankhamun. Actually, it is possible that because Tutankhamun was not her son, she never permitted him to appear at all at Amarna. We are sure from the al-Ashmunayn blocks that he was the son of a king and lived at Amarna.[18]

We do not know the name of the Younger Lady because Amenhotep and Tiye had five daughters whose names are known and others whose names are unknown.[19] Did the Younger Lady, the sister of Akhenaten, change her name to Kiya when she married him? Dennis Forbes[20] has also suggested that the Younger Lady could be Princess Sitamun, oldest daughter of Amenhotep and Tiye.

After eliminating the Younger Lady from contention, the Egyptian Mummy Project began its quest for the mummy of Queen Nefertiti and her daughter Ankhesenamun, the wife of Tutankhamun.

The KV21 Mummies

There were two mummies of possible relevance from tomb KV21 that were examined in this study, as well as the DNA of the two fetuses found in Tutankhamun's tomb.

KV21 was originally discovered by the Italian explorer Giovanni Belzoni on October

9, 1817. The two mummies inside (figs. 58a–b) were rediscovered by Donald Ryan in 1990. Belzoni described the finding of the mummies in the burial chamber as follows:

> At one corner of this chamber, we found two mummies on the ground quite naked, without cloth or case. They were females, and their hair pretty long, and well preserved, though it was easily separated from the head by pulling it a little.[21]

Both James Burton and Edward Lane confirmed that these mummies were still intact and in the tomb in the mid-1820s. Also, graffiti on the ceiling of the small room off the tomb's burial chamber gives a date of 1826. The tomb seems to have been covered up by flood debris and buried deeply sometime in the decades that followed. A trench may have been dug down to the tomb's entrance around 1896, and this too was later covered over. When Ryan began to re-excavate this tomb in 1989, it was difficult for him and his team to find the tomb's entrance because it was hidden in flood debris.[22]

Ryan's aim in searching for this tomb was actually to locate these two mummies

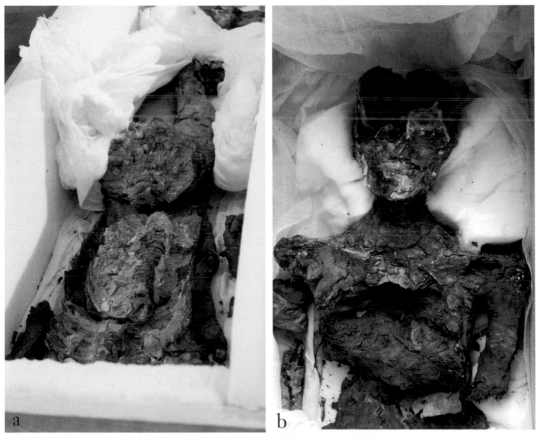

Figs. 58a–b: The remains of the unknown female mummies KV21 A (a) and KV21 B (b). Egyptian Museum, Cairo.

described by Belzoni. Ryan was surprised to find a head and torso face down in the debris of the first corridor. Other body parts were found on the interior stairs and especially in the burial chamber, where Ryan found on the floor a pile of snapped-off hands and feet. As Ryan has suggested, the destruction of the two mummies could only have been caused by human vandals who tore them apart. When Ryan collected all of the pieces in the tomb, there were several missing parts and one mummy was missing its head. He suggested that its long hair had perhaps made it an attractive souvenir for the violators of the tomb.[23]

As Ryan has noted, these mummies are quite interesting. Both of the left hands are clenched and the left arms might have been bent diagonally across the chest in the royal female pose. The tomb itself appears to be a small royal tomb; thus its occupants could be queens or princesses.

Ryan reconstructed the two mummies and constructed a custom wooden case to hold the remains. Mark Papworth did an initial description of the mummies, and made the following observations in an undated report to the SCA made by Ryan:

Mummy No. 1 [21 A]: This mummy is represented by the posterior elements of the torso, with most of the vertebral column intact. The left shoulder and left arm were missing. A left hand, however, minus the thumb, has been associated with this mummy, as the second mummy has a hand definitely identified with it. The left hand is clenched. An articulated radius and ulna, which are partly unwrapped, are attributed to this mummy because of distinctive mud stains. The abdominal cavity is, in fact, completely filled with flood debris. This is on as well as under the skin and wrappings of the cavity, indicating that the abdomen was open at the time of the flood.

Two femurs are associated with this mummy. . . . The left foot has been painfully distorted, flexed across its plantar surface to approximately 90 degrees. The right foot is even more distorted in the same way.

The various indicators of the history of this mummy suggest that it was unwrapped, and the abdominal and other cavities were open prior to the flood event. The articulations suggest that the mummy was not disarticulated at the time of its unwrapping and opening, but rather lay on the floor of the burial chamber more or less intact until it was partially filled with debris and thoroughly soaked with water for a considerable length of time by the flood event.

The missing skull, cervical vertebrae, and visible diagnostic bony elements make it difficult to discern the stature and age of this mummy beyond a general impression. It is likely that it represents an adult female, probably more than twenty-five years of age, of slender build and medium stature, perhaps 1.62 meters tall.

Mummy No. 2 [21 B]: This mummy provides much more information than Mummy No. 1. The upper torso, neck, and greater part of the skull lay face down in corridor "B" (the upper corridor). She was partially covered by rocks and debris displaced from the slope above. Her skull is smooth and round and her nose, now missing, was apparently small and narrow. The lack of destruction of the area of the post-nasal air sinuses does not indicate that this was an avenue of entry for the removal of the brain. Her left eye is in place and intact, and unadorned. The right eye is missing. Newspaper and flood debris are plastered to the skin of her right cheek.

On the nape of the neck on the left side of the skull, there are tufts of dark hair, brown in color. Some dark hair was also found of the floor of the burial chamber.

The proximal half of the left humerus is in situ, as well as both clavicles and scapulae. The chest is open from the upper sternum down. The manubrium and sternum are absent, as are the frontal aspects of all the ribs. The vertebral column is somewhat intact. Copius amounts of wadded wrapping fill the pleural cavity.

The head of the right humerus with the shaft of the long bone is broken off at its inferior dorsal margin. This appears to be a relatively recent break from rough handling over the past century. The left humerus is shattered medially, apparently a complex compression fracture associated with crushing. The articulating joints of the partial left radius and ulna and partial humerus match nicely when the wrappings of the elbow are brought into alignment. This gives us a left arm acutely flexed at the chest. A left hand that appears to belong to these other fragments is loosely clenched, with a small finger missing. If this interpretation is correct (and it appears to be, judging from similarity in the fit of the wrapping materials and foreign incrustations on their surfaces), then the left arm is embalmed in the Eighteenth Dynasty "queen" or "royal female" position.

The lumbar vertebrae are articulated with a pelvis that was apparently intact until recently. Both femurs are fixed in their sockets by the heavy wrappings covering most of this area. The left illia and ischium are fractured irregularly throughout their dorsal height. The os pubis is neatly separated. The surface presented by both sides of the pubic symphysis is considerably smoother than could be expected in a young girl. Without cleaning and careful comparison to symphyseal aging standards, an estimated age could only be approximated. The woman represented by this mummy was definitely over forty years of age.

The flesh of the upper legs appears to have been greatly shrunken prior to the wrapping of the mummy. They appear very thin. There are suggestions of osteoarthritis in the lumbar vertebral margins that are visible. Similarly, the disarticulated right knee joint suggests arthritic deformity to some extent. The right foot is tiny and delicate. The digits are missing and the foot is partly distorted. There is none of the marked deformity of Mummy No. 1.

A rough estimate suggests that the lady represented by Mummy No. 2 was probably older and was somewhat taller than Mummy No. 1, perhaps 1.68 m tall.

It is unfortunate that both of these mummies have not survived intact since their discovery in 1817. Enough remains, however, to suggest some interesting possibilities. As mentioned above, there is at least one left arm with a flexed position and clenched hand that strongly suggests the 'royal position' found in the mummy of Queen Tiye and the mummy in Tomb 60 (now identified as Hatshepsut; see chapter 3, "The Discovery of the Mummy of Queen Hatshepsut, and Examination of the Mummies of Her Family"). There is also a clenched left hand that has survived from the other mummy. If these mummies were indeed posed this way, then perhaps they represent two more royal females buried in the Valley of the Kings. A complete study of this pose is needed to examine whether it is truly an exclusively royal one in the Eighteenth Dynasty.

Considering the questions raised by Dr. Papworth's preliminary examination of the two mummies from KV21, it was decided to examine them by CT and DNA analysis to investigate whether they could be associated with Ankhesenamun and Nefertiti. The CT studies of KV21 A and B were reported by Sahar Saleem. CT images provided more details of the mummies and corrected several findings in the previous forensic observation report.

CT Scans of the KV21 Mummies
Mummy KV21 A
General CT findings
The headless mummy is very poorly preserved. It is formed of incomplete body parts that belong to at least two identities assembled incorrectly in several places (plate 48).

Gender
The morphological appearance of the body fragment containing the pelvis is likely for a female. The relatively small size of the femoral head (the anteroposterior diameter of the right femoral head is 36.6 mm) suggests a female mummy.[25]

Age at death
Based on epiphyseal union of all bones, the parts that comprise the studied specimen are of a mature skeleton older than twenty-one years. There are no significant age-related degenerative changes of the skeletal remains, which suggest a relatively young age at the time of death.

Detailed CT findings
Head and neck are missing.

Torso
The torso is torn transversely and is separated into three parts: upper to mid-thoracic region, lower thoracic to upper lumbar region, and lower lumbar to pelvis.

The anterior wall of the torso is markedly defective, and most of the anterior parts of the ribs are missing. The right lower ribs (ninth to twelfth) are missing. The manubrium, sternum, left clavicle, and left scapula are missing. Only the posterior part of the right clavicle and right scapula are present.

The opened torso cavity contains multiple embalming linen packs and multiple dense structures with irregular surface measuring from 2 cm to 4 cm in diameter (likely stones) (fig. 59).

Spine
There are fragments from the seventh cervical vertebra and the upper seven thoracic vertebrae. The eighth to twelfth thoracic vertebrae are present. The lumbar and sacral vertebrae are present, except for the third lumbar vertebra, which is missing.

Table 16. CT measurements of long bones of Mummy KV21 A

Right femur	39 cm
Left tibia	31.8 cm
Right tibia	33.5 cm
Right fibula	33.1 cm

Estimated stature of the individual as inferred from the femur length is 148 cm ± 2.517 cm.[24]

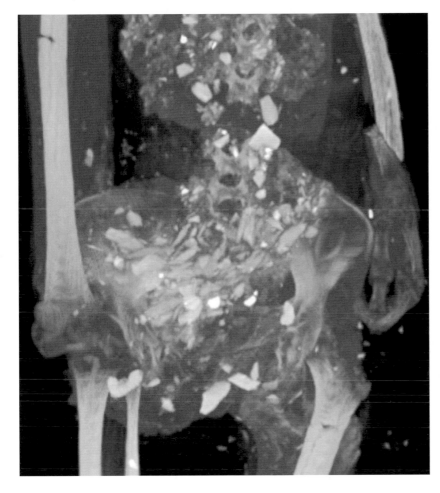

Fig. 59: Three-dimensional reconstruction of the lower torso of mummy of KV21 A using MIP shows multiple irregular, dense objects within the opened body cavity. This was interpreted as flood debris.

Shoulder girdle bones are missing: only part of the right clavicle and left scapula are present.

Limbs

The limbs are composed of different bones belonging to different identities assuming the wrong position in some parts (table 17; fig. 60).

Mummification style

Due to the poor preservation, missing head, and markedly destroyed torso, we could not determine the style of mummification.

Mummy KV21 B
General CT findings

The mummy is poorly preserved, with its body dismantled into several segments and missing some of its parts (plate 49).

Gender

With fractured skull and pelvis, it is difficult to assign with certainty the gender of the mummy. However, the morphology of the remaining cranial and facial bones and the relatively small size of the femoral head may suggest a female.

Table 17. CT findings of arrangements of upper and lower limbs of Mummy KV21 A

Right upper limb	Proximal (arm)	A forearm of a right limb is placed upside down with its back facing up. The ulna is thus seen at the outer side (instead of the usual inner or medial side). The distal ends of both forearm bones are tapering.
	Distal (forearm)	A right arm is placed upside down with its back facing up. The humeral head and proximal shaft are sharply cut off.
	Hand	A disarticulated left hand along with about 5 cm stump of the distal forearm bones. The hand is clenched and is placed with its back up, and the thumb is missing.
Left upper limb	Proximal (arm)	Both bones of a left arm placed with their back facing up. The ulna is fractured, and its olecranon process is missing. The distal ends of both bones are fractured with tapered end points (tapering ends indicative of amputation that would fit the missing hand).
	Distal (forearm)	A left thigh bone and its patella
	Hand	Missing
Right lower limb	Proximal (thigh)	A right femur with multiple fractures involving the trochanters and neck.
	Distal (leg)	A right leg with both leg bones present.
	Foot	A left foot is markedly distorted with severe plantar flexion. Multiple toes are missing.
Left lower limb	Proximal (thigh)	A right leg with both bones (tibia and fibula). The upper end of the tibia is impacted in the acetabulum of the hip bone.
	Distal (leg)	Missing
	Foot	A right foot is placed upside down. The foot is distorted; the metatarsal bones show osteoporosis. Several bones of the forefoot are missing; amputated distal ends of the proximal phalanges from 2 to 4; middle and distal phalanges of all toes are missing. Only part of the soft tissues of the 5th toe is present.

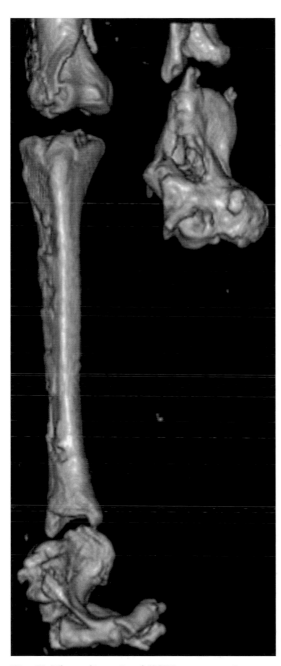

Fig. 60: Three-dimensional (SSD) reconstruction CT images in frontal projection of the lower limbs of mummy KV21 A show the wrongly placed bones and markedly deformed feet.

Table 18. CT measurements of the bones of Mummy KV21 B

Right femur	39.6 cm
Left femur	39.9 cm
Right tibia	32 cm
Left tibia	32.1 cm

Stature inferred from femoral length is about 151 cm ± 2.517 cm.[26]

Age at death

Based on epiphyseal union of all bones, the parts comprising the studied specimen are of a mature skeleton. The presence of mild to moderate degenerative changes of the spine and joints indicate a relatively older age of forty-five years.

Detailed CT findings
Skull

There are large bony defects involving the frontal part and most of the vault of the skull, as well as the right orbit and partially the adjacent part of the cribriform plate (figs. 61a–b). The cranial cavity is almost empty except for a small remnant of brain and fragments of fractured skull (fig. 62). Multiple maxillary teeth are missing; the other teeth show moderate wear.

Torso

There is complete separation of the body transversely at the level of the first lumbar vertebra. The anterior chest wall is opened below the level of the upper sternum; the lower sternum and anterior chest wall are missing. The torso cavity is partially filled with linen packs impregnated with resin; no viscera or heart are seen within the body cavity. Marginal degenerative osteophytes

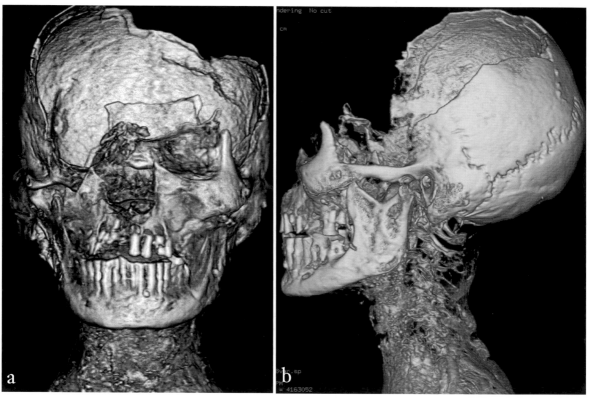

Figs 61a–b: SSD reconstruction of the head and neck of the KV21 B mummy in frontal (a) and lateral (b) projections shows the fractures and missing bones of the skull and face. Also note the poor dental condition and lack of several maxillary teeth.

and Schmorl's nodes are seen at multiple vertebral levels. The sacrum is fractured and opened, with most of its parts missing, except for a small part of the left alum. Multiple fractures of the right and left hip bones, and separation of the pubic bones, are noted.

Limbs

Multiple soft tissues and bony defects of the limbs are detected in CT images. The details are given in table 19.

Mummification style

Due to the partially destroyed skull and lack of most of the cribriform plate, we could not identify the style of mummification of the head. However, we identified remnants of tissues and probably resin intracranially, as well as resinous material in the naso- and oropharynx. The absence of viscera and presence of linen packs stuffed within the torso cavity indicated a high-quality evisceration and embalming process.

Table 19. CT findings of arrangements of upper and lower limbs of Mummy KV21 B

Right upper limb	Proximal (arm)	Missing most of the humerus, except for its head, which articulates in the shoulder socket (glenoid).
	Distal (forearm)	An anatomical right forearm; both bones are present.
	Hand	The hand is disarticulated and fractured, with missing little finger.
Left upper limb	Proximal (arm)	Only the upper two-thirds of the humerus is present and articulated in the shoulder. The rest of the limb is missing.
	Distal (forearm)	Missing except for a small part of the upper end of the ulna, which is loosely present close to the right side of the chest.
	Hand	Missing
Right lower limb	Proximal (thigh)	An anatomical right femur articulates in the acetabulum. The patella is present, in place.
	Distal (leg)	The leg is disarticulated at the level of the knee and displaced downward.
	Foot	The right foot is disarticulated at the ankle; part of the forefoot is missing.
Left lower limb	Proximal (thigh)	Present and articulating with the corresponding acetabulum.
	Distal (leg)	Present
	Foot	The left foot is misplaced at the level of the right knee, between the thigh and leg bones. Only the hind and mid foot bones are present.

The Two Fetuses in Tutankhamun's Tomb: DNA Analysis

We also did a preliminary DNA study of the two fetuses found in Tutankhamun's tomb, who are presumably the children of Ankhesenamun, and mummy KV21 A. The data obtained from the latter suggest that this was the mother of the fetuses. We cannot, however, identify the mummy as Ankhesenamun. More time is needed to analyze the data.

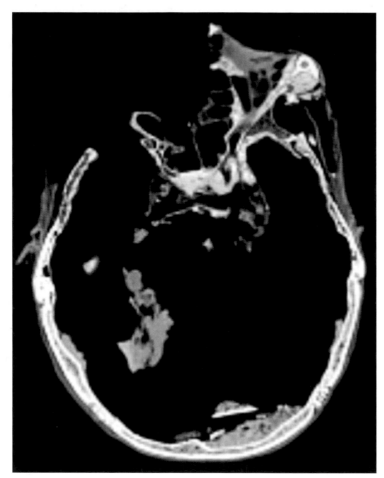

Fig. 62: Axial CT image of the skull of mummy KV21 B shows multiple craniofacial fractures. The right orbit and the adjacent cribriform plate are missing. The skull cavity is empty except for a few bony fragments and soft tissues (brain remnants). However, transnasal route of embalming the head cannot be confirmed.

Conclusions

The tomb of Ankhesenamun may be in the Valley of the Monkeys in the Western Valley, near the tomb of Ay. Our excavation in this area unearthed four intact foundation deposits and also some limestone stairs. The foundation deposits were full of pottery dated to the Eighteenth Dynasty, knives, tools, animal bones, and other objects. It is known that the ancient Egyptians created a foundation deposit before they began to construct a temple, but after the construction of a tomb, four or five foundation deposits were made. These recently discovered foundation deposits could indicate the existence of a tomb nearby, which we hope to pursue in a future line of research.

The mummy KV21 B is in very poor condition, with many missing parts, but we think that this mummy is a candidate for Nefertiti. As we saw in the case of KV35, the priests of Dynasties Twenty-one and Twenty-two placed Queen Tiye near her daughter. The two mummies of KV21 could be a mother and daughter as well. We hope that our future research will lead us to the mummy of Nefertiti.

Mutnodjmet

Another objective of this project is to find the remains of Nefertiti's sister, Mutnodjmet, the wife of Horemheb, the army commander under Akhenaten and Tutankhamun who eventually assumed the kingship. DNA analysis from her mummy could prove conclusive when comparing it to a possible candidate for Nefertiti's mummy. Mutnodjmet was buried in the private tomb in Saqqara prepared for Horemheb before he became king, excavated by Geoffrey Martin in 1975.[27] Unfortunately, there is no record of the current location of the queen's skeleton found by Martin. There are no bones remaining in the chamber, but it has been said that they were moved to the storage magazine at Saqqara. The magazine was checked, but the bones were not located. I hope that these remains have not left the country without the knowledge of Geoffrey Martin.

We do know that the queen was buried inside a hidden room in the tomb, beyond two old shafts. The shaft of Mutnodjmet was dug between two pillars in the rock and is uninscribed. A sarcophagus was found in the chamber and also some funerary equipment belonging to the queen. There was also a large quantity of pottery vessels once filled with food and wine for Mutnodjmet's use in the afterlife. A canopic jar inscribed with her name is now in the British Museum.

When Martin excavated the shaft, he found animal bones in the tunnel that led to the burial chamber. Eugen Strouhal studied a skull and other bones and concluded that they belonged to the queen. According to his analysis, the queen lost her teeth at an early age. She died at about age forty, possibly in childbirth, as the remains of a fetus were found with her body.[28]

Z. H.

9

The Nineteenth Dynasty

Historical Introduction

The end of the Eighteenth Dynasty witnessed a new era in kingship, because the ruler who took the throne after the death of Ay was Horemheb, the army commander in the reign of Tutankhamun.[1] He had no royal blood; he was born in Hut-nesut in Middle Egypt[2] and spent most of his life at Memphis. He built a tomb for himself there (fig. 63), which was discovered south of Saqqara in 1975 by an English expedition.[3]

Horemheb was married to Mutnodjmet, who may have been the daughter of Ay and sister of Nefertiti (see sidelight, "Mutnodjmet," in chapter 8). Among her monuments is a fragmentary statue naming her as a "God's Wife," a rare title at this time, indicating the continuation of the strong queens of the late Eighteenth Dynasty.[4] Horemheb disavowed completely the period that began with the death of Amenhotep III, razing monuments of the Amarna Period, chiseling out the names of his predecessors, and

appropriating Ay's mortuary temple. After he was crowned as king in Thebes, he returned to Memphis to rule, whereupon he issued a decree, preserved in a stela set up in Karnak temple, to save the country from chaos. His actions and rulings began to stabilize Egypt. Horemheb's reforms included restoring the temples and priesthood of Amun, the fair collection of taxes, halting corruption, and abolishing some abuses of appropriations of slaves and property. He also divided the command of the army into the two geographical divisions of Upper and Lower Egypt.

His foreign policy included military campaigns in Asia and a victory in Nubia. All of these were recorded in the rock-cut temple sanctuary of Gebel Silsila and the Ninth and Tenth Pylons at Karnak.

The length of Horemheb's rule has long been in dispute; scholars have endorsed reign lengths from fourteen to twenty-seven to fifty-nine years. Recent evidence has established it

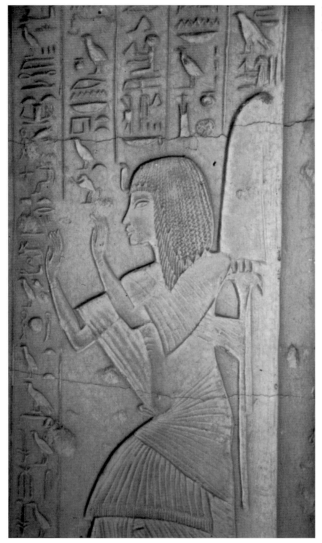

Fig. 63: Figure of Horemheb from his Memphite tomb.

as fourteen years,[5] but there are other factors that would suggest a nearly thirty-year reign.[6] He was buried not in his tomb at Memphis, but in an unfinished tomb in the Valley of the Kings (KV57),[7] which is notable for its spectacular decoration and architecture that is transitional between the Eighteenth and Nineteenth Dynasties. It may also have been a third cache of royal mummies.[8]

In the succeeding Nineteenth and Twentieth Dynasties, the kingship and the capital passed to families from the Delta, who moved the chief residence to the north but continued to be buried in the south at Thebes. Horemheb died without any living progeny; he apparently had selected Ramesses I,[9] who was a vizier and held the same military title as Horemheb, as his successor.

Ramesses was already in old age, however, and reigned for only two years. He chose a capital in the Delta called Per-Ramessu (Qantir in the eastern Delta). His family worshiped the god Seth, but he also built the beginning of the hypostyle hall devoted to Amun in Karnak, as well as other temples in the north and in Nubia.

The tomb of Ramesses I lies in the Valley of the Kings (KV16),[10] but his mummy was removed from the Deir al-Bahari cache and moved to Niagara Falls, Ontario, Canada (see introduction), from whence it was retrieved and returned to Egypt with the cooperation of the Michael C. Carlos Museum. It now resides in the Luxor Museum.

Seti I,[11] the son of Ramesses I, took the throne upon the death of his father when he was about forty years old. He was an officer on the eastern border of Egypt. The Four Hundred Year Stela, erected in the eastern Delta by his son Ramesses II, gives his titulary and celebrates the worship of the god Seth. Though his name ("of Seth") emphasized his connection to this god, he honored other deities as well, building an exquisite temple dedicated to Osiris at Abydos.[12] His reign is considered a period of restoration of traditional temples after the disruptions of the Amarna Period.[13]

Seti I followed in the tradition of Eighteenth Dynasty rulers by undertaking an extensive building program at home and military expeditions abroad. He conducted a campaign into Syria and in areas where the Hittites were threatening Egyptian interests. Seti I battled the Bedouin while crossing the Sinai, restored Egyptian dominance in Syria and Canaan, and fought the Hittites on several occasions. His most important achievement was the capture of the Syrian city of Qadesh.

He also conducted campaigns against the Libyans and Nubians. These military successes were commemorated on the walls of the hypostyle hall in Karnak. The scenes here are on a large scale, a new style for the king. His building program was supported economically by the opening of quarries and gold mines.

Seti I built a palace at Qantir. He married Tuya, who was the mother of his successor Ramesses II. The length of his reign has been debated, but may have been eleven years.[11] His tomb,[15] discovered by Belzoni in 1817, is perhaps the most magnificent in the Valley of the Kings (plate 50). It is the longest and deepest tomb in the valley, and the first tomb to have all of its chambers and passages decorated. Its program of decoration was innovative and set the stage for all royal tombs in the valley afterward. There were religious texts from the Book of Gates, the Litany of Re, the Amduat, a complete version of the Book of the Celestial Cow, an astronomical ceiling (plate 51), and an Osiris shrine.

Giovanni Belzoni found a tunnel in the tomb of Seti I, and this was excavated in 1960 by Ali Abdel Rasoul, who reached a depth of 100 m. In 2005, Zahi Hawass led an expedition with Tarek El Awady, who was the director general of the Egyptian Museum, Cairo, archaeologist Mostafa El Hoksh, and soil mechanical engineer Ayman Hamed, along with *rais* Saad El Gassab. The expedition excavated and restored the tunnel to a depth of 174.5 m. The tunnel came to a dead end, and this mystery has now been solved.[16]

Seti I's son, Ramesses II, was chosen as crown prince in his mid-teens[17] and succeeded his father on the throne several years later. He ruled for sixty-six years and had eight wives, the best known of whom is Nefertari. He built for her a great temple at

Abu Simbel (plate 52) and a beautifully decorated tomb in the Valley of the Queens. His other wives included two of his daughters (Merytamun and Bintanath), a sister (Henutmire), and the daughter of the king of the Hittites (Maathorneferure).[18]

Ramesses II carried out numerous military campaigns to take back territory previously held and to secure the borders of Egypt. His most important campaign was against the Hittites in Year 5. The Egyptian source for this is found on the walls of the king's temples at Abu Simbel (fig. 64), Luxor, Karnak, Derr, Abydos, and the Ramesseum (plate 53), where Ramesses proclaimed victory in the battle of Qadesh. However, a Hittite source also claimed victory for that side. Though it appears that Ramesses may have lost this war, he built a temple for himself at Abu Simbel as a king worshiping himself as a god. For the king to be a god, he had to be victorious over his enemies. Therefore, his construction of the temple ensured his divinity. Later in his reign, he fought against his Hittite foes once again and was more successful. In Year 21, he signed the world's first known peace treaty with the Hittites, copies of which are extant in hieroglyphs on the temple of Karnak and in Akkadian on a cuneiform tablet. The deal was further sealed through the marriage of Ramesses to the daughter of the Hittite king.

Ramesses II was a prolific builder, with temples, statues, and chapels almost everywhere in Upper and Lower Egypt, and into Nubia,

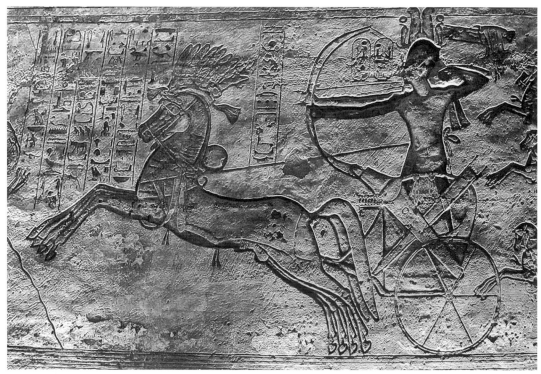

Fig. 64: The battle of Ramesses II against the Hittites at Qadesh. Temple of Ramesses II at Abu Simbel.

many on a monumental scale (fig. 65). His family was prolific as well; evidence indicates that he fathered around one hundred children—forty-eight to fifty sons and forty to fifty-three daughters.[19] In the Valley of the Kings, tomb KV5 was rediscovered in 1995 by Kent Weeks and the Theban Mapping Project. The largest tomb in the Valley of the Kings, it is thought to have been the burial place of many of his sons and consists of more than 130 chambers and corridors.[20] On the contrary, Hawass believes that this tomb was a cenotaph for the family of Ramesses II.[21] Ramesses himself was buried in a large tomb in the Valley of the Kings (KV7, fig. 66),[22] sadly damaged by flooding.

Several sons of Ramesses II predeceased him, and his thirteenth son, Merenptah, was appointed prince regent[23] and took the throne at the end of his father's long reign. He was in at least his late sixties upon his accession and reigned for about ten years.

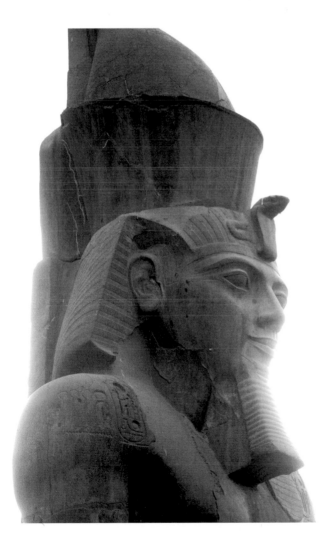

Fig. 65: Statue of Ramesses II from Luxor Temple.

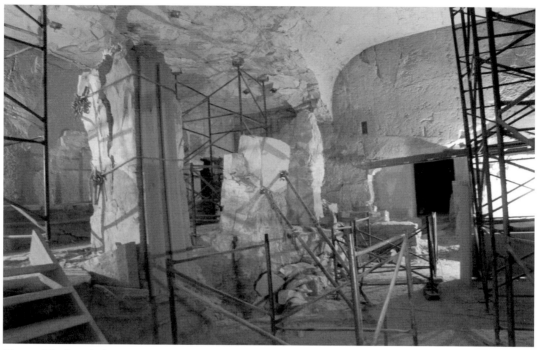

Fig. 66: The burial chamber of Ramesses II inside his tomb (KV7), Valley of the Kings.

Merenptah undertook military campaigns in Palestine and Nubia in the first years of his reign. The "Israel stela" is his most famous monument, which records his victory over Libya and the "Sea Peoples"; it claims that the people of Israel were destroyed, the first mention of Israel in an Egyptian text (see sidelight, "The Exodus). He was buried in KV8 in a tomb with a simplified single axis (fig. 67). His burial equipment included four stone sarcophagi (fig. 68).

Merenptah was followed by Amenmesse, amid a great disturbance in the succession.[24] Although the situation is not clear, Amenmesse appears to have been a usurper who reigned for several years in at least the southern part of Egypt, at the beginning or in the middle of the reign of Seti II, the eldest son of Merenptah. After a six-year reign, Seti II was followed by Siptah, who ruled for another six years with his regent, Queen Tawosret.[25] She reigned as sole ruler for another two years, the third queen of the New Kingdom to rule as king. Amid such dynastic difficulties, the Nineteenth Dynasty came to an end.

CT Examination of Selected Mummies of the Nineteenth Dynasty

The CT scanning of the mummies of this period was done by Ashraf Selim and Hany Abdel-Rahman, and CT image reconstructions, analysis, and reporting were provided by Sahar Saleem. The mummies in question are those of Seti I, Ramesses II, and Merenptah.

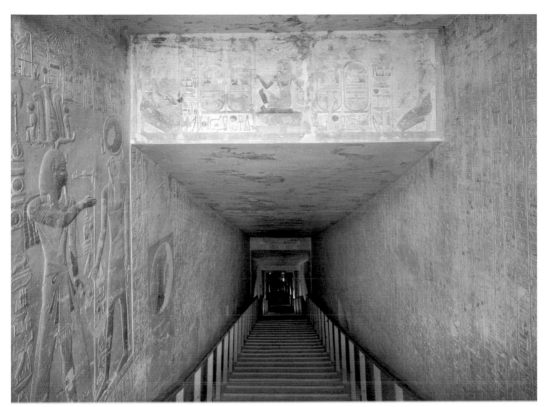

Fig. 67: The tomb of Merenptah (KV8), Valley of the Kings.

The mummy of Seti I

Genealogy of Seti I
Father: Ramesses I
Mother: Sitre

Identification of the mummy
The mummy of Seti I was found in tomb
DB320 in one of his original coffins, with several dockets on the coffin and mummy wrappings bearing his name.

General CT findings
The CT study shows that the head and face of
the mummy are perfectly preserved (fig. 69),
while the body was damaged, likely by ancient
plunderers. The body is dismantled, with

Table 20. General CT findings for the mummy of Seti I

Preservation status	Fair
Age	40–50 years
Gender	Male
Stature (vertex–heel)	About 167 cm

total separation into three parts at the attachment of neck and body as well as above the
iliac crests.

The morphological appearance of the skull
supports the known gender of a male.

Based on the epiphyseal union of all bones,
the mummy has a mature skeleton. The

SIDELIGHT:
The Exodus

We do not have any archaeological evidence about the Exodus, and the written texts from this period in Egypt do not shed any light on Moses or the Exodus. The same is true for Joseph and Abraham, who also came to Egypt.

The sacred texts of the Torah (Old Testament) and Qur'an are our sources on this matter, but they do not give dates or names of the pharaohs who were involved. The biblical story of the Israelites' departure from Egypt can be found in the second book of the Torah, Exodus. According to this familiar story, Moses's mother, in order to save him, put him in a basket and set it adrift on the Nile. Moses was found by an Egyptian princess, who adopted the child. Moses thus grew up in the palace of the pharaoh. As an adult, he killed an Egyptian overseer and was forced to escape to the desert. He later had an encounter with God, who commanded him to return to Egypt in order to save his people from the persecutions of the pharaoh. When Moses and his people attempted their escape, the pharaoh and his army pursued them, but the Egyptians were drowned in the Red Sea. The Hebrews stayed forty years in the Sinai, where Moses received the Ten Commandments.[26]

The Old Testament scriptures imply that there were two pharaohs connected with the Exodus (the pharaoh of the oppression and the pharaoh of the Exodus). The word 'pharaoh' is derived from the hieroglyphic word $pr-\varsigma$, meaning 'great house,' and referred to the king. It is mentioned only with regard to Moses; in the Qur'an's stories of Abraham and Joseph, the word 'pharaoh' is not used.

There have been many attempts by scholars to confirm the details of the holy books regarding the Exodus and the pharaoh connected with it. There are theories that the Exodus occurred in the time of the Hyksos occupation of Egypt, and others suggest that the pharaohs could be

Thutmose III or Amenhotep II.[27] Christiane Desroches-Noblecourt believed that Moses returned to Egypt during the reign of Ramesses II.[28] Others are of the opinion that it was Merenptah, perhaps because of the "Israel stela" that dates to Year 5 of his reign.[29] The stela itself does not mention the Exodus, but the word 'Israel' appears, written without the city determinative that would indicate that it refers to a geographical location.[30] Other scholars believe that the name does not refer to Israel because the text has no verb of 'leaving' or 'dismissing.' The text also does not mention the miracle of the Exodus as related in the scriptures.[31]

The stela records military victories of Merenptah in Year 5, but all of the holy books tell us that the pharaoh was drowned. The writer of the text, detailing the great victories and efforts made by the king, would never have written this if the king were dead. In addition, there are monuments of Merenptah dating to the tenth year of the reign. The stela of Merenptah can confirm that the Exodus took place before the reign of this king.

The Old Testament mentions two kings in connection with the Exodus.[32] It is impossible to identify them. The Qur'an mentions only one; this has led many to believe that this pharaoh could be Ramesses II, due to his long reign of sixty-six years. This would have been long enough for Moses to be born, to escape Egypt after killing the Egyptian, to return to Egypt, and to leave with his people, but there is no Egyptian evidence for this.

In 1975, Maurice Bucaille, a French surgeon and archaeologist, received permission to examine the bodies of Ramesses II and Merenptah in Cairo. Bucaille's forensic report stated that Merenptah died of asphyxiation or drowning, and that the presence of salt crystals in the mummy favored him as the drowned pharaoh of the Exodus. According to Bucaille's report, the mummy of Merenptah bears the traces of fatal blows that may have been inflicted during his drowning or after the recovery of his body that had washed ashore.[33]

However, the presence of salt in the body is not proof of his drowning, as mummification required the use of natron, a natural salt, to remove all moisture from the corpse. CT identified a defect at the back of the skull of Merenptah; this could be what Bucaille referred to in his report as a fatal blow that happened during drowning. In CT images, the lack of sclerosis or other healing signs suggests that the lesion was likely post-mortem. The defect has beveled, sharp edges with pointed margins that are longer in the outer than inner skull plate. These findings indicate that a sharp, pointed, solid tool (similar to instruments used by the embalmers) was used to induce the defect. We suggest that the embalmers deliberately induced this defect to introduce linen inside the skull, rather than its being accidental.[34]

A fundamental question is: why is there no archaeological or textual evidence for the Exodus? The answer is very simple. The ancient Egyptians had a basic religious concept: for the king to be a 'good god,' or to be equal to the universal god, it was necessary for him to accomplish certain duties, such as conquering the enemies of Egypt, building temples to the gods and making offerings to them, unifying the Two Lands, and celebrating the sed-festival, or jubilee. Scenes recording these duties and focusing on the king emphasized the domination of the king over his enemies. In such a context, the Exodus could never have been recorded inside a temple or tomb of the king. He was defeated on this occasion, which negated his divinity. Therefore, it is impossible that any royal text exists to inform us about this event, but among the multitude of objects yet to be discovered, perhaps there is a text written by a student in a temple school that can yet inform us about the Exodus.

Z.H. and S.N.S.

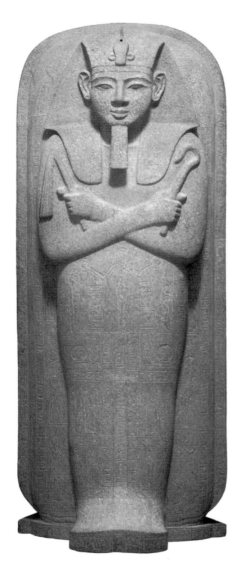

Fig. 68: The lid of Merenptah's sarcophagus in his burial chamber.

degree of union of the ectocranial sutures indicates that the age was over forty years at the time of death. The presence of moderate degenerative changes of the lumbar spine, mild lippings of the knee, tooth wear, and attrition all support what is known about his age at death of about forty to fifty years.[35]

Because the body was dismantled into pieces, the height from vertex to heel could only roughly be measured at about 167 cm. The measured height of the mummy was also close to the stature of 169 cm (± 4.4 cm) as extrapolated from the length of the humerus (32.8 cm), using the following equation:

Stature (cm) = 3.26 x (length of humerus: 32.8) + 62.1 = 169 cm ± 4.4 cm.

CT findings in different regions
Head (fig. 70)
A large defect detected at the base of the ACF indicates removal of the brain via transnasal excerebration. The skull defect measures 26 mm in transverse and 56 mm from front to back. There is partial interruption of the bony walls of the ethmoidal air cells, which are partly filled with resin. The nose is stuffed with embalming materials, mainly resin. The posterior half of the skull is filled with embalming materials of different CT features. From posterior to anterior, there is a homogeneous, moderately dense material (solidified resin or resin-like); a heterogeneous, low-density material containing multiple moderately dense objects with their long axes ranging between 0.9 cm and 1.75 cm (likely hardened soil); and linen threads.[36]

There is also a small scalloping at the inner occipital skull table, just to the right of the midline (1.2 cm x 0.7 cm), which likely represents part of the lambdoid suture.

There are subcutaneous homogeneous moderate-density packs of comparable widths seen in both sides of the mid- and lower face. The packs involve the front plane of the face around the nose and mouth, cheeks, lateral jaw, and superficial temporal regions.[37]

The orbits contain dry eye globes and are filled with heterogeneous linen impregnated

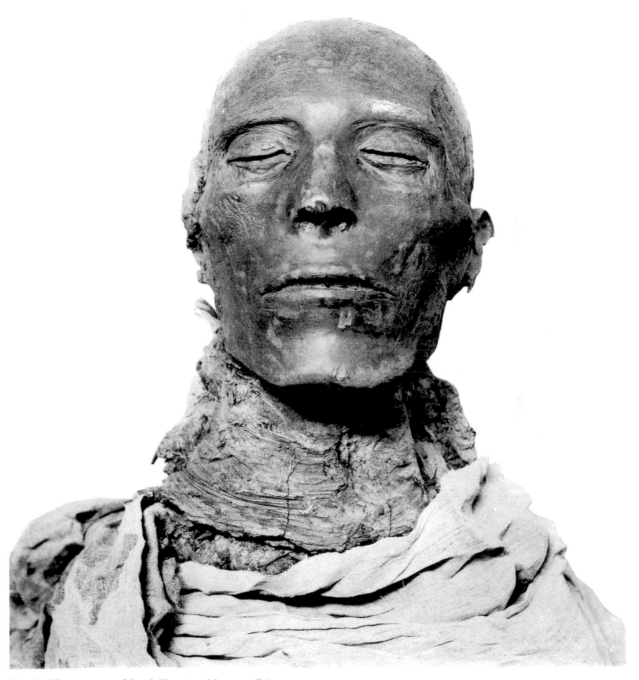

Fig. 69: The mummy of Seti I. Egyptian Museum, Cairo.

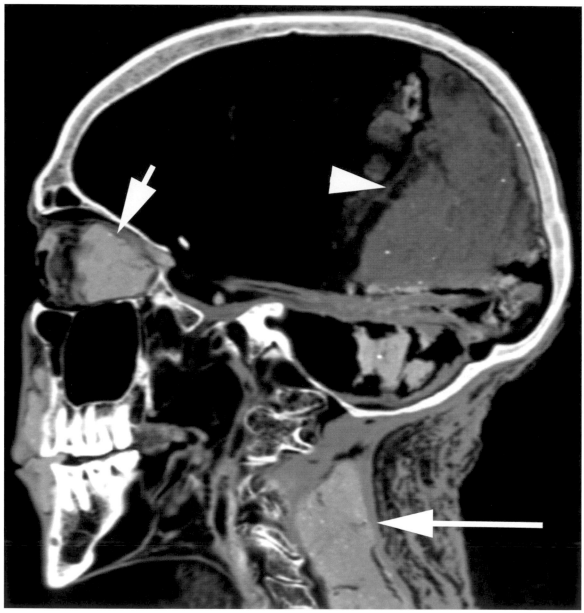

Fig. 70: CT image in sagittal plane of the head and neck of the mummy of Seti I shows a well-preserved head with meticulous mummification and ample amounts of embalming materials and resin placed in the orbit (short arrow), inside the skull (arrowhead), and underneath the skin of the neck (long arrow).

with resin (–130 HU to 250 HU); the resin was likely introduced in its hot liquid state, as it is seen smearing the optic foramina and the nearby meninges.

The right auricle is malformed (likely was detached and remodeled during mummy restoration). The lobule of the left auricle is missing. The throat of the mummy (oropharynx and hypopharynx) is partly filled with embalming materials, probably linen bits soaked in resin.

Teeth (plates 54a–b)
Generally, the dental condition of the mummy of Seti I was reasonably good. There is moderate tooth wear, alveolar resorption, attrition, and fair periodontal health. Changes are consistent with the estimated age of the king at time of death.

A single supernumerary tooth is seen in the right anterior aspect of the maxilla. The tooth lies obliquely within the confinement of the maxillary bone opposite the palatal surface of the right maxillary incisors. The impacted supernumerary tooth is of the supplemental-tooth type, being well formed and composed of a cusp and root. It is likely a duplication of the maxillary right lateral incisor (mesiodens). There are no detectable complications resulting from the supernumerary tooth, which indicates that this dental condition was likely asymptomatic for the king. The impacted tooth did not cause maleruption, displacement, or crowding of the related teeth. There was no associated dentigerous cyst or resorption of roots of the adjacent teeth.

A focal bony loss and depression is seen at the alveolar margin of the left side of the mandible at the origin of the first molar tooth (#19). The depression is well defined with a sclerotic margin indicating its chronicity.

Tooth #19 is missing and most likely had fallen out during the king's life; this caused the second premolar (#20) to flip out of its position toward the buccal cavity. The alveolar bony defect could be the end result of a chronic process like periodontosis at the nineteenth tooth. The remaining teeth are well spaced and properly aligned; no protrusion of incisors is noted.

Spine (fig. 71)
The neck (cervical) vertebrae are intact. The body of the mummy is severed at the upper back level (between the third and fourth dorsal vertebrae). There is a gap of about 2.5 cm between the severed body parts; the upper vertebral column is displaced anteriorly and 3 cm to the right in relation to the lower part. The fractured vertebrae are likely postmortem, with no sclerosis or attempt of healing. Patches of moderately high, resin-like density are seen within the cancellous vertebral bones, especially noted from sixth to eighth thoracic vertebrae. The height of the intervertebral discs is not reduced. No CT evidence of fused zygapophyseal or sacroiliac joints or ossified spinal ligaments could be detected.

Torso (chest and abdomen)
The walls of the torso are interrupted at multiple locations. The embalmers placed layers of linen soaked in resin outside the torso wall as well as beneath the skin in several locations. There is CT evidence that the superficial soft tissues of the torso are formed of multiple layers of linen soaked in resin, as well as subcutaneous packing. The cavity of the torso is partially stuffed with folded linen packs immersed in resin in the right side of the body and loose linen folds in the left hemithorax. There is also a homogeneous layer of

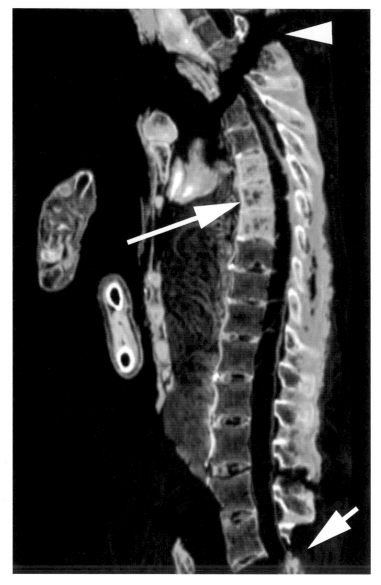

Fig. 71: Sagittal CT image of the torso of Seti I shows that the body is dismantled at the attachment of neck and body (arrowhead) as well as in the lower back (short arrow). There is resin-like increased density inside the vertebral cancellous bones (sixth to eighth thoracic vertebrae) and the discs (long arrow).

solidified resin lining the posterior of the body cavity.

Upper limbs

The arms are flexed at the elbows, and the forearms are crossed over the chest, right over left. The fingers of both hands are flat.

There are multiple focal bony interruptions of both upper limbs that are postmortem and postembalming, likely caused by tomb robbers. The fractures involve the proximal and distal shaft of the right ulna, the proximal shaft of the left humerus, and bones of the left elbow (medial humeral condyle and olecranon process). There are also mild degenerative changes of both shoulders in the form of osteophytic lippings at the glenoid labra.

Lower limbs

There are mild degenerative changes of both hip joints (acetabular osteophytic lippings). There is no CT evidence of fusion of the joints (ankylosis), or abnormal calcification of the tendons or the joints. The bones and soft tissues have heterogeneous CT densities (a mix of air and resin), likely caused by pouring the hot liquid resin during mummification.

There is a comminuted fracture of the anteromedial aspect of the distal shaft of the right tibia. The fracture is about 8 cm above the ankle talo-tibial joint. It is likely post-mortem and before one of the later embalming restorations (see below), as resin is seen entrapped within the bony fragment.

Both feet show fractures. The right foot has irregular fractures at the proximal phalanges of the first to fourth toes and the middle phalanx of the fifth toe. The left foot shows disarticulation of the first and second toes, and fractures of the mid-shaft of the proximal phalanges of the third, fourth, and fifth toes.

The superficial soft tissues of the upper and lower limbs are thickened and have homogeneous moderate CT densities (120 HU); this was likely caused by hot poured resin that infiltrated the skin and the underlying soft tissues. In addition, there are heterogeneous dense packs placed beneath the skin of the upper and lower limbs. The subcutaneous fillings are seen also in the palms of the hands and soles of the feet. This resulted in the restoration of the girth of the limbs.[38]

Comments on mummification

Although the mummy of Seti I was badly affected by tomb robbers, it exhibits an excellent mummification job. The mummy was a subject of several later restorations by embalmers, as the series of linen and coffin dockets associated with his mummy attested: the first occurred during Year 6 of *wḥm mswt*, the period of 'renaissance' under the high priest Herihor; a second took place after Year 10 of Smendes I, when the king's body was rewrapped with dated linen of Pinudjem I, possibly in Year 15, when the mummy of Ramesses II was cached with that of his father in KV17; and again in Year 7 of Psusennes I, when it was rewrapped again. A coffin docket documents the mummy's removal from KV17 in Year 10 of Siamun.[39]

These restorations of the mummy in later dynasties may explain the abundance and heterogeneity of embalming materials detected by the CT study. CT findings indicate that the outer surface of the mummy is covered by multiple layers that could be linen layers from different restorations.

The mummification style of Seti I's body is consistent with that commonly seen in the Nineteenth Dynasty: transnasal removal of the brain, different embalming materials placed inside the skull, and the torso stuffed with materials of different CT properties, most likely resin, linen, and soil.

However, there were aspects of the mummification of Seti I that were unusual for that time.

1. The king's arms were crossed with hands flat, not clenched, a finding that was common later, in the Twentieth Dynasty.[40]
2. Ample amounts of resin (or resin-like) substances were used in mummification. It was previously believed that

more reliance was placed on the use of resin only after the Twenty-fifth Dynasty.[41] CT study showed that the soft tissues and bones of the mummy are impregnated with layers of homogeneous, moderately high-CT-density (130–160 HU) material that extended to the body cavities and infiltrated the adjacent bones and spinal canal. The thoracic vertebral bodies from the sixth to the eighth thoracic vertebrae showed a peculiar distribution of resin. When it was applied in a molten state, the resin invaded the cavity and penetrated into the cancellous structure of bone. The resin material formed a horizontal level at the back of the body, filled the soft tissues, and penetrated into the bones and spinal canal. The horizontal level at the posterior aspect of the torso indicates the liquid status of the resin at the time of embalming, and that the body lay recumbent and flat at the time of mummification.[42]

3. Another atypical point in mummification is that the skin of the mummy's face and body was likely painted with resin, a treatment usually found in later times. Over the millennia, the resin became altered to acquire a black, glistening appearance, which explains the external dark appearance of the mummy of Seti I. Based on the adherence of superficial wrappings to the body surface, it seemed that resin seeped into the most superficial wrappings of the mummy.

4. The presence of elaborate subcutaneous packing is another notable aspect in the mummification of Seti I. Subcutaneous packs presented in the face, neck, and multiple regions in the torso and limbs.[43] This resulted in the lifelike appearance of the mummy's face and enhanced the contours of the body. Subcutaneous filling is also seen in other regions in the mummy of Seti I that are not usually filled in other mummies, such as the axilla and the palms of hands and feet.[44]

A heart amulet, wrapped within a linen pack that likely contains heart residue, is detected within the right upper part of the mummy. A *wedjat* amulet is detected at the back of the left arm of Seti I. A small amulet with geometric openwork designs, possibly another *wedjat*, was found in the wrappings outside the body of Seti I at the left side of his back (opposite the third lumbar vertebral level). Multiple rounded structures (likely beads) are seen at the medial surface of the lower shaft of the right femur of the mummy.[45] (For further details, see chapter 12, "Amulets, Funerary Figures, and Other Objects Found on the Mummies.")

Manner and cause of death
The mummy offers no definite explanation for the manner or cause of death of King Seti I.

The mummy of Ramesses II
Genealogy of Ramesses II
Father: Seti I
Mother: Tuya

Identification of the mummy
The mummy of Ramesses II was found in tomb DB320. Its linen bandages, as well as the wooden coffin into which the body had been transferred, were inscribed with the king's name and epithets in hieratic script.

General CT findings

The mummy was fairly preserved but had suffered from multiple mutilations caused by tomb robbers in antiquity, as well as the public unwrapping that took place on June 1, 1886, staged by Gaston Maspero.[46]

The morphological appearance of the bones of the skull and hip supports the known gender of a male, despite the absence of male genitalia at the groin region.[47]

The mummy has a mature skeleton with united long bones and fused sutures of the skull. The marked attrition of the dental arc, spine, and joints (especially hips and shoulders) all indicate geriatric diseases found in individuals over seventy years of age. The suggested age of death coincides with the historically known age of about eighty-seven to ninety-two years.[48]

The CT measurement of the stature from vertex to heel is 170 cm. Electronic CT measurements of the long bones are: right and left humerus 33 cm, right femur 44.7 cm, left femur 44.6 cm, right tibia 37 cm, and left tibia 36.6 cm.

CT findings in different regions
Head (fig. 72; see also fig. 4d in chapter 1 and fig. 103 in chapter 11)
There is a defect at the front of the skull base (ACF) that measures 1 cm in transverse and 3.2 cm from front to back. This bony defect indicates removal of the brain via transnasal excerebration, likely via the right nare. The posterior two-thirds of the skull is filled with resin, signifying that the body was lying supine during the process. The resin is compartmentalized within dural remnants.[49]

The contour of the nose is hooked in appearance and is almost totally stuffed with different embalming materials: a small animal

Table 21. General CT findings for the mummy of Ramesses II

Preservation status	Good
Age	Over 70 years
Gender	Male
Stature (vertex–heel)	170 cm

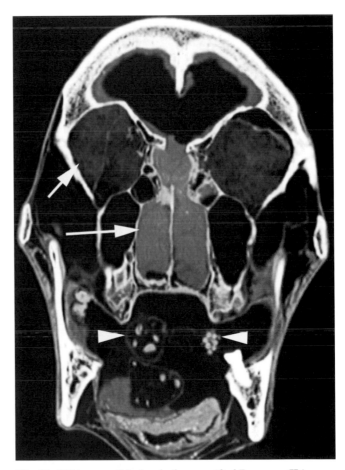

Fig. 72: CT image of the head of mummified Ramesses II in coronal plane shows that the embalmers used different materials: the orbits are filled with linen packs (short arrow), the nasal cavities are filled with resin (long arrow), and parcels of plant seeds are placed in the mouth (arrowheads).

bone, plant seeds, and resin. The orbits contain dry globes and are filled with heterogeneous, low-density material (–660 to –300 HU), probably linen. The throat of the mummy (oropharynx and hypopharynx) contains multiple dense, oblong plant seeds that measure 2–4 mm in diameter; the seeds are arranged in clusters, likely within parcels.

Teeth

The dental condition of the mummy of Ramesses is generally poor, with marked tooth wear and alveolar resorption; changes are consistent with the estimated advanced age of the king at time of death. The periodontal health is poor, with evidence of a large cavity in the mandible at the root of the left second molar. This represented an abscess that must have caused the king marked pain.

Spine (figs. 73a–b)

The neck is fractured at the level of the disc between the fifth and sixth cervical vertebrae, with mild forward displacement of the distal spine. There is no evidence of soft-tissue collections or bony healing related to the neck fracture, suggesting that this injury could have happened postmortem. There is moderate hunchback (dorsal kyphosis), and scoliosis with its convexity to the right.[50]

The body of the mummy is also severed at the upper back level between the third and fourth dorsal vertebrae. The fractured vertebrae have an irregular outline, and their posterior elements are interrupted. There is a gap of about 2.5 cm between the severed body parts; the upper vertebral column is displaced anteriorly and 3 cm to the right in relation to the lower part. The fracture is most likely postmortem.

The CT study identified ossifications at the right side of the anterior longitudinal ligament (ALL) associated with multiple bridging osteophytes at multiple levels in the cervical and thoracic spine. The ossified ALL flows continuously along the vertebrae and the intervertebral discs to form blocks at the following levels: between the third and fifth cervical vertebrae, between the seventh cervical and fifth thoracic, and between the sixth and ninth thoracic vertebrae. A low-density rim can occasionally be detected between the anterior vertebral body and the ossified ALL. The intervertebral discs have normal or slightly reduced heights, with no evidence of severe degenerative changes. Additional findings include ossifications or calcifications of the supraspinous and ligamenta flava at multiple levels, and osteoarthritis of the uncovertebral and costovertebral joints without bony ankylosis. There is no fusion or ankylosis of the posterior vertebral elements or sacroiliac joints.[51] In addition to the spinal changes, there are extraspinal calcifications or ossifications at the attachments of tendons in the axial and peripheral skeletons. The CT findings fulfill the diagnostic criteria of DISH disease.

Torso

The chest cavity is filled with linen and linen impregnated with resin. The desiccated heart is seen in place, slightly to the left side of the thorax (fig. 74). Calcified plaques are identified within the aorta, indicating atherosclerosis.

The rest of the viscera were removed, and the cavity of the torso is partially stuffed with different embalming materials of variable densities that ranged between –200 and +600 HU. The embalming materials include linen

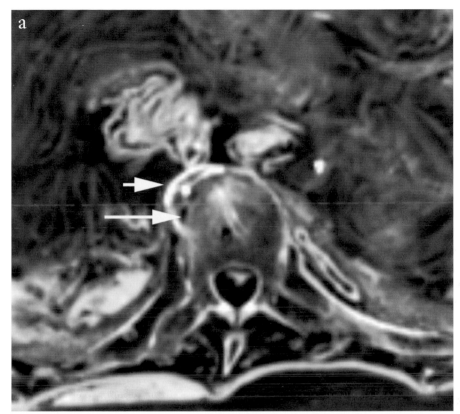

a

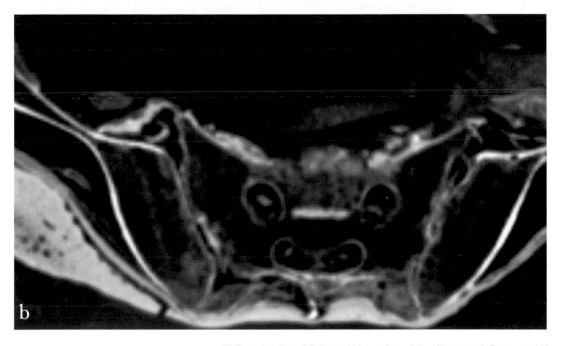

b

Figs. 73a–b: Axial two-dimensional CT images of the thoracic spine and sacroiliac joints of Ramesses II. (a): There is a bulky ossification at the right anterolateral aspect of the eighth thoracic vertebral body (short arrow). Note the low-density line that separates the ossified ligament from the underlying vertebra (long arrow). (b): The sacroiliac joints show no erosions or bony fusion.

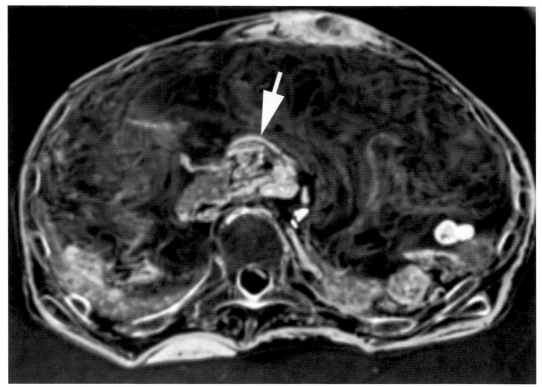

Fig. 74: Axial CT image of the chest of Ramesses II shows the desiccated heart (arrow) in place, surrounded by linen packs.

packs impregnated with resin, and loosely packed material containing small, very dense particles, likely sand or small stones. The left lower quadrant of the torso cavity is empty.

A dense object that measures 67 mm x 14 mm x 120 mm in transverse, front-to-back (AP), and upper-to-lower respectively, occupies the left upper chest cavity of Ramesses II. The object is oblong shaped, and may represent an amulet with two upper and lower hooked processes.[52] (For further details, see chapter 12.)

The male organ and the scrotum are missing. The skin and soft tissues at the pubic region are interrupted, as well as the resin layer that covers the skin. The suggested scenario is that the genital structures were bro-ken after the completion of the embalming process, likely by vandalism or possibly as a result of the public unwrapping.

Upper limbs
The arms are flexed at the elbows, and the forearms are crossed over the chest, left over right. The fingers of the hands are flexed as if clenching something.

There are moderate degenerative changes of both shoulders in the form of osteophytic lip-pings at the glenoid labra. There is calcification of the tendons of the cuff muscles of both shoulders, as well as mild thickening of the lig-ament of the right shoulder (coracoclavicular). There are multiple postmortem fractures that involve the ulnar bone of both elbows, likely induced by the tomb robbers.

Lower limbs

There are moderate degenerative changes at both hip joints, with large lippings at the acetabulum.

Multiple bony projections are seen in the bones of the thighs:

1. A small bony excrescence or outgrowth (1.6 cm x 1 cm in transverse and AP dimensions) is projecting medially from the junction of the neck and great trochanter of the right femur.
2. In the left femoral neck region, a sessile bony excrescence (2.2 cm x 1.4 cm) is seen at the anterior border of the greater trochanter, close to the insertion of the gluteus minimus muscle.
3. A well-defined bony excrescence is outpunching from the posterior sur-

face of the medial condyle of the left femur. The lesion has a short pedicle, and it is corticated with its cortex continuous with that of the parent bone. The bony cortex underlying the excrescences is intact, without associated deformity or dysplastic changes of the bones (fig. 75).

There are bilateral calcifications (enthesopathies) in the pelvis at the iliac crests and ischial tuberosities; around the knees in the quadriceps tendon insertion and patellar ligaments; and in the feet at the insertion of the Achilles tendons and peronii muscles (longus and brevis). Degenerative changes of the ankles are visible, with bilateral calcaneal spurs.

Two sesamoid bones (about 17 mm in diameter each) are seen at the plantar surface of the head of the first metatarsal of both feet, along the path of the tendons of the tibialis posterior and flexor digitorium muscles. A

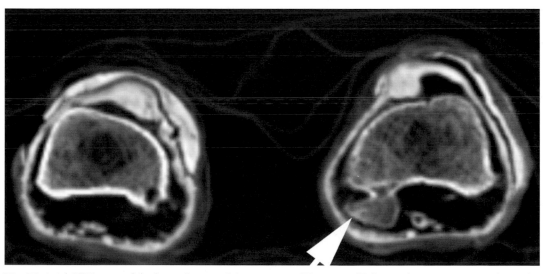

Fig. 75: Axial CT image of the lower femurs of the mummy of Ramesses II shows a bony excrescence (arrow) outpouching from the posterior surface of the medial condyle of the left femur. The lesion has a short pedicle and it is corticated, with its cortex continuous with that of the parent bone.

linear fracture is detected at the proximal phalanx of the second toe of the left foot.

Multiple calcified plaques involve the walls of the arteries of the lower limbs, denoting atherosclerosis of the arteries.

Resin-like material surrounds both lower limbs. The skin and soft tissues at the lateral aspect of the left lower leg are interrupted.

Comments on mummification

The quality of the embalming process was excellent, as expected for a king. The mummification style is comparable to that commonly seen in the Nineteenth Dynasty. The brain had been removed via the transnasal route. The viscera were removed, and the abdomen is fully stuffed with different embalming materials.

Unusual aspects of the mummification of Ramesses II consist of the introduction of unique embalming materials inside the nose and throat, including a bone of a small animal and plant seeds, as well as the use of resin for superficial contouring of the body.[53] The embalmers did not apply the procedure of subcutaneous packing, except in a localized region in the right cheek.[54]

Manner and cause of death

The preservation status of the mummy is good. Ramesses II was probably crippled with arthritis and walked with a hunched back for at least several years of his life. He also suffered from painfully poor dental health. However, there were no definite CT findings to suggest the cause of death.

Conclusions

The CT findings of the mummy of King Ramesses II reflect various systemic effects of a condition of abnormal bone diathesis (ten-

dency)[55] that involves the axial and peripheral skeleton. It manifests by calcification or ossification at different regions of the skeleton, such as at the insertion point of a ligament, tendon, and joint capsule (enthesopathy). The process is also accompanied by new bone growth (hypertrophic new bone formation) in the form of osteophytes, enthesophytes, and exostosis, as well as overgrowth of sesamoid bones. For a detailed discussion of the diagnosis of the spine of Ramesses II, see sidelight, "Questions about Ramesses II and Merenptah."

The Mummy of Merenptah
Genealogy of Merenptah
Father: Ramesses II
Mother: Isetnofret

Identification of the mummy

The mummy of Merenptah was discovered in KV35, in a replacement coffin, the base of which was inscribed for the Twentieth Dynasty king Sethnakht; the upturned lid held remains that may be Queen Tawosret. The identity of Merenptah's mummy was proved by a linen docket.

General CT findings

The general condition of the mummy is good (fig. 76), although there is evidence of multiple mutilations, likely inflicted by tomb robbers in antiquity. The morphological appearances of the bones (the skull and hip) as well as the presence of the phallus at the groin region support the known gender of a male. Based on CT findings, the epiphyseal union of all bones indicates a mature skeleton. The coronal and sagittal ectocranial sutures are closed, while the lambdoid is patent. The moderately degenerated dental arc, spine, and joints, as well as the morphology of the symphyseal

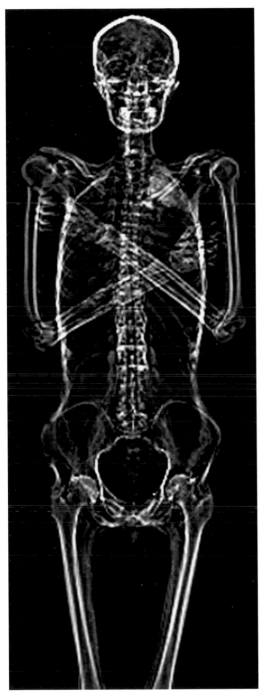

Fig. 76: A scout CT image of the mummy of Merenptah gives a rapid impression of the good preservation status and the crossed-arms royal position.

Table 22. General CT findings for the mummy of Merenptah

Preservation status	Good
Age	50–60 years
Gender	Male
Stature	171 cm

surface, all indicate an age of fifty to sixty years at time of death.

The stature of the mummy as measured from vertex to heel is 171 cm. The length of the left humerus is 32.1 cm; the right humerus is fractured and its length cannot be assessed. The length of the right femur is 46 cm, while the left is 45.9 cm.

Findings in different regions
Head (plates 55a–b)
There is evidence of transnasal excerebration through a defect inflicted in the cribriform plate that measures 28 mm x 32 mm in transverse and anteroposterior dimensions, respectively. The skull had been almost evacuated, with only minimal brain residue. Convoluted linen threads impregnated with resin of CT density between –830 HU and 35 HU are seen filling the anterior two-thirds of the skull cavity. The bulk of the cranial filling is more on the right side, pushing the interhemispheric fissure to the left side. An additional irregular defect (41.6 mm x 30 mm in transverse and anteroposterior dimensions respectively) was likely deliberately inflicted by the embalmers in the right posterior parietal bone to introduce the linen into the skull cavity.[56]

The orbits contain the atrophic globes with optic nerves and are filled with heterogeneous low-density material (–500 to –200

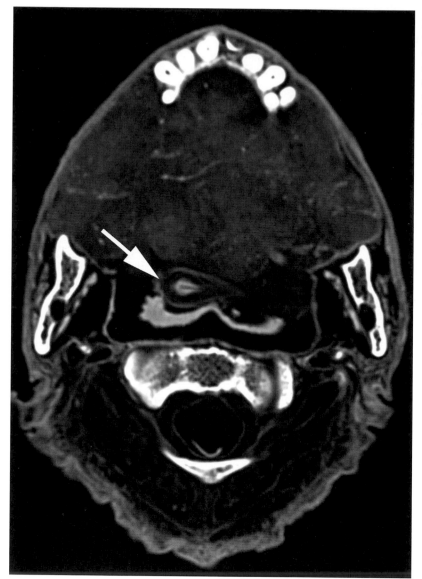

Fig. 77: Axial CT image at the level of the oropharynx of Merenptah reveals oblong-shaped, low-density structures showing central denser laminations, likely linen tampons impregnated with resin (arrow).

HU), likely representing linen. The outer contour of the nose is flattened, probably caused by pressure from the bandages. The nasal cavities contain packs of convoluted linen impregnated with resin.

Both ear auricles are preserved. The right shows a large piercing in its lobule. The lobule of the left ear auricle is missing. Heterogeneous low-density fillings (450 to –127 HU) are seen beneath the skin of the mid and lower face (right and left cheeks) and the front plane of the face around the nose and mouth.

Teeth (plates 56a–b)

The dental condition of the mummy of Merenptah is poor, with moderate to severe tooth wear and marked alveolar resorption. There are multiple missing teeth and multiple fractured teeth with only fragments present. No CT evidence supported the possibility that the missing teeth were deliberately removed by surgical extraction. Some teeth had fallen out and are seen within the pharynx. Most of the remaining teeth show cavities, irregular occlusal surfaces, attrition, and marked periodontal destruction.

Pharynx

The throat of the mummy (oropharynx and hypopharynx) is stuffed with amorphous embalming material of low to moderate density (–600 to 178 HU). There are multiple oblong-shaped, low-density structures showing central denser laminations, likely linen tampons impregnated with resin (fig. 77). Multiple fallen teeth are also identified within the throat.

Spine (figs. 78a–b)

There are ossifications of the right side of the ALL associated with osteophytes that extend continuously along several contiguous cervical (third to seventh) and thoracic (fifth to tenth) levels, giving the spine a bumpy appearance. The intervertebral discs in the involved regions do not show significant height reduction. In addition, there are ossifications of the posterior longitudinal and supraspinous ligaments in the cervical region. The zygapophyseal (facet) joints are not fused. No erosions or ankylosis could be related to the sacroiliac joints. CT findings excluded the diagnosis of ankylosing spondylitis and suggested DISH.

Torso

There are multiple large defects involving the front, back, and right side of the chest and abdomen; they are likely postmortem, inflicted by tomb robbers in antiquity. The viscera were removed, with only thin tissue remnants in the chest and no evidence of heart tissues. Only the left upper thoracic cavity is stuffed with embalming materials of variable CT densities measuring between –200 and 600 HU. The abdominal and pelvic cavities are loosely filled with embalming materials of threadlike morphology, likely linen, with a wide range of CT densities.[57] There are lacerations of the soft tissues at the left groin associated with bony fractures of the left pubic bone, left superior pubic ramus, and left anterior inferior iliac spine.

Genital organs (plates 57a–b)

The base of the penis is preserved and measures 41 mm in length and 22 mm in diameter. The free edge of the organ is beveled, denoting that its tip is missing. The anterior penile tissues have moderate high density (325 HU), and the posterior has lower density. The scrotum is missing. A transverse dimple (scar line) is seen in the perineal region between the penis base and anus.[58]

Upper limbs and pectoral girdle

The arms are flexed at the elbows, and the forearms are crossed over the chest, left over right. The fingers of the hands are flexed as if clenching something. A complete transverse fracture is observed at the right humeral neck; the bone fragments are in place.

There are comminuted fractures of the mid shaft of the right forearm bones (radius and ulna), likely postmortem. Mild to moderate degenerative changes of both shoulder

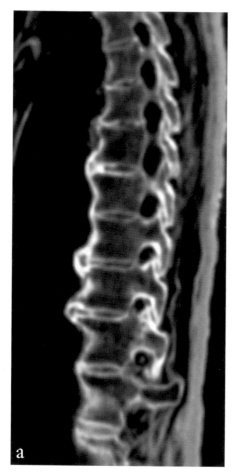

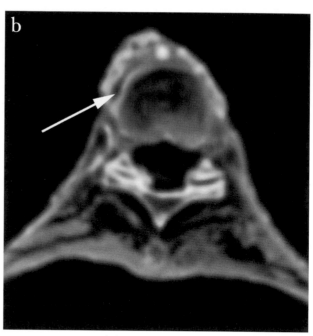

Figs. 78a–b: Two-dimensional CT images of the spine at the thoraco-lumbar region of Merenptah. Right parasagittal CT image (a) shows dense anterior longitudinal ligament (ALL) and exuberant bony outgrowths continuously flowing over a long spinal segment. Note the relatively preserved height of the involved discs. These findings are suggestive of DISH disease. Axial CT image (b) shows a low-density rim (arrow) between the dense bony mass and the right anterolateral border of the vertebral body; this indicates an ossified ALL.

joints are seen. There is calcification at the left elbow, probably involving the musculotendinous junction of the left brachioradialis muscle. The inner (medial) one-third of the right clavicle is missing, along with the adjacent sternum (the right sternoclavicular joint) and the overlying skin, likely caused by tomb robbers.

Lower limbs

There are multiple bony fractures seen in the lower limbs that were apparently inflicted postmortem by tomb robbers in antiquity.

The injuries involve the right iliac blade, the left acetabulum, the left superior pubic ramus, and the anterior part of the left pubic bone. There is also an incomplete fracture of the anterior cortex of the upper shaft of the right tibia. The bones of the left forefoot (distal to the metatarsophalangeal joints) are missing. There are multiple irregular fractures at the base of all of the proximal phalanges of the left foot, and mild degenerative changes involving the hip and knee joints of both lower limbs.

There are enthesopathies and calcifications at the insertion of the tendons at the hip region, knee, and calcaneus (heel bone); these changes are part of the extraspinal changes of DISH disease.

There is CT evidence of atherosclerosis of the right and left femoral arteries.

Comments on mummification

The embalming process of Merenptah was excellent, as expected for a ruler. The mummification style has some unique or unusual features that differ from that commonly seen in mummies of this period:

1. Unique intracranial embalming materials: Resin was not used intracranially in this mummy (resin has a characteristic homogeneous, moderately high CT density that assumes a fluid level when solidified). Instead of resin, the skull was stuffed with inhomogeneous material of mixed densities that contains tortuous linear low densities, likely linen or similar fabrics.

2. Additional intracranial routes: There are apparently two routes that were used in mummification in this case. The transnasal route was likely used for excerebration, supported by the fact that the nasal septum and the cribriform plate are defective. An additional small hole at the back of the skull (right posterior parietal) was likely carefully induced by the embalmers and used to stuff the skull with the heterogeneous embalming material that would have been very difficult or impossible to introduce using the transnasal route. In support of this assumption, the right half of the skull (where the defect lies) contains more embalming material than the left side, and the anterior interhemispheric fissure is deviated to the contralateral side (left).[59]

Unfortunately, the destruction imposed upon the torso by tomb robbers masked the mummification features in this part of the mummy, such as the location of embalming incisions or the type of embalming material employed.

Manner and cause of death

The mummy offers no definite explanation for manner or cause of death of Merenptah, but documents that the king had suffered from degenerative skeletal diseases, poor dental health, and arterial atherosclerosis. The multiple injuries detected in the mummy were likely inflicted postmortem, either deliberately by the embalmers (as the skull defect), accidentally during mummification (absent scrotum and tip of penis), or by tomb robbers in antiquity. There are no CT findings to support or deny that the king was drowned, or that he was the pharaoh of the Exodus (see sidelight).

Questions about Ramesses II and Merenptah

1. *Did Kings Ramesses II and Merenptah have ankylosing spondylitis disease?*

Several studies have suggested that among the pharaohs of the Eighteenth and Nineteenth Dynasties, at least three had ankylosing spondylitis: Amenhotep II, Ramesses II, and Merenptah. Ankylosing spondylitis (AS) is a progressive inflammatory disease of the joints of the spine that affects young men and is characterized by pain and progressive vertebral fusion resulting in stiffness (ankylosis) and diminished mobility of the spine. A prerequisite for radiographic diagnosis of AS is involvement of the sacroiliac joints; changes start with bilateral and symmetrical erosions and end with bony fusion. The diagnosis of AS in pharaonic mummies was based on plain x-ray findings of ossified ligaments along their lumbar spines and supposed fusion of their sacroiliac joints.[60]

Rethy Chhem and colleagues described DISH (diffuse idiopathic skeletal hyperostosis) in Ramesses II based on the re-examination of a limited collection of x-rays of the upper cervical vertebrae and pelvis; CT scannning was thus recommended to confirm the condition from which the king suffered.[61] Radiographic evaluation of the spine in the royal mummies was limited by the presence of dense embalming materials within the torso that obscured the thoracic and lumbar spine as well as the sacroiliac joints. Moreover, usually only the upper cervical spine could be examined in the lateral view of the head.[62]

Unlike with plain x-rays, the whole spine and related structures could be well evaluated in CT studies. Our CT findings excluded the diagnosis of AS in Ramesses II and Merenptah based on the absence of sacroiliac erosions, or bony fusion of sacroiliac or facet joints. We suggested the diagnosis of DISH based on the presence of continuous thick ossifications of the right side of the ALL of the cervical and thoracic spine that extended for four or more contiguous vertebrae. The preserved height of the discs in the regions involved in ossifications fulfilled the diagnostic criteria of DISH disease[63] and excluded the diagnosis of spondylosis deformans (fig. 78). Spondylosis deformans is a degenerative disease resulting in focal (noncontinuous) osteophytes and severely degenerated intervertebral discs.[64] The extraspinal bone formation and calcifications of the tendons at their bony attachments in the peripheral joints and pelvis (enthesopathies) also fulfilled DISH diagnosis using other criteria, including Utsinger's.[65]

Patients with DISH disease tend to be asymptomatic. However, clinical symptoms in DISH may result, usually at an advanced age, from decreased range of motion and stiffness of the fused spine.[66] This was most evident with the presence of hunchback in Ramesses II. DISH is also correlated with risk factors that included diabetes mellitus, obesity, and high serum level of uric acid.[67] The results of our CT study accord well with what history tells us about the lifestyles of Ramesses II and Merenptah. AS, which begins at a younger age (twenty to forty years) than DISH, is a painful ailment that can cause progressive stiffening of the spine, leading to immobility at a young age. However, history tells us about the active, long life of Ramesses II, who died at the age of approximately eighty-seven years, and the vitality of Merenptah, who traveled to the land of Canaan during the fifth year of his reign, probably at the age of sixty years.[68]

2. *Was the bony defect in Merenptah's skull the act of tomb robbers or the embalmers?*
The literature has dealt with the defect at the back of the skull (right parietal bone) of Merenptah by postulating two theories. The first suggested that the hole was made by thieves who carelessly chopped through the bandages in their search for valuables. Similar skull defects were also found in other mummies of KV35, where the mummy of Merenptah was buried, including those of Ramesses IV, Ramesses V, Ramesses VI, Seti II, Siptah, the Younger Lady, and the Unknown Boy. It was thus postulated that all of these skull defects were inflicted by the same robber (or group of robbers) who had employed the same kind of tool (most likely an axe) in the same fashion in order to first cut through the bandages of the head in an attempt to strip the mummies of their outermost wrappings.[69] In addition to the aforementioned mummies, x-ray studies done by Harris added Ramesses IX and Queen Sitkamose to the list of mummies with this skull defect.[70]

The other theory maintained that the cranial opening may have been deliberately made by the embalmers for occult reasons in order to allow evil spirits to escape from the skull.[71]

We suggest that each cranial defect should be examined and considered on an individual basis. In the case of Merenptah, the CT study showed that the skull defect is relatively small (about 4 cm in diameter) at the back of the skull to the right (plate 55). Its nonsclerotic, beveled margins (longer in the outer than the inner skull plate) indicate that the defect was inflicted by a sharp, pointed, solid tool after death. We assume that the embalmers deliberately induced this defect and utilized it in the unique brain treatment of Merenptah's mummy, in addition to the usual anterior cranial fossa defect. The brain was removed using the usual transnasal route. However, instead of the resin fluid that was commonly used in the other royal mummies dated to the same period, the embalmers introduced linen threads inside the skull of Merenptah's mummy. Unlike resin fluid, it would have been extremely difficult or impossible to fill the interior of the skull with linen via the transnasal route. The embalmers seem to have deliberately inflicted the defect at the back of the skull for the purpose of stuffing the linen fibers into the skull through it. The fact that the stuffed material is bulkier at the front and on the right side of the skull (where the defect lies), and that the remnant of the anterior interhemispheric fissure is deviated to the left, all support the suggestion that filling took place from the right side of the back of the skull.[72]

3. *The missing scrotum of the mummy of Merenptah: Was the king castrated?*

G.E. Smith reported what he called a very curious feature of the mummy of Merenptah: the complete absence of the scrotum, although the penis was present. Smith noted a transverse cut between the base of penis and anus and that this area had been coated with balsam. Smith concluded that this injury had been inflicted prior to the completion of the embalming process, although he was not sure if Merenptah was castrated either after death or within a short time of death. The missing tip of the penis, Smith explained, was likely done by tomb robbers long after the body was mummified.[73]

In CT images, the penis measured 36.5 mm in length and 20 mm in diameter, and its free edge looked beveled, denoting a missing tip. The reconstructed images documented the missing scrotum and identified a transverse dimple at the perineal region midway between the root of penis and anus; this is the place from which the scrotal sac was cut, then smeared with resin (plate 57). In addition, CT images showed the full-thickness, soft-tissue lacerations that involved the left side of the lower pelvic region in association with comminuted bony fractures of the left hip bone (body of the left pubic bone, the left superior pubic ramus, and left anterior inferior iliac spine).

The CT findings do not contradict the theory that a postmortem accident could have happened to the scrotum before the completion of mummification by the embalmers, who used resin to disguise the tissue loss.[74] CT study also provided evidence of a brutal trauma to the soft tissues (including the tip of the penis) and bones of the pelvic region that must have happened after mummification, likely by the hands of tomb robbers.

Some researchers suggested other explanations of the missing scrotum in Merenptah's mummy, including the removal of the hugely enlarged diseased scrotum of the king by the embalmers *before* mummification. However, in mummies within a reasonable time frame of King Merenptah, the embalmers did not have the convention of treating genital organs during the mummification process. For example, in King Ramesses V, the embalmers did not remove the hugely enlarged scrotum, possibly caused by a hernia, but instead folded the baggy skin on his perineum.[75]

Another alternative was that Merenptah's scrotum had been removed during his life by surgery as a treatment for hernia. This theory was based on the presence of a large wound in the groin, with the scrotum separated from the body that was not part of the procedure of mummification, but of surgery.[76] Although the ancient Egyptian physicians were familiar with the diagnosis of hernia (the Ebers Papyrus, circa 1552 BC, contains some observations on the subject), there is no textual evidence that surgery for hernia was done in the time of Merenptah. In the medical literature, Praxagoras in Alexandria (fourth century BC) suggested a surgical operation for the treatment of a strangulated hernia, as reported by Caelius Aurelianus (25 BC to AD 50).[77] However, this was centuries after King Merenptah. Even assuming that the Alexandrian physician had learned the surgical technique from older Egyptian medical writings, the wounds in King Merenptah did not likely match the ancient surgical technique as first described by Aurelianus.

S.N.S.

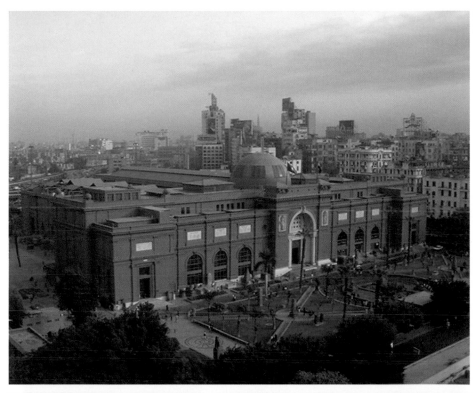

Plate 1: The Egyptian Museum in Cairo.

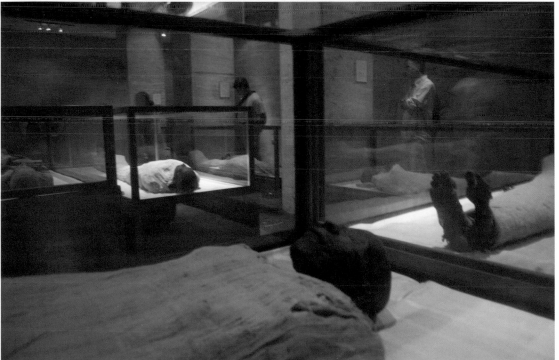

Plate 2: The so-called royal mummies room in the Egyptian Museum, Cairo.

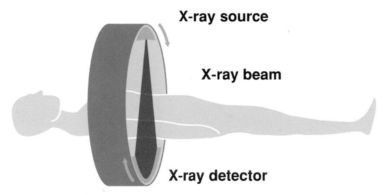

X-ray source

X-ray beam

X-ray detector

Plate 3: An illustration of the principle of computerized tomography (CT) imaging. A motorized table moves the mummy through a circular opening in the CT machine body (gantry). As the mummy passes through the CT machine, an x-ray source rotates around the circular opening and produces a narrow beam to irradiate a thin section of the mummy's body, to be received by opposing detectors. The detectors send the data to a computer to create a cross-sectional image of the body.

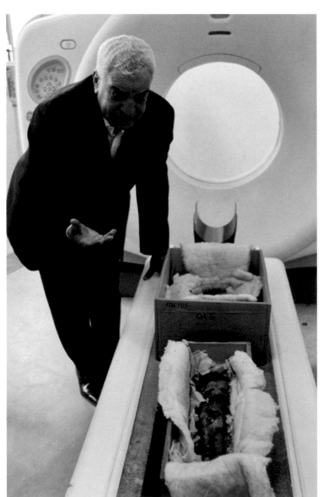

Plate 4: CT scanning of a mummy. Two mummified fetuses (daughters of King Tutankhamun) are placed on the CT table in the stage of preparing to move through the gantry. Zahi Hawass is seen beside the table supervising the examination.

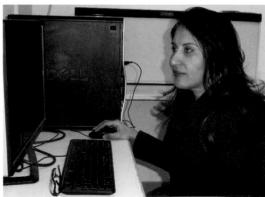

Plate 5: The reconstruction stage of the CT images takes place in a separate workstation. Sahar Saleem is handling the CT images on the workstation.

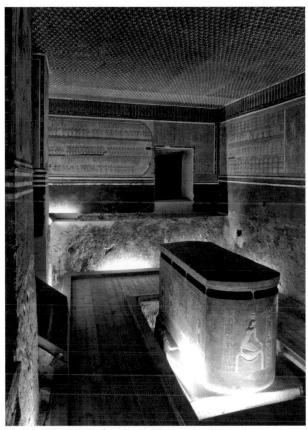

Plate 6: The burial chamber of the tomb of Amenhotep II.

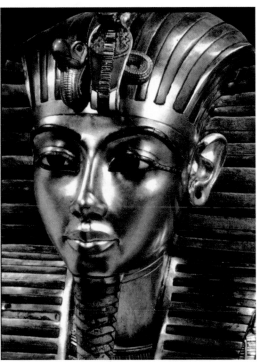

Plate 7: The funerary mask of Tutankhamun. Egyptian Museum, Cairo.

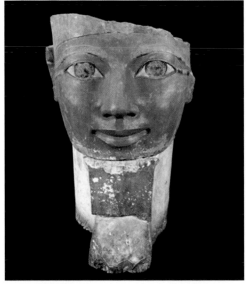

Plate 8: Colossal limestone head of Queen Hatshepsut from her temple at Deir al-Bahari. Egyptian Museum, Cairo.

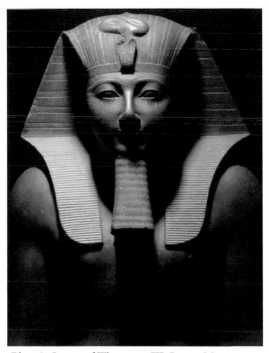

Plate 9: Statue of Thutmose III. Luxor Museum.

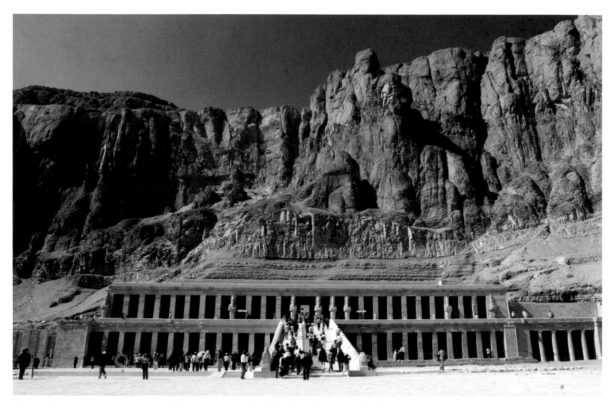

Plate 10: The mortuary temple of Hatshepsut at Deir al-Bahari, west bank of Luxor.

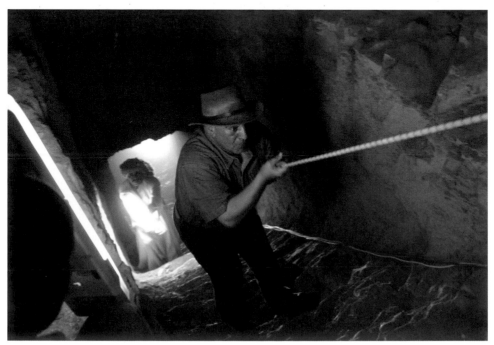

Plate 11: Inside the tomb of Hatshepsut, KV60, Valley of the Kings.

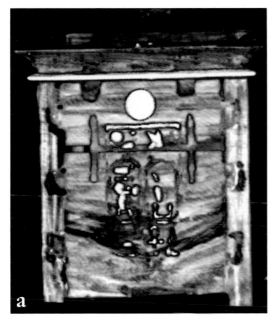
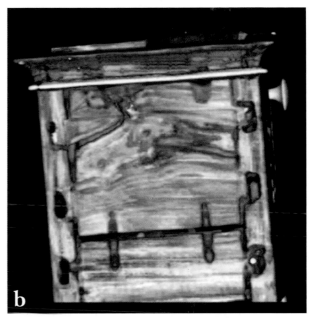

Plates 12a–b: Three-dimensional CT images of the box in front (a) and lateral (b) projections show the details of the box shape and surface.

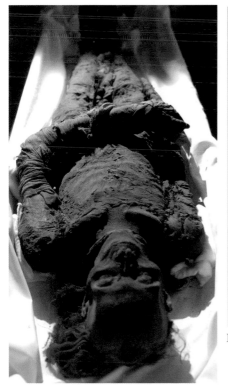

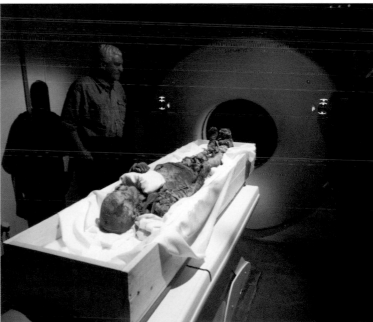

Plate 14: The CT scanning of mummy KV60 A.

Plate 13: The mummy of Sitre-In (KV60 B), the wet nurse of Queen Hatshepsut.

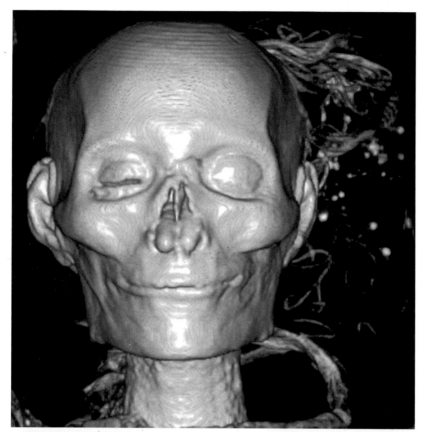

Plate 15: Three-dimensional CT image of the face of mummy of KV60 B, Sitre-In.

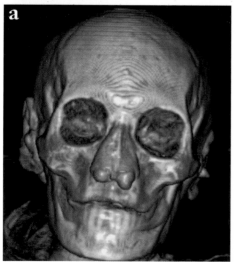

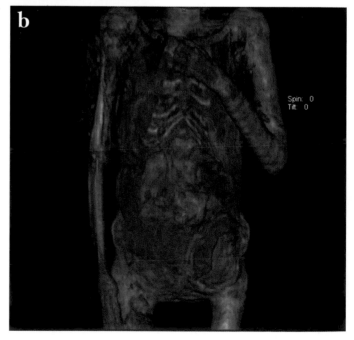

Plates 16a–b: Three-dimensional CT image of the face of mummy of KV60 A (Hatshepsut) (a). Three-dimensional image of the torso of the mummy of Hatshepsut (b).

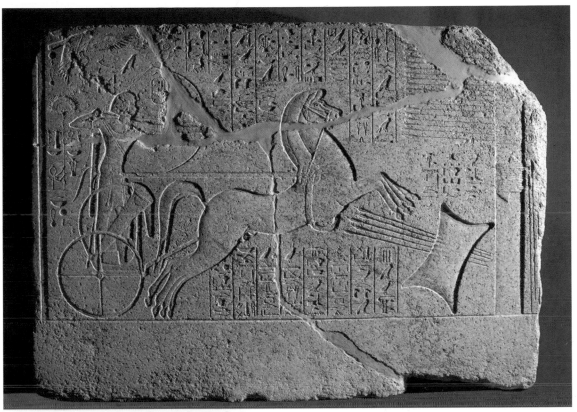

Plate 17: Amenhotep II shooting arrows at a target as part of his military training. Luxor Museum.

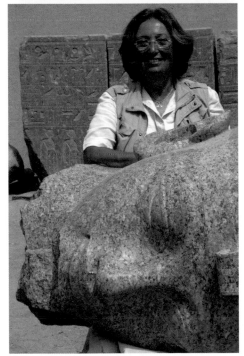

Plate 18: Hourig Sourouzian with finds from the excavations of the German Archaeological Institute.

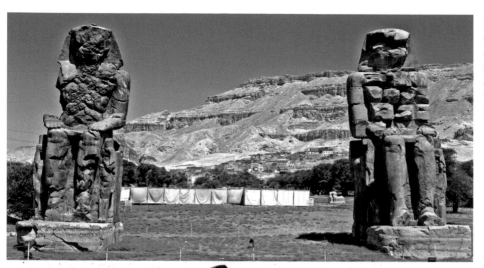

Plate 19: The two colossal statues of Amenhotep III known as the colossi of Memnon. Mortuary temple of Amenhotep III, west bank of Luxor.

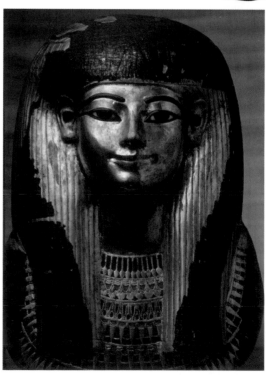

Plate 20: Innermost gilded anthropoid coffin of Yuya. Egyptian Museum, Cairo.

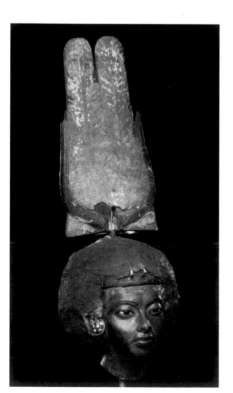

Plate 21: Nefertiti's mother-in-law, Queen Tiye. Neues Museum, Berlin.

Plate 22: Gilded funerary mask of Thuya. Egyptian Museum, Cairo.

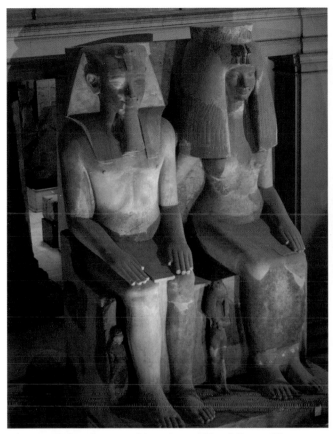

Plate 23: Colossal statue of Amenhotep III and Queen Tiye. Egyptian Museum, Cairo.

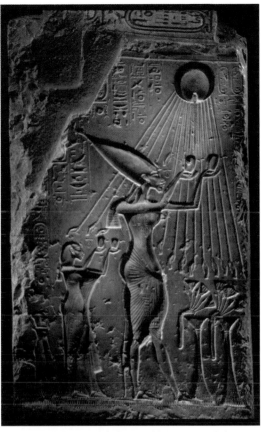

Plate 24: Nefertiti with King Akhenaten and their daughters making an offering to the Aten, on a red quartzite altar from Amarna. Egyptian Museum, Cairo.

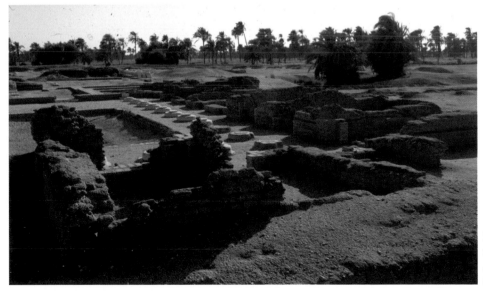

Plate 25: The remains of the northern palace at Amarna, residence of the royal family of Akhenaten.

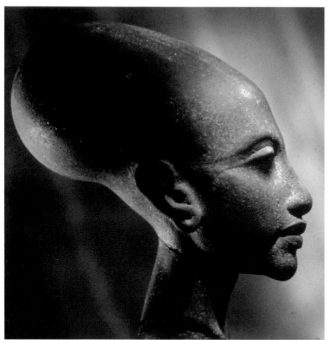

Plate 26: The quartzite head of a princess, from Amarna. Egyptian Museum, Cairo.

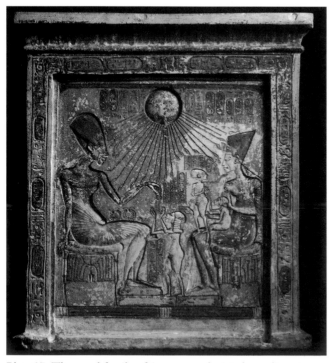

Plate 27: The royal family of Amarna, as depicted on a limestone stela from Amarna. Egyptian Museum, Cairo.

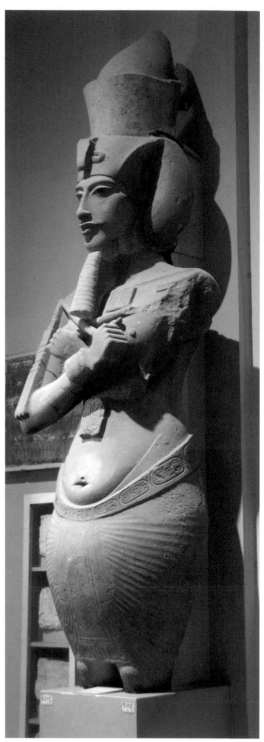

Plate 28: Sandstone colossus of Akhenaten, from the temple of Aten at Karnak. Egyptian Museum, Cairo.

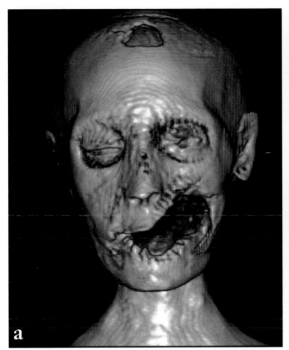 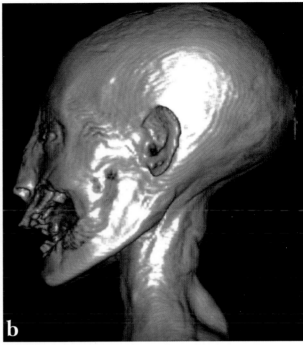

Plates 29a–b: Three-dimensional reconstructed CT images of the head of the mummy of the Younger Lady of KV35, in frontal (a) and profile (b) projections, show a large defect in the left side of the lower face involving the left cheek and mouth. A small bony defect is also seen at the top of the skull.

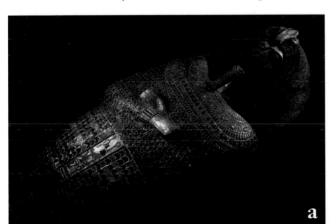

Plates 30a–b: The lid of the anthropoid coffin found in KV55, now confirmed to be that of Akhenaten. Egyptian Museum, Cairo.

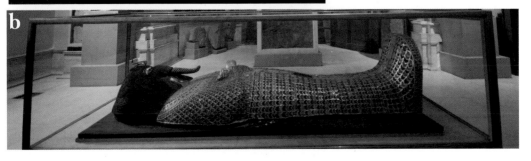

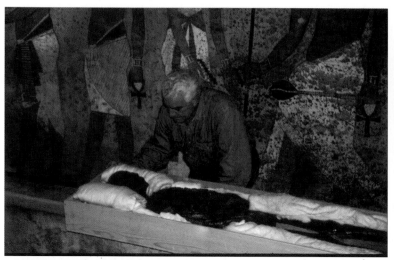

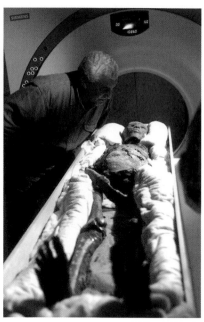

Plate 31: Reopening the king's sarcophagus in order to carry out the new research on the king's mummy, seen here in its tray.

Plate 32: CT scanning the mummy of Tutankhamun in the Valley of the Kings.

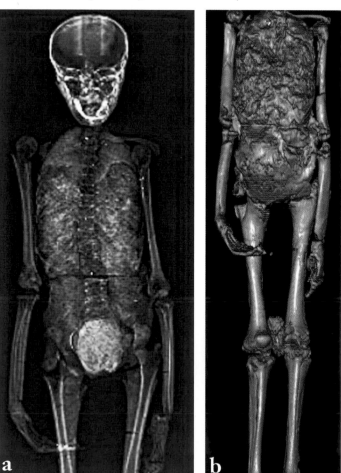

Plates 33a–b: CT scout views in AP projection (a) and three-dimensional reconstructed frontal CT image of the body (b) of Tutankhamun permit all-over evaluation of the multiple postmortem fractures and mutilation of the body.

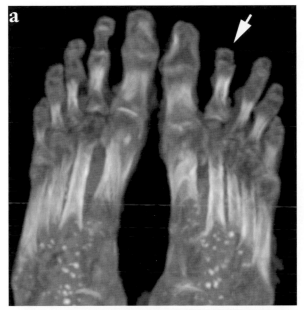

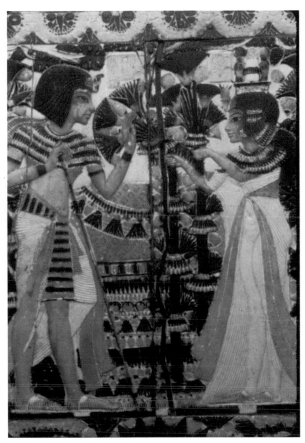

Plate 35: Tutankhamun leaning on a walking stick while in a garden with his queen, Ankhesenamun. Egyptian Museum, Cairo.

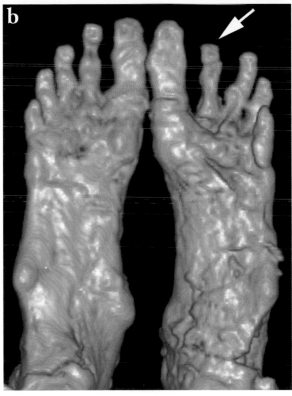

Plates 34a–b: Two-dimensional (a) and three-dimensional (b) CT images of the feet of Tutankhamun, seen from below, show a left-foot deformity in the form of wide separation of the toes in addition to shortness of the second toe (arrows).

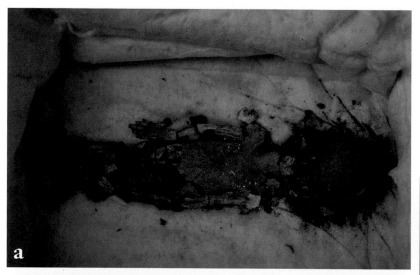

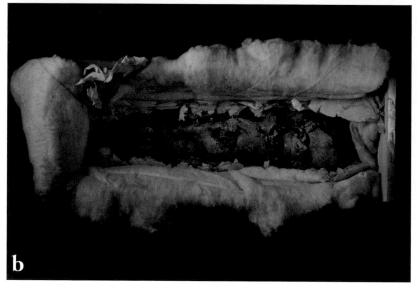

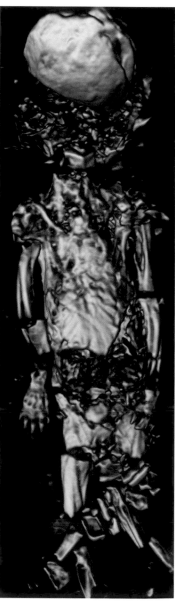

Plates 36a–b: The mummified fetuses (a) 317a and (b) 317b. Kasr Al-Ainy Hospital, Cairo.

Plate 37: Three-dimensional reconstructed frontal CT image of the mummy of the smaller fetus (317a) in frontal projection shows the very poor preservation due to multiple postmortem bony and soft-tissue injuries.

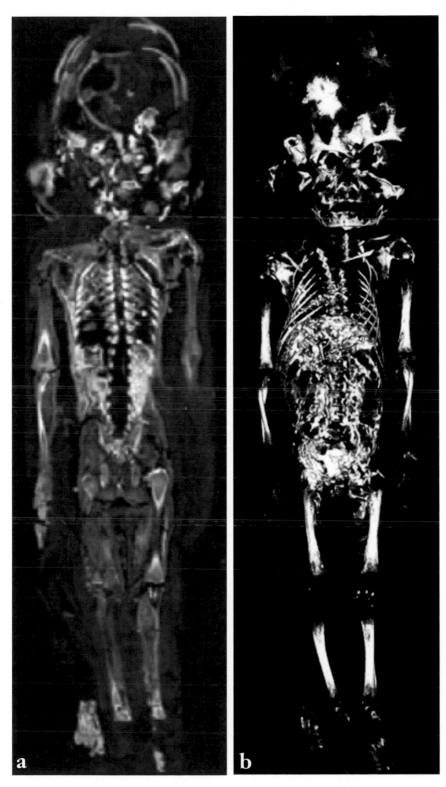

Plates 38a–b: Two-dimensional reconstructed CT image (a) of the body of mummified fetus 317b in coronal plane. The full-body image allows an overview of the preservation status of the mummy and shows multiple postmortem bony injuries.

Three-dimensional reconstructed frontal CT image (b) of fetus 317b in coronal plane documents the extensive bony and soft-tissue injuries of the mummy.

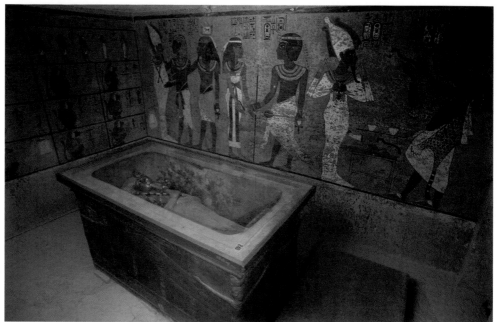

Plate 39: The burial chamber of Tutankhamun, Valley of the Kings.

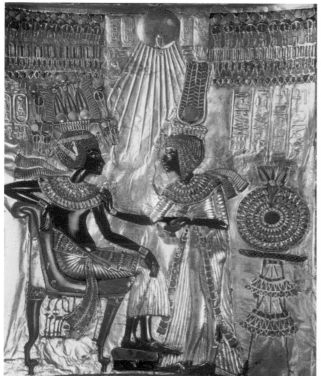

Plate 40: Tutankhamun and his queen Ankhesenamun are strongly believed to be the father and the mother of the two mummified fetuses. Detail from the throne of Tutankhamun found in his tomb. Egyptian Museum, Cairo.

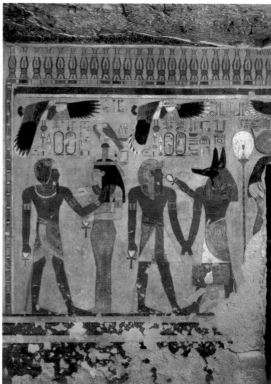

Plate 41: Amenhotep III being received by the gods and goddesses of the netherworld, from his tomb (WV22) in the Western Valley, known as Valley of the Monkeys.

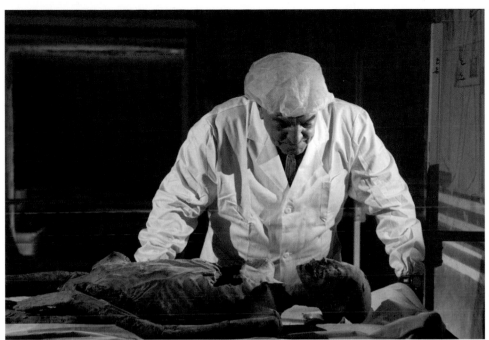

Plate 42: Preparing the mummy of the Younger Lady for extracting DNA samples.

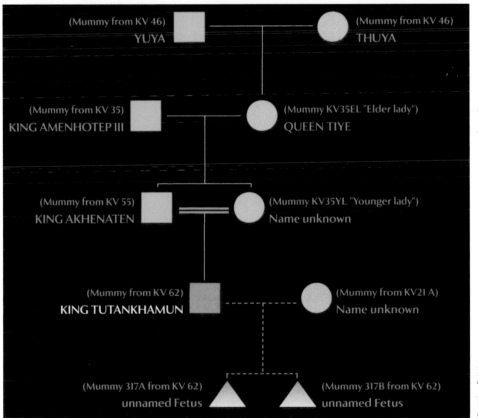

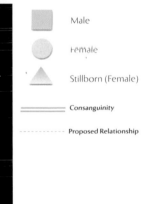

(Mummy from KV 46) YUYA

(Mummy from KV 46) THUYA

(Mummy from KV 35) KING AMENHOTEP III

(Mummy KV35EL "Elder lady") QUEEN TIYE

(Mummy from KV 55) KING AKHENATEN

(Mummy KV35YL "Younger lady") Name unknown

(Mummy from KV 62) KING TUTANKHAMUN

(Mummy from KV21 A) Name unknown

(Mummy 317A from KV 62) unnamed Fetus

(Mummy 317B from KV 62) unnamed Fetus

Male

Female

Stillborn (Female)

Consanguinity

Proposed Relationship

Plate 43: King Tutankhamun's pedigree, based on the DNA and CT scan analysis.

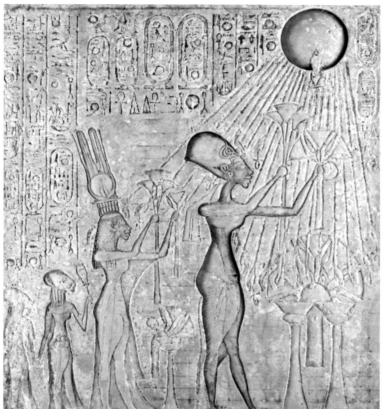

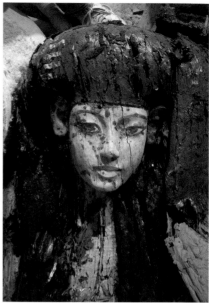

Plate 45: The lid of an anthropoid coffin of a woman found inside KV63.

Plate 44: Akhenaten with his wife Nefertiti and two of their daughters making offerings to the god Aten. Limestone stela from Amarna. Egyptian Museum, Cairo.

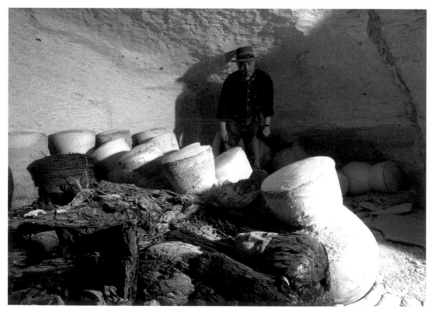

Plate 46: Inside the sole chamber of KV63, Valley of the Kings.

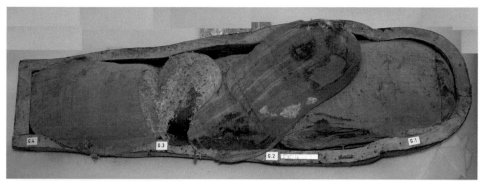

Plate 47: Linen pillows filled with straw from a coffin in KV63.

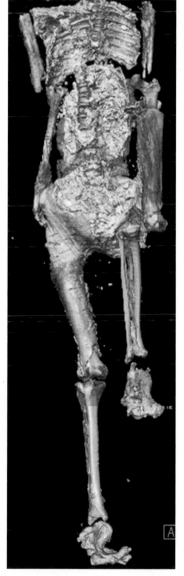

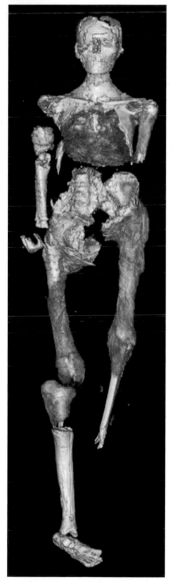

Plate 48: Three-dimensional CT of mummy KV21 A. The image permits overall evaluation of a headless mummy that is composed of an assembly of misplaced bones and body fragments.

Plate 49: Three-dimensional CT of the KV21 B mummy enables rapid evaluation of its poor preservation and destruction.

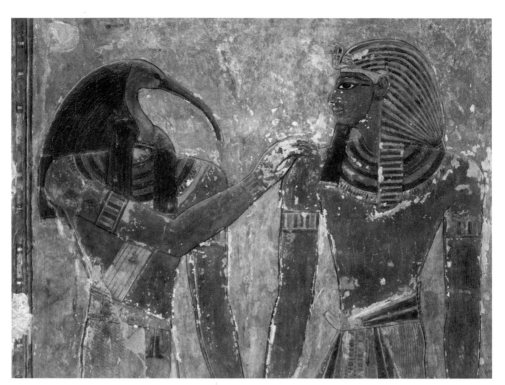

Plate 50: Seti I and the god Thoth. Tomb of Seti I (KV17), Valley of the Kings.

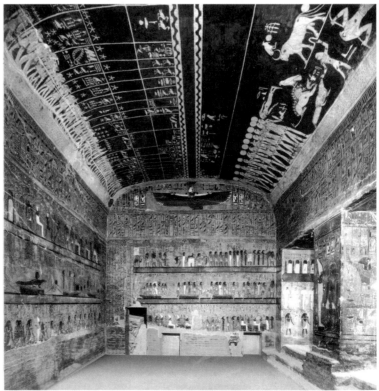

Plate 51: The burial chamber inside the tomb of Seti I, Valley of the Kings.

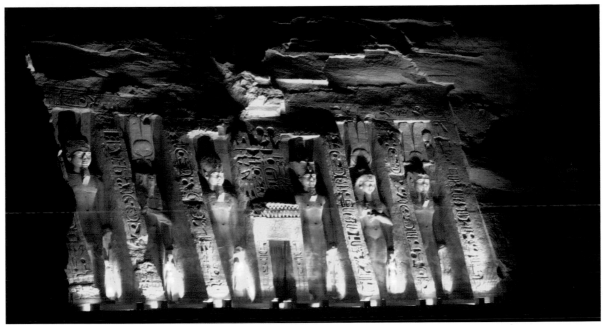

Plate 52: The rock-cut temple of Queen Nefertari at Abu Simbel.

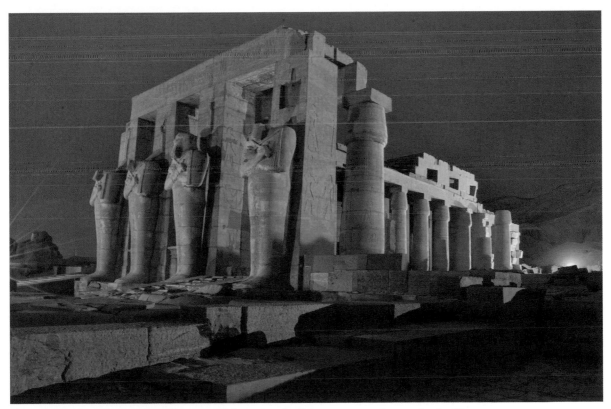

Plate 53: The funerary temple of Ramesses II, known as the Ramesseum, on the west bank of Luxor.

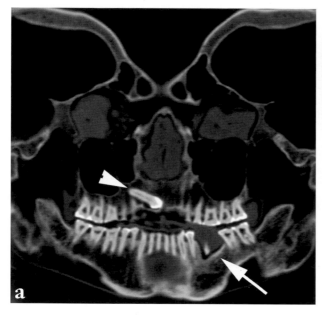

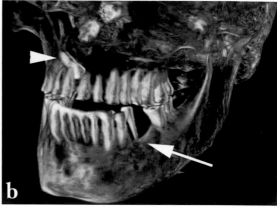

Plates 54a–b: CT of the mummy of Seti I: panorama for teeth (curved MPR) (a) and 3D left frontal oblique (b) images show the good condition of the teeth, with fair periodontal health. A supernumerary tooth lies obliquely in the maxilla (arrowhead). A well-defined bony depression with sclerotic margin at the alveolar margin of the mandible is likely due to a chronic process (periodontosis) (arrow).

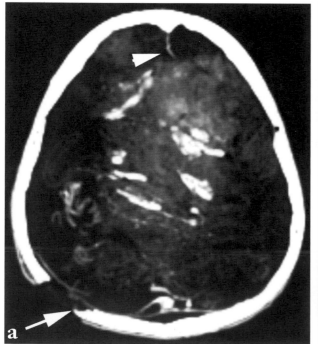

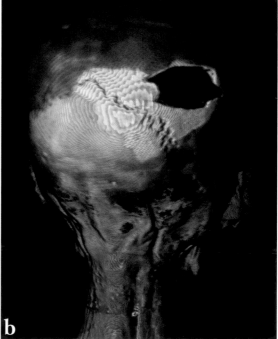

Plates 55a–b: Two-dimensional and 3D CT images of the head of Merenptah's mummy.

Axial CT image (a) shows convoluted linen threads impregnated with resin filling the skull cavity. In addition to an anterior cranial fossa defect (not shown), there is a defect in the right posterior parietal bone (arrow), with beveled edges longer on the outer than the inner skull tables that was likely deliberately inflicted by the embalmers to introduce the linen fibers. As a result, the bulk of the filling is more in the right side, causing displacement of the interhemispheric fissure to the left (arrowhead). Three-dimensional (SSD) CT image (b) of the right lateral oblique view of the head demonstrates the bony defect at the back of the skull.

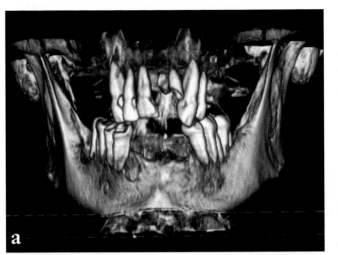
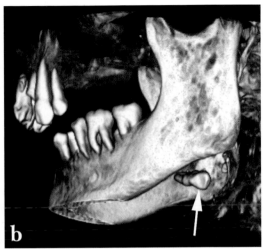

Plates 56a–b: Three-dimensional (SSD) CT images of the maxillary and mandibular teeth of the mummy of Merenptah in frontal (a) and right lateral (b) views show the poor condition of the teeth. Many teeth are missing; others are fractured or have irregular occlusal surfaces. A tooth had fallen and is seen within the pharynx (arrow in b).

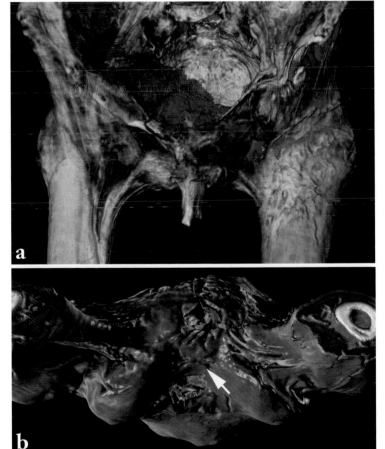

Plates 57a–b: Three-dimensional reconstructed (SSD) CT images of the pelvic region of the mummy of Merenptah in frontal projection (a) and basal view of the perineal region (b) show that only the base of the penis is present, while its tip and the scrotum are missing. A depressed transverse line is seen at the perineum (arrow).

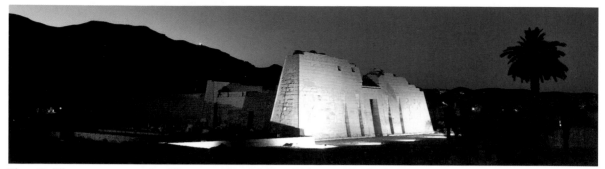

Plate 58: The mortuary temple of Ramesses III at Madinet Habu, west bank of Luxor.

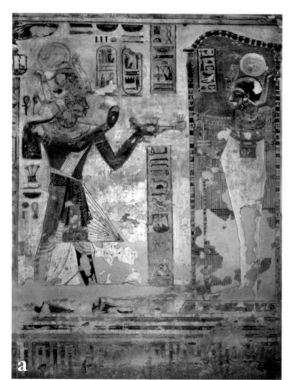

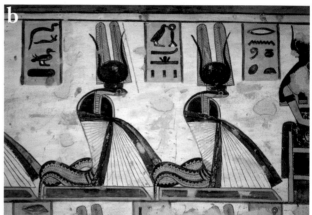

Plates 59a–b: Ramesses III offers incense to the god Ptah (a), and female deities depicted as crowned cobras (b). Tomb of Ramesses III (KV11), Valley of the Kings.

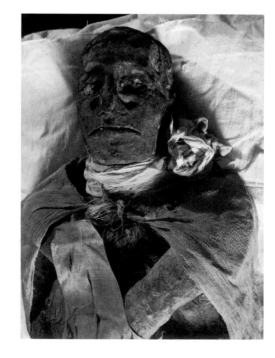

Plate 60: The mummy of Ramesses III. Egyptian Museum, Cairo.

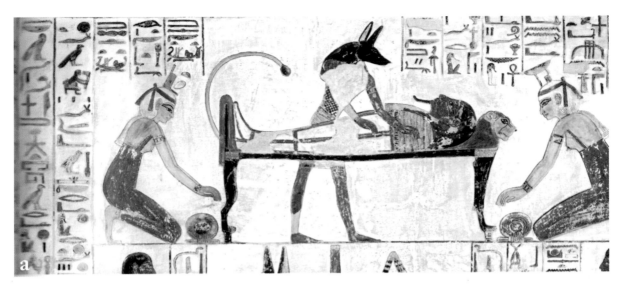

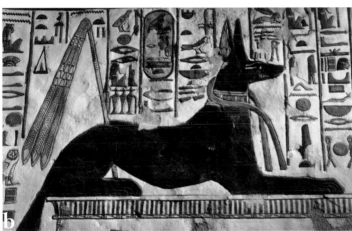

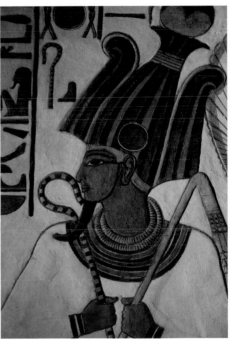

Plates 61a–b: Anubis embalming King Siptah (a), with the protective goddesses Isis, the wife of Osiris (left), and her sister Nephthys (right). Tomb of Siptah (KV47), Valley of the Kings. The jackal god Anubis (b), guardian of the necropolis and lord of embalming. Anubis was said to have performed the wrapping of the mummy of Osiris. From the tomb of Queen Nefertari, Valley of the Queens.

Plate 62: The god Osiris, ruler of the afterlife. According to Egyptian mythology, Osiris was murdered and dismembered by his brother Seth, and was magically reassembled, becoming the first mummy. From the tomb of Queen Nefertari (QV66), Valley of the Queens.

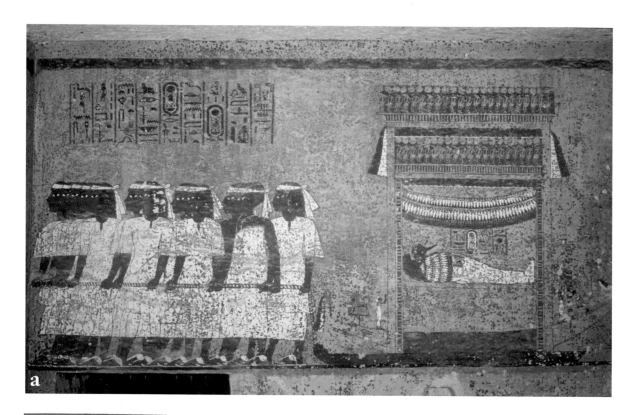

a

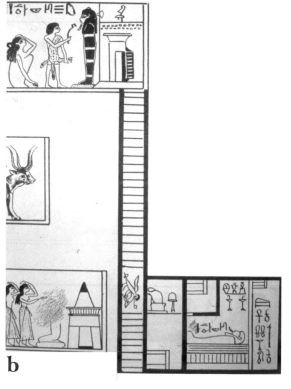

b

Plates 63a–b: The funeral of Tutankhamun (a) as depicted in his tomb; the king's mummified body is taken to his last resting place. From Tutankhamun's tomb (KV62), Valley of the Kings. The Opening of the Mouth ceremony (b) is performed on the mummy, in which an adze touched to the mouth would restore the faculties of the deceased. Here the coffin is shown in front of the tomb entrance; a long shaft links it to the burial chamber.

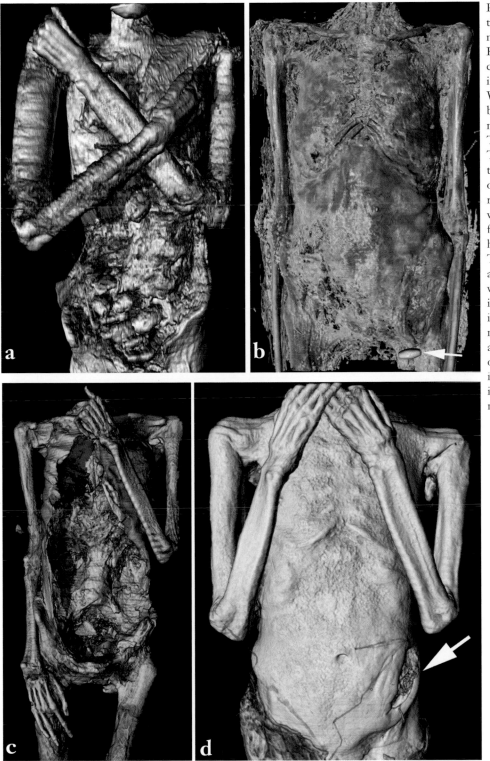

Plates 64a–d: The position of arms of the mummies varied in the study. Kings had forearms crossed over the chest, as in Thutmose II (a). Women's arms were beside the thighs, as in the mummy of Thuya (b). The mummy of Queen Tiye had a unique position of left arm crossed over the chest while the right arm is extended (c), while her mummified father, Yuya, had his hands under the chin (d). The arrow in (b) points to a bead placed just below a vertically oriented visceral incision at the left inguinal region in the mummy of Thuya. The arrow in (d) points to the obliquely oriented visceral incision at the left inguinal region in the mummy of Yuya.

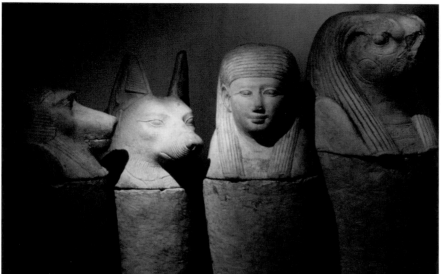

Plate 65: Four canopic jars with the heads of the Four Sons of Horus. Egyptian Museum, Cairo.

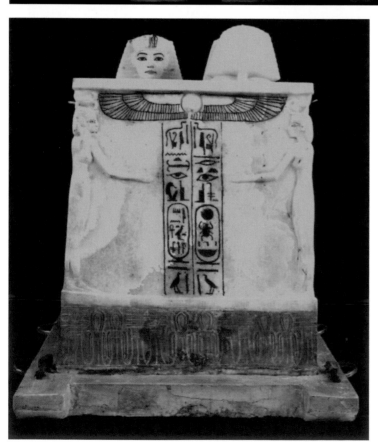

Plate 66: The calcite (Egyptian alabaster) chest for Tutankhamun's canopic containers, which consisted of miniature gold coffins inlaid with glass and semi-precious stones. Egyptian Museum, Cairo.

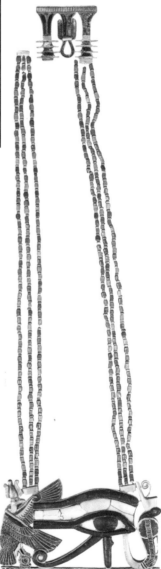

Plate 67: Necklace with *wedjat*-eye pendant, from the treasure of Tutankhamun. Egyptian Museum, Cairo.

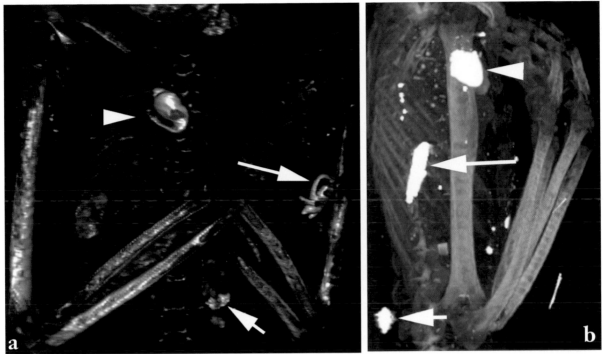

Plates 68a–b: Reconstructed CT images of the torso of Seti I in frontal (a) and lateral (b) projections help to determine the exact position of three foreign objects in the mummy. The first, a heart amulet (arrowhead), is within the chest cavity; the second, a *wedjat* amulet (long arrow), is in the wrappings behind the left arm; and the third, likely a *wedjat* amulet (short arrow), is in the wrappings at the lower back of the mummy.

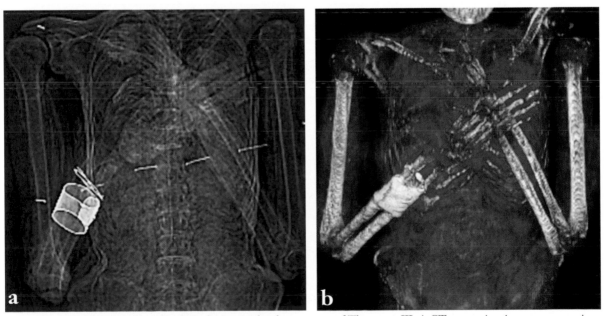

Plates 69a–b: CT images of jewelry (bracelets) worn by the mummy of Thutmose III. A CT scout view in anteroposterior projection (a) and a 3D CT reconstruction in frontal view (b) of the crossed forearms of Thutmose III show both broad and narrow metallic bracelets worn at the distal right forearm.

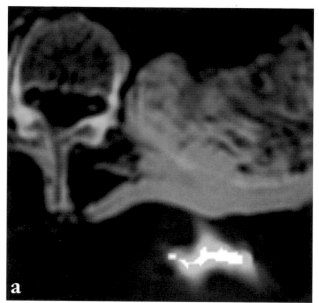

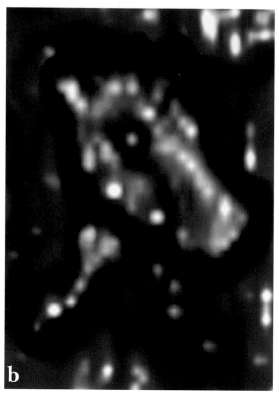

Plates 70a–b: CT images of the Eye of Horus amulet placed within the wrappings in the left side of the back of Seti I. The axial CT image (a) of the left side of the lower torso shows a flat, irregular, dense metallic object. This image was processed using MDT for removal of metallic streak artifacts. The 3D reconstructed CT image of the object (b) shows the characteristic shape of an Eye of Horus amulet. The lower curved line and teardrop are evident. (The colors of the amulet and the background are generated by the computer software and do not represent the reality.)

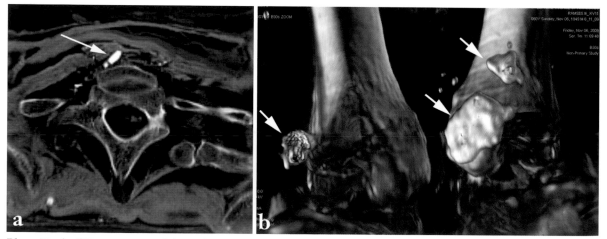

Plates 71a–b: CT appearances of the *wedjat* amulets in Ramesses III placed at injured body parts, presumably for the purpose of healing. Axial 2D image of the neck of the mummy at the level of C7 (a) shows a dense metallic object placed at the cut throat. The dash-and-dot appearance of the object represents the eye and tear components of the Eye of Horus. Three-dimensional reconstructed image of the ankles (b) shows three solid plates with processes (arrows) that resemble Eye of Horus amulets. The amulets are placed at the anterolateral aspect of the right ankle, left medial malleolus, and anteromedial aspect of the left ankle. The amulets are condensed in the region of the partially amputated left big toe.

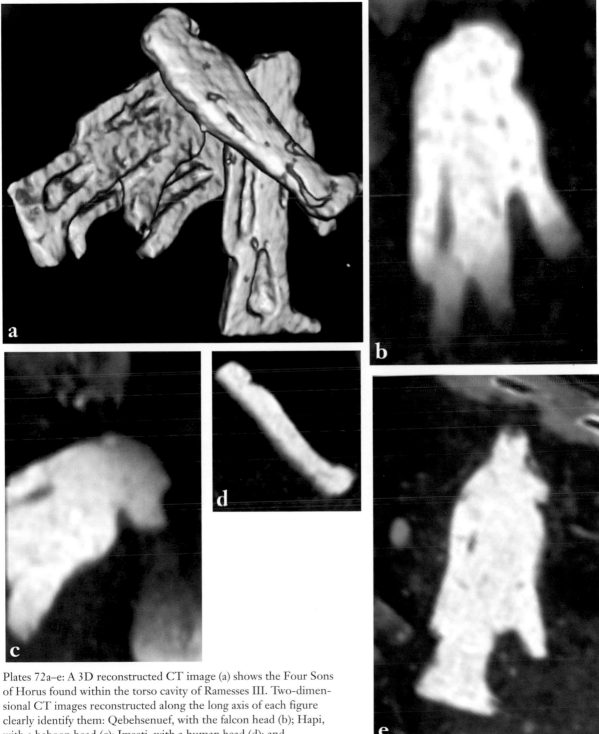

Plates 72a–e: A 3D reconstructed CT image (a) shows the Four Sons of Horus found within the torso cavity of Ramesses III. Two-dimensional CT images reconstructed along the long axis of each figure clearly identify them: Qebehsenuef, with the falcon head (b); Hapi, with a baboon head (c); Imseti, with a human head (d); and Duamutef, with a jackal head (e).

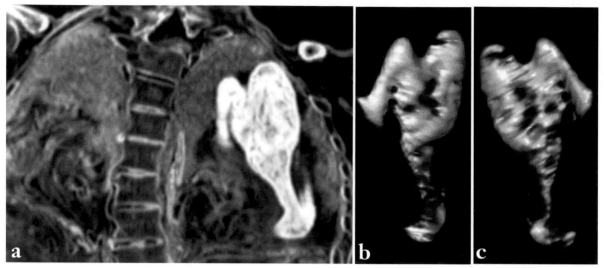

Plates 73a–c: CT images of an oblong amulet within the left side of the upper chest cavity of Ramesses II. Two-dimensional reconstructed CT image in coronal plane (a) shows the location of this dense oblong object with processes. Three-dimensional reconstructed CT images show the details of the front (b) and back (c) of the amulet.

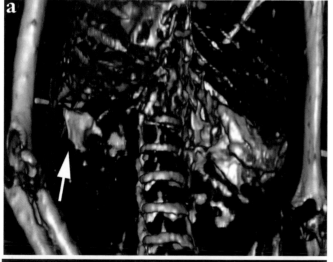

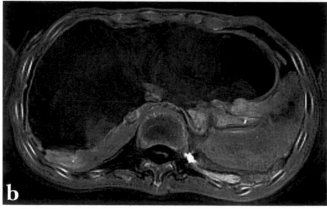

Plates 74a–b: CT images of a foreign object in the lower right side of the mummy of 'Thutmose I.' A 3D reconstructed CT image in frontal projection (a) for the same object seen in fig. 108 shows that the object has the shape of an arrowhead with its tip directed upwards and laterally (arrow). This could be part of a weapon that injured 'Thutmose I' and probably caused his death. An axial CT image at a lower level (b) shows a small metallic fragment below the head of the left eleventh rib. This could be another injury or an entry point of the arrowhead in the right side of the chest cavity.

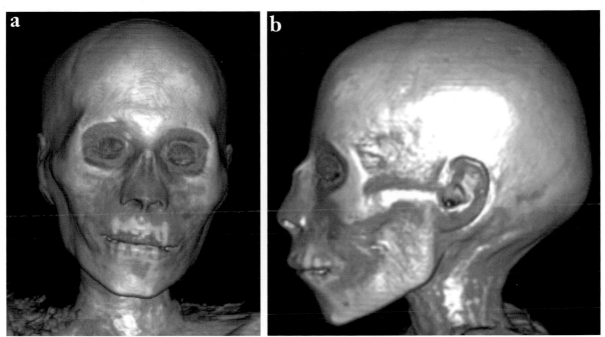

Plates 75a–b: Three-dimensional CT image of the head of so-called Thutmose I in frontal projection (a) and left profile (b).

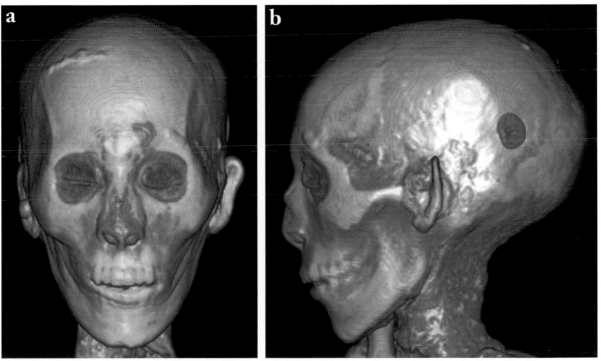

Plates 76a–b: Three-dimensional CT image of head of Thutmose II in frontal projection (a) and left profile (b).

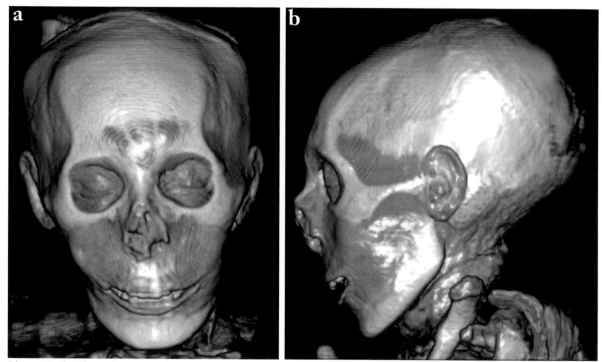

Plates 77a–b: Three-dimensional CT image of head of Thutmose III in frontal projection (a) and left profile (b).

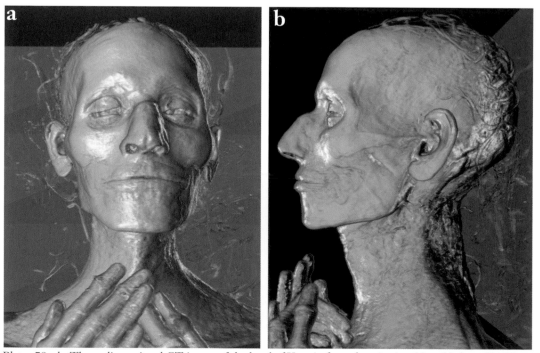

Plates 78a–b: Three-dimensional CT image of the head of Yuya in frontal projection (a) and left profile (b).

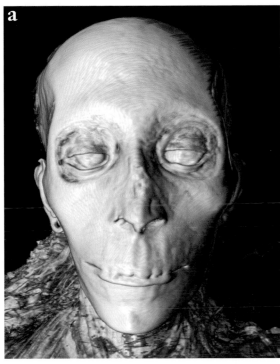

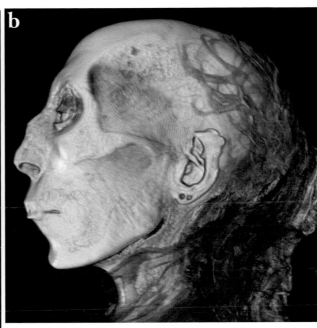

Plates 79a–b: Three-dimensional CT image of the head of Thuya in frontal projection (a) and left profile (b).

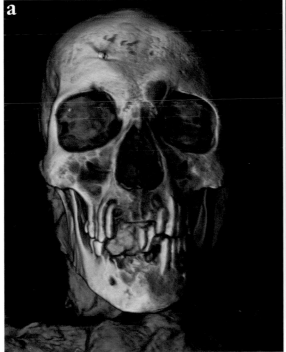

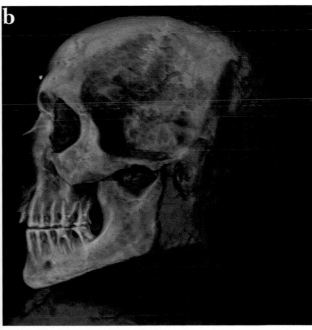

Plates 80a–b: Three-dimensional CT image of the head of Amenhotep III in frontal projection (a) and left profile (b).

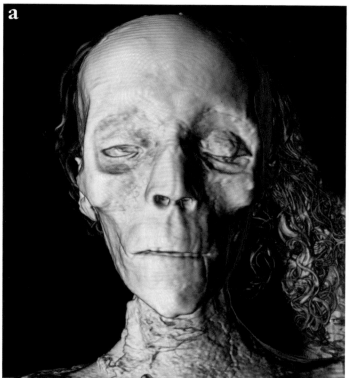

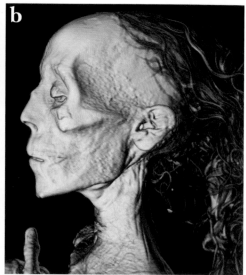

Plates 81a–b: Three-dimensional CT image of the head of Tiye in frontal projection (a) and left profile (b).

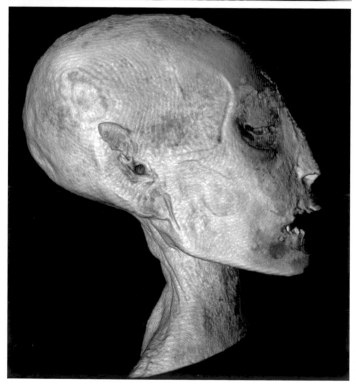

Plate 82: Three-dimensional CT image of the head of the mother of Tutankhamun (Younger Lady of KV35) in right profile.

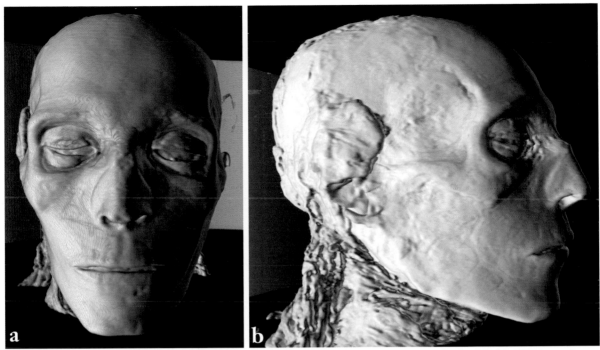

Plates 83a–b: Three-dimensional CT image of the head of Seti I in frontal projection (a) and right profile (b).

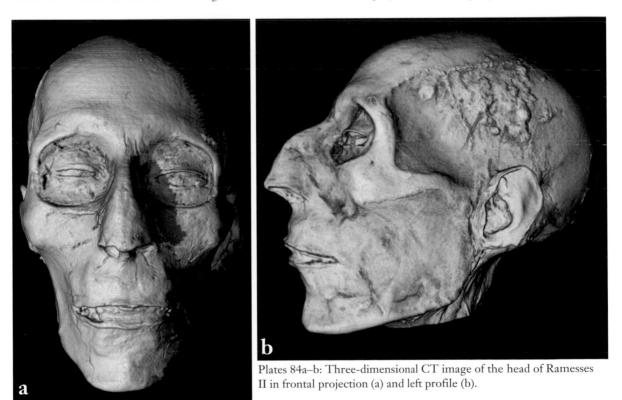

Plates 84a–b: Three-dimensional CT image of the head of Ramesses II in frontal projection (a) and left profile (b).

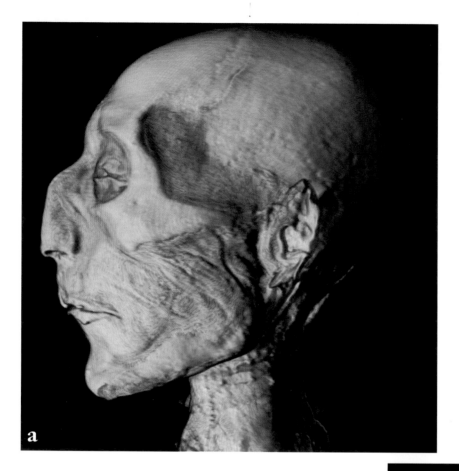

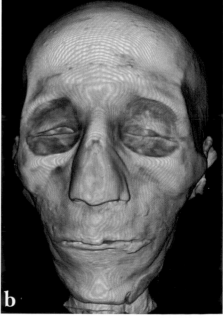

Plates 85a–b: Three-dimensional CT image of the head of Merenptah in left profile (a) and frontal projection (b).

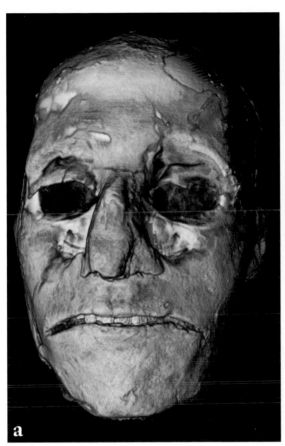

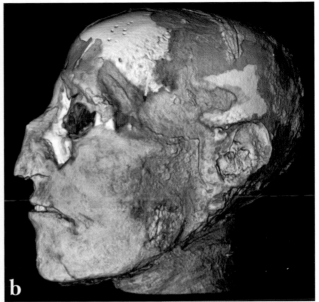

Plates 86a–b: Three-dimensional CT image of the head of Ramesses III in frontal projection (a) and left profile (b).

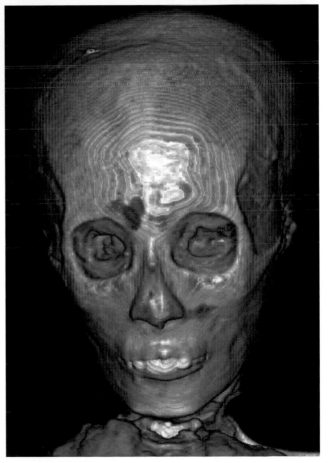

Plate 87: Three-dimensional reconstructed frontal CT image of the head of Tutankhamun shows the characteristic facial features of the king.

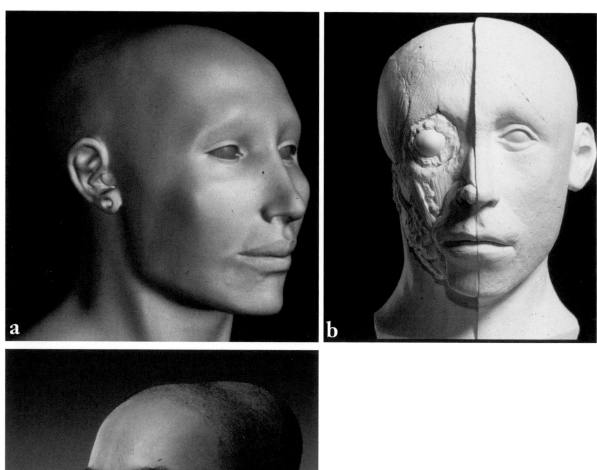

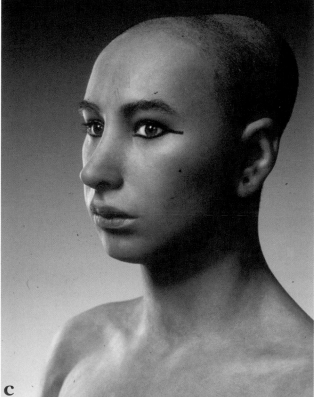

Plates 88a–c: Facial reconstruction of Tutankhamun, rendered by the Egyptian team (a); the American team's work on the reconstruction (b); and the final product of the French team: this silicone-skinned bust brings the king's features to life (c).

10

The Twentieth Dynasty:
Ramesses III, Pentawere, and the Harem Conspiracy

Historical Introduction

The Twentieth Dynasty began with a short reign of only four years by Sethnakht; a stela was recently discovered in the avenue of the sphinxes in Luxor dated to the fourth year of his reign. He was followed by his son, the great ruler Ramesses III, who ruled for thirty-one years.[1] Ramesses III was a formidable military leader, fighting major battles against the Libyans and waging a naval and land battle against the Sea Peoples, but he was burdened by domestic problems, which culminated in a workmen's strike and ultimately an assassination attempt upon his life (see below).

Ramesses III's heirs tried in vain to imitate his military successes, but external events were against them. Movements of landless people in the eastern Mediterranean, the Sea Peoples, were disrupting trade and stability, and though their attacks against Egypt in the thirteenth and twelfth centuries BC were

unsuccessful, economically the country was in decline. By the end of the period, there are references to civil unrest, incursions by desert raiders, fraud, and repeated tomb robbery. Outside Egypt, control over Syria–Palestine was lost as the city-states there were overrun and destroyed by newcomers. To the south, Nubia broke away under the leadership of the former Egyptian viceroy, Panehesy. The New Kingdom came to an end with the last king of the Twentieth Dynasty, Ramesses XI.

The reign of Ramesses III

The life of Ramesses III has been a mystery to Egyptologists. Most scholars maintain that he survived the assassination plot against him, designated in papyri as a harem conspiracy. A few others assert that the plot was successful, as discussed below.

Ramesses III was the son of Sethnakht and Tiye-Mereniset. He may have had a short coregency with his father.[2] Ramesses III had several wives, including Queen Iset Ta-Hemdjeret, owner of tomb QV51 in the Valley of the Queens, and possibly a secondary wife named Titi, owner of tomb QV52.[3] A third wife, Tiye, was implicated in the plot against his life, to be discussed below. He had many children, borne by more than one queen. A procession of family members is portrayed in his mortuary temple in western Thebes, though the identity of many of these has been debated, as the names were added posthumously.[4]

Ramesses III can be considered the last great warrior king of the golden age, the New Kingdom. The two most important sources informing us about his religious and political activities are the Great Harris Papyrus[5] and his mortuary temple in western Thebes, Medinet Habu[6] (plate 58). The papyrus, one of the longest papyri in existence from ancient Egypt, was found in 1855 in a tomb near this temple. Though dated to the day of the king's death, it is thought to have been composed afterward, in the reign of his son, Ramesses IV. It is a retrospective of the reign of Ramesses III, and sheds light on the political, religious, social, and economic situation of the country.

For example, the papyrus documents large land grants that the king made to the major temples, the system of the temple administration, and the wealth of the priests. There is also an account of the new buildings constructed under the king, such as Medinet Habu; a temple at Karnak dedicated to Khonsu, as well as a shrine to house the barques of the Theban triad of Amun, Mut, and Khonsu; and additions to Luxor Temple. Detailed descriptions are given of each temple, as well as stelae, statues, and vessels. Also included is a list of the monuments left by

Ramesses III at Serabit al-Khadim in the Sinai; in Lower Egypt at Tanis, Tell al-Yahudiya, al-Qantara, Heliopolis, and Almaza; and in Upper Egypt at Abydos, Qift, Qus, Medamud, and Armant.[7]

Ramesses III also left us a complete record of his military campaigns, which were chronicled on the walls of his temple at Medinet Habu. He undertook a campaign to Nubia early in his reign, but greater threats came from the west and north. Infiltration into the western Delta by the Libyans, or Tjehenu, was halted through two campaigns, in Years 5 and 11.[8] In Year 8, action by the king was necessitated by another imminent invasion, this time by the Sea Peoples. This group of tribes occupied Mediterranean islands, such as Cyprus, and destroyed the Hittite capital, Hattusa, setting into motion the fall of the entire Hittite Empire. Other cities in the Levant were razed. They turned next to Egypt, which they attempted to infiltrate by land in oxcarts and by sea. In Year 8, Ramesses undertook a heroic land and naval battle against the Sea Peoples, preparing a strong fleet and winning a decisive victory, recorded on the walls of Medinet Habu and in the Harris Papyrus.[9]

At the end of Ramesses III's reign, foreigners played a greater role in the court, including the royal harem.[10] Scenes at Medinet Habu portray the king relaxing with ladies of the harem in a particularly intimate way. The king boasted of the opulence of his Theban palace in the Harris Papyrus.[11] However, severe domestic problems arose during these final years. The king's wars, along with the grants to the temples, had depleted the royal treasury, and the Nile floods, which were crucial for irrigating the fields, were poor during this period. This caused a drought and destroyed the crops; famine spread. The workers who toiled on the estates of Ramesses III were paid in grain,[12] but the grain had run out.

In Year 29, this economic crisis caused a strike among the workmen of Deir al-Medina who constructed and decorated the royal tomb[13] (plates 59a–b). The Deir al-Medina workmen had not collected their salaries for two months, and they attempted in vain to bring their complaints to the attention of the authorities. They met in front of the storerooms of the Ramesseum (the mortuary temple of Ramesses II), protesting that they were hungry. After repeated demonstrations and strikes, the vizier finally intervened and provided them with some, though not all, of their rations. The unstable situation caused one of the king's two viziers to revolt from Athribis, in the Delta, but the attempted revolution did not succeed.[14] The circumstances of the strike have been recorded in a papyrus known as the Strike Papyrus, which paints a disturbing picture of an aging pharaoh who seems to be losing control of his empire.[15]

This is the first recorded instance of a labor strike. It shows the level of public resentment toward Ramesses III; normally, it would have been unthinkable for the ancient Egyptians to actually put in writing a negative action against the pharaoh. With the unprecedented undercurrent of ill feeling against him, the climate was perfect for conspirators to carry out an attempt on the king's life.

The harem conspiracy

The Judicial Papyrus in the Museo Egizio, Turin[16] documents the conspiracy against Ramesses III, in which all thirty-eight conspirators, among them harem women, officials, and even army members, were apprehended and brought to trial.[17] Part of a larger document now broken into fragments, it is the best textual evidence available for understanding these events. The section in Turin is the largest remaining piece, and lists all of the conspirators involved in the plot against the pharaoh, but of course, it does not provide all of the details that would be desirable. Other parts of the papyrus are the Rollin Papyrus at the Louvre and the Lee Papyrus at the British Museum,[18] as well as Papyrus Varzy, Papyrus Rifaud I (A, B, and C), and Papyrus Rifaud II (E).[19] The court transcripts of the trial are recorded in the Turin papyrus. In this document, the names of the accused are listed, followed by the crimes with which they were charged, and their punishment. The sentences were harsh: most were sentenced to death, and the most prominent compelled to commit suicide. It provides a fascinating glimpse into the makeup and power structure of the royal court.

The main culprit in the conspiracy was Queen Tiye, whose motivation in plotting against the king was the placement of her son Pentawere on the throne in place of the legitimate successor, Ramesses IV.[20] The conspirators acted with the aid of ten harem officials as well as the supervisor of the treasury, a Nubian official, an overseer of the army, and three royal scribes. The text gives specifics of each criminal's name and titles, such as the pantry chief Pebekamen, the butler Mesedsure, and the superintendent of the harem, Panouk. The names, which usually would incorporate the name of a deity, were modified with substitutions that rendered them as shameful.[21] The conspirators had contact with their relatives outside the palace, intending that the plot would expand into a revolution affecting the entire country. They even resorted to the use of magic figures representing gods and people, with the hope that their magical power could be applied against the palace guards.[22]

The attack on the king himself was to be carried out while he was in the harem. At the same time, a revolt was to be staged from outside. This was arranged through messages that were sent out from the harem to overseers of workmen and military commanders, including Bonemwese, captain of the Nubian archers, whose sister was a member of the harem. One such message is recorded in the Turin Papyrus: "Stir up the people! Incite enemies to hostility against their lord."[23]

The plot was discovered, and the king issued an order for all of the perpetrators to be judged by the court. He appointed the twelve members of this court, which included overseers of the treasury, Mentemtowe and Pefrawa, and others. The court took direct orders from the king and was given the authority to carry out all penalties.[24]

The main text of the Judicial Papyrus of Turin focuses on the four separate trials that took place. Twenty-eight people were sentenced to execution, and ten were allowed to take their own lives. We do not know what happened to Queen Tiye, as the text does not address her situation.

The fourth trial involved charges that were brought against three judges of the court itself who misused their power. They, along with two police officers, were accused of cavorting with some of the female conspirators. Four of them were condemned to lose their noses and ears.[25]

If we examine the Turin papyrus carefully, we discover that one name comes up again and again: Pebekamen, the man in charge of food for the royal court. He seems to have been Tiye's connection to the outside world.

An important clue to the extent of the conspiracy can be found in the names of two high-ranking military officers, Pasai and Bonemwese, who planned to lead the armed rebellion against Ramesses IV after his father was killed. The women of the harem needed the help of the military for the plot to lead to an armed revolt, a coup d'état, if they were to stand any chance of putting Pentawere on the throne after the planned assassination of Ramesses III.

The official death date of Ramesses III is Year 32 of his reign, the third month of Shemu, day 15. This is recorded in an ostracon from Deir al-Medina, which states that "the hawk has flown to heaven."[26] The Turin Papyrus leaves out one key piece of information: Did the conspirators succeed in killing the old king?

There has traditionally been disagreement as to the success of the plot. J.H. Breasted noted that Ramesses III was referred to as the "great god" in the text, an epithet given only to deceased kings, and came to the conclusion that Ramesses III gave instructions to the court but died before the trials. This would suggest that Ramesses III was alive at least long enough to appoint these magistrates. This also suggests that their attempted regicide failed. Breasted stopped short of stating that the king was wounded.[27]

The text has been studied again, and it is now thought that the story of the attack as described in the papyrus was not rendered in the present tense, but put into the mouth of the deceased king. Some believe that Ramesses IV is the author of the text.[28] Papyrus Rifaud makes mention of Ramesses III as the "father of the king," indicating that his son, Ramesses IV, was already the pharaoh at the time of the trials. It has also been suggested that an allusion to the royal barque being overturned is a metaphor for the murder of the king.[29]

Due to the inconclusive nature of this textual evidence, and the lack of any obvious cause of death found in previous forensic studies of the king's mummy, scholars have argued a variety of positions: that the king was injured as a result of the plot and later died of his wounds; that the plot failed entirely; or that the attempt was successful. It was not clear from the texts, therefore, whether the harem conspiracy was successful in its plot to kill Ramesses III.

Examination of Ramesses III and Unknown Man E

We studied the mummy of Ramesses III using forensic, anthropological, radiological, and genetic methods. We also studied the 'Unknown Man E,' a possible candidate for Pentawere.

CT examination of the mummy of Ramesses III[30]
Genealogy of Ramesses III
Father: Sethnakht
Mother: Tiye-Mereniset

Identification of the mummy
Ramesses III was originally buried in KV11. His mummy was rewrapped and placed in a replacement coffin by Twenty-first Dynasty priests of Amun and moved to the Deir al-Bahari cache, where it was found in a cartonnage coffin placed inside the massive coffin of Queen Ahmose-Nefertari, which also contained the queen's remains. The mummy had been rewrapped in orange-colored linen. It was partially unwrapped by Maspero in the presence of Khedive Tewfik on June 1, 1886.[31] The mummy was later examined by G. Elliot Smith, but he produced little information

about it in the absence of x-rays.[32] Dockets on the wrappings confirmed its identity.

General CT findings
The mummy of Ramesses III is generally in good condition (plate 60) and likely escaped the mutilations by tomb plunderers often noted. The body is encased in its resinous bandages. The morphological appearances of the skull and hip bones support the known gender of a male.

Epiphyses of all of the bones are united, indicating a mature skeleton. Evidenced by the closure of the cranial vault sutures, the age at death is over fifty years. The morphology of the pubic symphysis indicates an age of twenty-five to eighty-three years with an average of about 46 years. The presence of moderate degenerative changes of the spine and joints, as well as atherosclerosis, indicate an age of about sixty years.

Electronic measurements of bones are: right humerus 31.5 cm; right femur 45 cm; right tibia 35.5 cm. The stature as measured from vertex to heel is 163 cm.

CT findings in different regions
Head (fig. 79)
Thickening of the skull diploe in the frontal and parietal region is likely an anatomical variant. There is evidence of excerebration as

Table 23. General CT findings for the mummy of Ramesses III

Preservation status	Good
Age	About 60 years
Gender	Male
Stature	163 cm

part of the mummification process, with only dural remnants seen in the posterior fossa. The interruption of the cribriform plate and disturbance of the nasal septum indicate a transnasal route of skull mummification, likely via the left nostril. Two-thirds of the posterior aspect of the skull is full of resin or resin-like material. The nose is deformed and flattened, probably by pressure from bandages. The nose is stuffed with embalming materials, mainly resin, and concentrated more in the left nasal cavity, causing deviation of the septum to the right side.

Subcutaneous packs are seen in the mid and lower face bilaterally with comparable widths.

The orbits contain atrophic globes with optic nerves and are filled with heterogeneous, low-density material, likely linen impregnated with resin.

Both auricles are preserved. The lobule of the right auricle shows piercings, while the lobule of the left auricle is partly missing.

The oral cavity and oropharynx are filled with linen impregnated with resinous material.

Teeth (fig. 80)
The absence of all maxillary and mandibular wisdom teeth, a congenital situation (oligodontia), was likely asymptomatic for the king. Oligodontia is not an uncommon condition

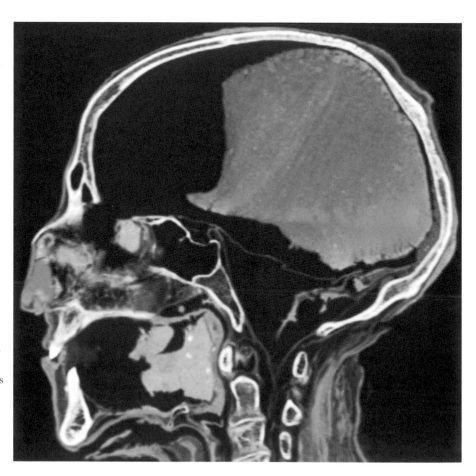

Fig. 79: Sagittal CT reconstruction in the midline of the head of Ramesses III shows almost complete excerebration through a defective cribriform plate. The posterior two-thirds of the skull cavity is filled with structureless, moderately dense resin material. The nasal cavity is filled with resin.

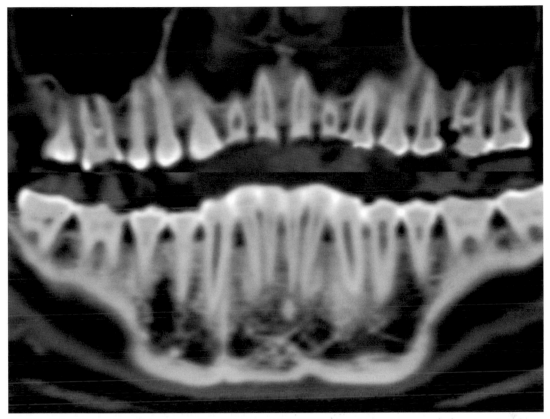

Fig. 80: CT of the teeth of jaw and maxilla of Ramesses III. CT image obtained in curved plane (teeth panorama) shows the absence of all four third molars. Note caries in the upper right first molar and second premolar, as well as dentin exposure on all molars, with localized bone loss between the teeth. The bone of the anterior region of the mandible is partially resorbed.

in any historical period. The teeth in general show fair periodontal health and moderate attrition consistent with the age of the king at time of death.

Dentin exposure is noted on all molars, especially the mandibular left first molar. Lack of space at the front of the mandible caused rotation of the right canine; mild rotation of the left central incisor caused widening between it and the adjacent lateral incisor. There is mild bone resorption at the front (anterior) of the mandible. Caries (cavities) are seen at the mesial wall of the maxillary

right first molar and the opposing surface of the adjacent second premolar, with a localized bone loss between the teeth.

Neck (fig. 81)

There is a cut wound in the soft tissues of the lower neck that extends from the lower end of the fifth to the seventh cervical vertebrae, causing a gap in the soft tissues of the neck that measures 35 mm and extends deeply to reach the bone. All the structures of the neck (trachea, esophagus, and large blood vessels) were severed. The extent and depth of the

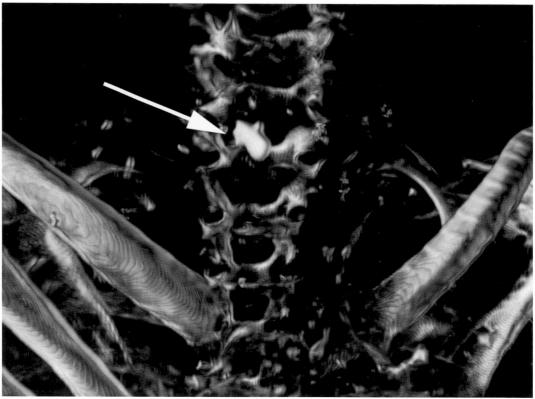

Fig. 81: Three-dimensional CT image of the front of the neck of Ramesses III shows an amulet in the shape of the Eye of Horus placed in front of the lower neck (arrow).

wound indicate that the injury was fatal. A small focal cortical interruption is seen at the front of the seventh vertebral body, more to the left side (antero-left-lateral); there is wide disc space between the sixth and seventh vertebrae. This may indicate that the wound was inflicted by stabbing with a pointed-tip, bladed weapon, such as a dagger. A dense, irregular, flat foreign object (Eye of Horus amulet; see chapter 12, "Amulets, Funerary Figures, and Other Objects Found on the Mummies") is lodged at the right lower rim of the wound that measures 15 mm in its widest diameter and 2166 HU in CT density.[33]

Upper limbs

The articulating bones at the sternoclavicular joints and scapulae have a normal configuration. Mild degenerative changes were observed in the form of small osteophytic lippings at the glenoid labra bilaterally.

The arms are flexed at the elbows, and the forearms are crossed over the chest, right over left. The fingers and the palms of the hands are flat. There is a comminuted fracture at the first metacarpal and first phalanx of the third finger of the left hand. There is also a linear transverse interruption of the soft tissues at the lateral aspect of the head of the right humerus, causing incomplete interruption of its anterolateral cortex. There is no evidence of healing attempts of these fractures; the injuries were likely inflicted postmortem.

Spine (fig. 82)

The right side of the anterior longitudinal ligament (ALL) is ossified continuously along a block that extends from the fifth to the eleventh thoracic vertebrae. The ossified ligament is associated with exuberant osteophytes at multiple discs that give the spine a bumpy appearance. However, the discs in the involved region preserve their normal height and show no significant degeneration. Additional findings include osteoarthritis of uncovertebral and costovertebral joints without ankylosis, as well as calcifications of the supraspinous ligament and ligamenta flava at multiple levels. There was no evidence of bony ankylosis of facet joints or severe sacroiliac changes (erosions or ankylosis). There is a small hyperostosis at the front of the atlantoaxial region. The findings favor the diagnosis of DISH, according to Resnick's criteria.[34] The normal height of the intervertebral discs excludes the diagnosis of a degenerative spine.[35] The absence of fusion or ankylosis of the spinal joints (zygapophyseal or sacroiliac joints) is inconsistent with the diagnosis of ankylosing spondylitis.[36]

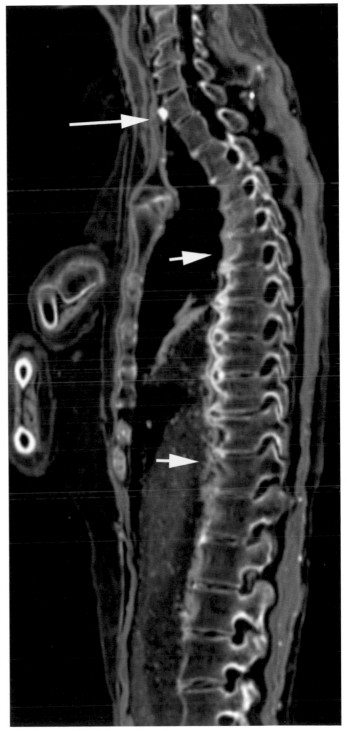

Fig. 82: Sagittal reconstructed CT image of the spine of Ramesses III (to the right of midline) shows the Eye of Horus amulet appearing as a dense plate beneath the linen tissues and overlying the body of the seventh cervical vertebra (long arrow). The thoracic spine shows an increased density that flows continuously along the right anterolateral aspect of the vertebral bodies and the intervertebral discs from the fifth to the eleventh thoracic vertebrae (between short arrows). There is no significant degeneration of the intervertebral discs in the involved region. No fusion of the posterior vertebral elements of the spine is noted. Findings are consistent with the diagnosis of diffuse idiopathic skeletal hyperostosis (DISH).

Torso (fig. 83)

The body cavities are eviscerated as part of mummification through a left oblique inguinal incision. Only the heart is seen in the thoracic cavity at the left side. The lower thoracic and abdominal cavities are stuffed with linen and resin, as well as a heterogeneous, low-density embalming material measuring –516 HU, with multiple small, dense objects within that could be soil or sawdust.

Four figures of the Sons of Horus are located in the lower left hemithorax (fig. 84; see chapter 12).

The male organs (penis and scrotum) are covered with superficial linen sheets impregnated with resin that are likely adherent to the male organ. Two- and three-dimensional CT images identified the penis (40 mm x 13 mm in length and width respectively) (fig. 85).

Lower limbs

The lower limbs are separately wrapped in several layers of linen impregnated with resin. There are subcutaneous packs in the legs of both sides. The girth of the wrapped left leg is bigger than the right side. There

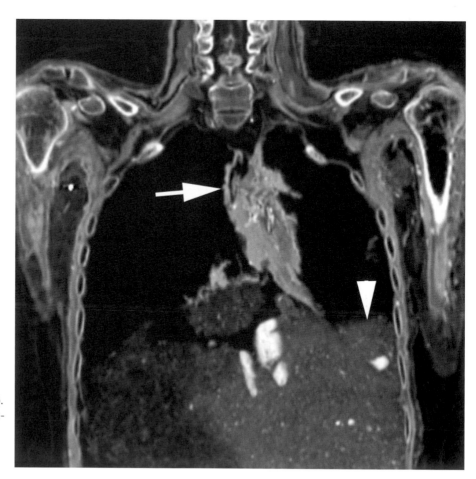

Fig. 83: Coronal reconstruction of the upper torso cavity of the mummy of Ramesses III documents evisceration sparing the heart (arrow). Heterogeneous, low-density embalming material fills the lower chest and abdomen (arrowhead).

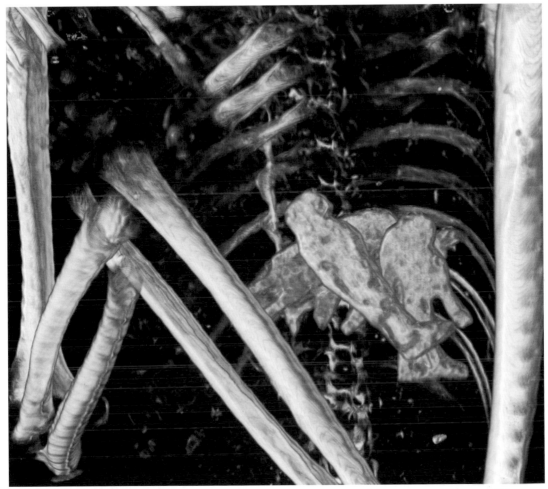

Fig. 82: Three-dimensional reconstructed CT image of the upper torso of the mummy of Ramesses III clearly shows the shapes of the figures of the Four Sons of Horus.

are mild acetabular osteophytes of both hip joints, without evidence of joint narrowing or ankylosis. Multiple enthesopathies at the level of hips, knees, and calcanei are noted as part of extraspinal manifestations of DISH. Atherosclerosis of the lower-limb arteries is noted.

Complex misalignment of both forefeet of King Ramesses III is evident. There is hallux valgus of the right big toe, and bilateral first metatarsus varus more evident in the right side. There are also claw deformities of the lesser toes (second to fifth) (fig. 86). The transverse metatarsus arches are also likely affected. There is mild to moderate rotational abnormality of the left foot (plantar eversion). Malalignments of the bones of the feet of the pharaoh could have been present during his life or resulted from the tight bandages applied during mummification. Two sesamoid

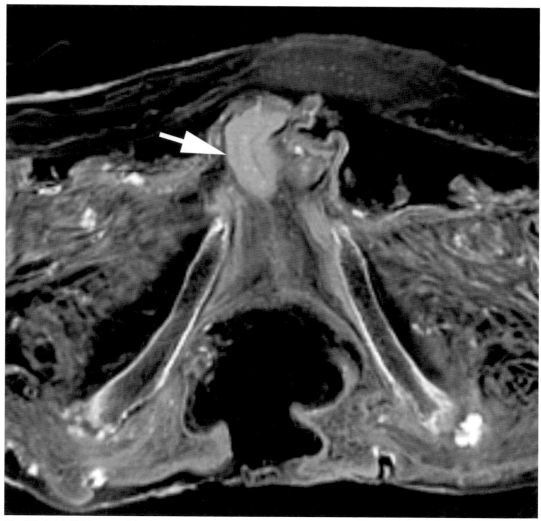

Fig. 85: Axial CT image of the lower pelvis of the mummy of Ramesses III shows the preserved phallus (arrow).

Fig. 86: Sagittal CT image along the left foot of the mummified Ramesses III shows a claw deformity of the imaged toe; this could be a deformity that the king suffered from during his life or the result of tight bandages of mummification.

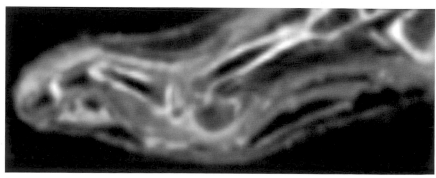

bones are placed at the plantar surface of the head of the first metatarsal of each foot.

For recent results of a re-examination of the evidence in the left foot, see sidelight, "New Evidence on the Death of Ramesses III."

Comments on mummification

The mummy of Ramesses III is well preserved and exhibits the excellent mummification job expected for a king. The mummification style is consistent with late Nineteenth and early Twentieth Dynasty royal mummies: transnasal removal of the brain, embalming material placed intracranially, and the torso almost fully stuffed.

There are notable CT findings in the mummification of Ramesses III:

1. Arms crossed with hands flat, not clenched: though the mummy of Seti I displayed the same arm and hand position, it was not common until after the reign of Ramesses III.

2. Orbital packings: The eye sockets had been packed with linen of low CT density. A denser substance (likely resin) was placed within the socket. The eyelids were left open by the embalmers. It is not certain if the substances inside the orbits were meant to be artificial eyes or merely to give a normal contour to the eyes. However, more elaborate artificial eyes have been noted only in the Twenty-first Dynasty (as in the mummy of Nodjmet) and later.

3. Layers of linen are still seen wrapping the mummy and adherent to its surface. This is the only royal mummy in the study that retained its wrappings. Upper and lower limbs were wrapped separately.

4. Several amulets were placed in and on the mummy (see chapter 12).

Manner and cause of death[37]

It has been postulated that Ramesses III died of cobra or other snake bite because in the trial transcripts some of the conspirators were called the "snake" and "lord of the snakes."[38] However, we believe that it is far more likely that the king died from a fatal cut wound to the throat by a sharp knife, as revealed by the CT examination.

There is textual and other Egyptological evidence to support this conclusion. The harem conspiracy papyrus implies this, but because of the divine nature of the king, the words 'kill' or 'murder' would be unthinkable. As mentioned above, an allusion in the text to the royal barque being overturned is a metaphor for the murder, and the reference to Ramesses III as the 'great god' further suggests that the king is deceased.

The embalmers inserted into the neck wound an Eye of Horus, or *wedjat*-eye amulet, one of the main protective amulets used in ancient Egypt. The name *wedjat* is derived from the hieroglyphic word for 'sound,' with connotations of healing and protection. Both eyes of the god Horus were used as protective amulets. The right eye was associated with Re and symbolized divine protection, while the left eye was associated with healing. It was the left eye that was said to have been torn out by the evil god Seth during his battle with Horus, and magically restored by the god Thoth.[39] The Eye of Horus was also used with reference to offerings. Temple and tomb offerings were referred to as an "Eye of Horus" in texts because of their association with divine protection and renewal for the deceased or the cult statue.[40]

It is clear that the embalmers provided the Eye of Horus so that Thoth would magically heal the wound, as he had healed the wounded Horus, in order to ensure the king's safe survival in the afterlife. The embalmers also covered the neck of Ramesses III with a collar composed of thick layers of linen, which prevented the detection of the deadly cut for more than three thousand years.

Unknown Man E (fig. 87)

There is a mummy that may possibly be identified as Pentawere, the son of Ramesses III who joined his mother, Tiye, in the plot against the life of his father. Unknown Man E[41] was found by Gaston Maspero at the Deir al-Bahari cache in 1886, inside an uninscribed cedarwood coffin. The mummy has several strange features that are not found in any other New Kingdom mummies. It was covered with a sheepskin that still retains its white color. Sheepskin was considered unclean and impure by the ancient Egyptians, as stated in the Middle Kingdom story of Sinuhe.[42] The hands and feet of the body were tied with leather thongs, and the face appears with mouth open, as though screaming. The body was not mummified and thus had no embalming incision.[43] Maspero's anatomist, Daniel Fouquet, and a chemist named Mathey examined the mummy and speculated that this person was poisoned or asphyxiated because he was buried alive.[44] In a 2006 re-examination of the mummy,[45] Bob Brier observed that the body was of a tall, stout young man in his twenties, who wore two gold earrings and a braided hairstyle, and whose toenails were trimmed and dyed red with henna. Natron had been sprinkled over his body and resin poured into his mouth, in an apparently hasty attempt at a basic mummification. The mummy and sheepskin were placed into a cedar coffin that was uninscribed and modified to fit the large body.

Some scholars have suggested that this mummy could be the Hittite prince who was sent to marry the widow of Tutankhamun[46] and was murdered before he arrived, but most theories suggest that the mummy is actually Pentawere.

The Egyptian Mummy Project team[47] estimated the age of the Unknown Man E to be about eighteen to twenty years old, based on the incomplete fusion of epiphyseal lines in the long bones. There was no evidence of removal of the inner organs. The team could not find any evidence of the cause of death of this young man, but they found that the compressed skin fold around his neck and the inflated thorax favored death by suffocation due to strangulation or hanging.[48]

The Judicial Papyrus reads:

> Pentewere who bore that other name. He was brought in because of his collusion with Teye, his mother, when she was plotting those matters with the women of the harem, and for making rebellion against his lord. He was placed before the judges, in order to be examined; they found him guilty; they left him alone; he took his own life.[49]

From these words, it is apparent that Pentawere was allowed to commit suicide. He did not use any weapon such as a knife; the only way to end his life was to hang himself. Because of this, the face was horribly frozen into a screaming expression. He was not fully mummified, because he would not have been considered as deserving of the proper postmortem treatment, having undergone the humiliation of an execution. The sheepskin

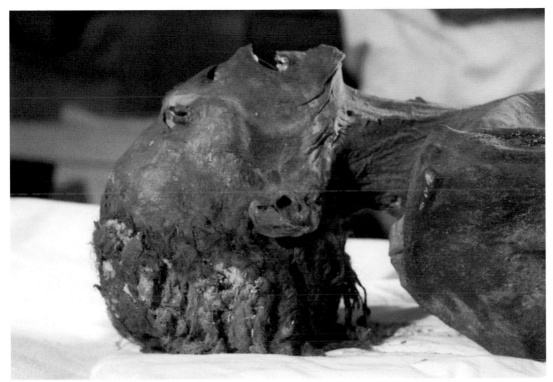

Fig. 87: The mummy of Unknown Man E.

covering his body was a further sign of his disgrace and an indication that he would never be accepted into the afterlife. Those wrapped in linen were the ones who met Osiris and journeyed safely to paradise. Therefore, the 'unclean' sheepskin, rather than the linen usually provided for mummies, could be an indication that the deceased was destined to journey to hell.

In order to discern the relationship between Unknown Man E and Ramesses III, a genetic analysis was performed. DNA was extracted from bone samples of the two mummies, according to the protocols described earlier. Sixteen Y-chromosomal short tandem repeats and eight polymorphic microsatellites of the nuclear genome were amplified using AmpF\STR Y filer, Identifiler, and the AmpF\STR Minifiler kit, according to the protocols of the manufacturer.[50] The genetic analyses revealed identical haplotypes of the Y-chromosome in both individuals. The testing of the polymorphic microsatellite loci provided concordant results in at least one allele of each marker.[51]

Although the mummy of Queen Tiye, mother of Pentawere and wife of Ramesses III, has not been located and thus could not be tested, the identical Y-chromosomal DNA and the autosomal half-allele sharing of the two male mummies suggest a great possibility of a father–son relationship. Unknown Man E appears to be Pentawere, and the truth of the harem conspiracy has been revealed.

SIDELIGHT:
New Evidence on the Death of Ramesses III

Recent further investigations and analysis of the CT images of the feet of Ramesses III done by the authors of this book have revealed an additional injury in the body of the king that supports the theory of an assassination attempt (figs. 88a–e). The left big toe has been partly chopped off; only part of the proximal phalanx is present and a small chip of bone distal to it. The bony cut is oblique, with the lateral border of the remaining part of the proximal phalanx longer than the medial. The bony edges are sharp, without any evidence of healing or sclerosis. The sharpness of the edges of the cut bone in the partially amputated left big toe indicates that it was inflicted by a sharp weapon such as an axe or a sword. The normal contour of the soft tissues of the amputated left big toe is preserved; it was likely restored by the embalmers using linen. The embalmers secured the feet by wrapping them individually, including the lower limbs, with layers of linen soaked with resin. There are six objects within the bandages of both feet and ankles; at least four of them are Eye of Horus amulets (see plate 185b). The absence of evidence of bone healing, restoration of the outer soft-tissue contour of the toe, and placement of amulets within the intact linen wrappings are all indicators that the injury happened shortly before death, before the embalming process. The circumstances of the injury of the left big toe are similar to those of the cut throat and indicate that both injuries may have resulted from the brutal fatal attack on the king, likely by more than one assassin using different weapons.

S.N.S. and Z.H.

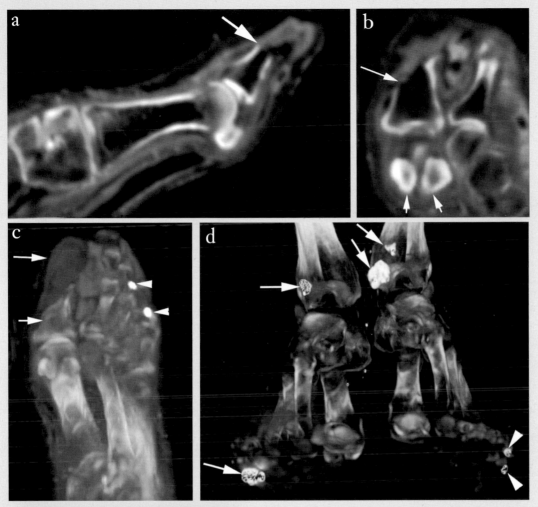

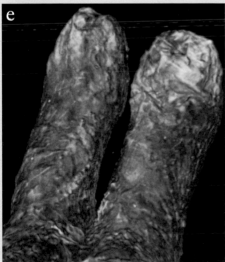

Figs 88a–e: CT images of the left foot of the mummy of Ramesses III. Sagittal reconstructed image of the first toe (a) shows sharp edge (arrow) of the fractured proximal phalanx. The distal part of the bone as well as the distal phalanx is missing. This denotes partial amputation of the toe. Note that the soft-tissue density contour of the big toe is preserved, which is likely remodeled with linen by the embalmers. Axial oblique view (b) shows well the oblique sharp edge of the fractured proximal phalanx; the lateral border of the remaining bone is longer than the medial (long arrow). The two shorter arrows each point to a sesamoid bone at the plantar surface of the first metatarsal. Three-dimensional reconstruction of the left foot (c) clearly identifies the partially amputated first toe (short arrow) and preservation of the soft-tissue density contour (longer arrow). The two arrowheads each point to a metallic (likely gold) bead placed close to the tips of the fourth and fifth toes. Three-dimensional reconstructed image of both ankles and feet (d) shows six dense metallic objects that were likely placed for healing and protection. The arrows point to four amulets probably representing the Eye of Horus, and the arrowheads point to two small beads. (e) Three-dimensional reconstructed CT image shows the intact wrappings of the feet.

191

11

CT Findings on the Mummification Process of Royal Ancient Egyptians, Eighteenth to Early Twentieth Dynasties

Mummification in Ancient Egypt

The ancient Egyptians believed in the resurrection of the body and everlasting life (plate 62).

Mummification was practiced in ancient Egypt over a period of more than thirty centuries with the aim of preservation of the body from decay, as well as maintaining the personal identity of the individual for the afterlife (plates 61a–b).[1] This, in combination with the proper funerary rituals (plates 63a–b), would help to ensure the survival of the deceased in the next world. There was very little textual evidence left behind to give insight into the mummification process, though embalming cachettes such as KV63 (fig. 89) give us an idea about materials used for mummification in the New Kingdom. The Rhind Magical Papyrus (ca. 200 BC) provides some information on the rituals associated with it. Three papyri (dating to about the first century AD) include some spells that were

to be recited during the wrapping of each part of the body. Another papyrus prescribes the order in which limbs were to be wrapped, amulets inserted, and spells recited.[2]

Much of the information we have available on the process of mummification comes from the writings of Herodotus, a Greek historian who visited Egypt during the fifth century BC. He stated that the mummification process varied depending on the financial status of the deceased. Wealthy citizens had the most lavish treatment, while for the middle and poorer classes, mummification was downgraded or minimally performed.[3]

According to Herodotus:

The most perfect process is as follows: as much as possible of the brain is extracted through the nostrils with an iron hook, and what the hook cannot reach is rinsed out with drugs; next the flank is laid open with a flint knife and

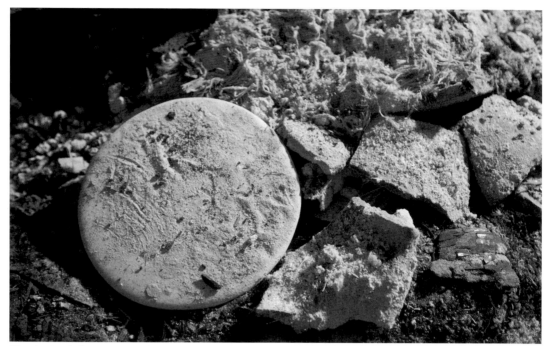

Fig. 89: Embalming materials (linen and natron) from the cachette of KV63, Valley of the Kings.

the whole contents of the abdomen removed; the cavity is then thoroughly cleansed and washed out, first with palm wine and again with an infusion of pounded spices. After that, it is filled with pure bruised myrrh, cassia, and every other aromatic substance with the exception of frankincense, and sewn up again, after which the body is placed in natrum, covered entirely over, for seventy days—never longer. When this period, which must not be exceeded, is over, the body is washed and then wrapped from head to foot in linen cut into strips and smeared on the underside with gum, which is commonly used by the Egyptians instead of glue. In this condition the body is given back to the family, who have a wooden case made, shaped like a human figure, into which it is put.[4]

Mummification of Egyptian bodies evolved through millennia of experimentation to reach its apex in the Twenty-first Dynasty, after which it gradually deteriorated. The changes in techniques provide dating criteria for the process.[5] The royal mummies are a unique and vital resource for our knowledge of ancient Egyptian funerary customs and mummification techniques. The royal mummies dating to the Eighteenth to Twentieth Dynasties in the Egyptian Museum belonged to the era of elaborate and 'classic mummification' and, as would be expected, must have had the best possible treatment.[6]

Although the archaeological literature demonstrates the basic outline of mummification in ancient Egypt, it is sometimes limited and inaccurate. Much information in the literature was derived from the forensic reports by G. Elliot Smith on the royal mummies of the Egyptian Museum more than a century ago.[7] These reports were neither detailed nor standardized, but rather narration that lacked modern statistical evaluation; failure to comment about the presence of a feature does not necessarily imply the absence of this feature. In addition, many bodies had not even been completely unwrapped when Smith examined them. At most, Smith was only allowed visual inspection with minimal dissection privileges.[8] These conditions must have limited reporting on processes such as excerebration and evisceration.

In their 1980 book, James Harris and Edward Wente described the x-ray examinations of the royal mummies at the Egyptian Museum. However, they admitted that the style of mummification could not be ascertained in many mummies. They faced difficulties in studying plain x-rays related to overlapping of the skull bones and ascertaining excerebration. Also, the radiographs could not indicate the presence of packing unless it contained radiopaque materials such as resin.[9] Another limitation of x-ray films is that the contents of a radiopaque mass cannot be differentiated as packing material or merely a desiccated organ.[10]

Analysis of ancient Egyptian mummies with CT and MDCT yielded a sum of information that is greater than that contributed by plain radiographic or forensic studies.[11] As part of the large MDCT study of the royal mummies, we selectively studied those mummies dating from the Eighteenth to early Twentieth Dynasties, with the aim to further investigate the mummification style in the royal social class during this time.[12]

Table 24 includes the identities as well as the general CT findings of the studied mummies. The table includes the estimated age at time of death, stature, current preservation status, and the position of the upper limbs of the mummies as revealed by CT studies.[13]

This chapter will discuss the following topics:
- Body position of mummies
- CT features of ancient Egyptian embalming materials
- Head mummification and excerebration
- Evisceration and visceral packs
- Cosmetic care: procedures done by the embalmers with the aim of restoration of a real-life form of the mummy, such as placing subcutaneous packs, artificial eyes, maintaining the shape of the nose, and support for external male genitalia

Body Position

All of the mummies in this study were lying recumbent with their bodies flat. Mummies dated to the Early Dynastic Period and earlier in the Old Kingdom were generally found in flexed, fetal-like position. However, mummies dated to later dynasties have all been found in a flat, supine position.[14]

The position of the arms of ancient Egyptian mummies varied according to the fashion of the time (dynasty), gender, and royal status. Predynastic mummies had flexed arms with their hands in front of their faces, while Old Kingdom and many Middle Kingdom mummies tended to have their arms beside their bodies. From the Seventeenth into the Eighteenth Dynasty, the arms were laid along the sides, with the hands often placed on the front of the thighs for women, and over the genitals for men. As the

New Kingdom progressed, both men's and women's arms lay along their sides, with their hands over their genitalia. In the Eighteenth Dynasty, beginning with Amenhotep I, the arms of kings were crossed over the breast with the hands clenched to hold the royal scepters, and in the Nineteenth and Twentieth Dynasties, the 'royal' crossed-arm position over the chest was the norm for the royal mummies. In the Twenty-first Dynasty, the arms of both royal and non-royal mummies returned to their sides, with hands over or near the pubic area (plates 64a–d).[15]

Among the Eighteenth Dynasty mummies we studied, the arms of Thutmose II and Thutmose III are in the 'royal' position, crossed over the chest (right above the left). Arm position is one of the reasons why there is significant doubt as to the identity of the mummy incorrectly attributed to Thutmose I, with his arms stretched down the side of his body. Despite the fact that both upper limbs of Thutmose III were broken and detached from the body, they were restored in ancient times to their original royal position. This indicated the significance of such posing. The arms of Yuya, father of Queen Tiye, were flexed at the elbows and crossed under the chin; this unique position could be due to his semi-royal status as the father-in-law of Amenhotep III. When his mummy was first found, Tutankhamun's arms were bent at the elbows, and the forearms were laid at right angles across his belly. This pose, however, is unique and not the norm for the New Kingdom royals, as Tutankhamun's forearms do not cross diagonally or reach the shoulders.[16]

We found the 'royal' position of arms more frequently in the Nineteenth and Twentieth Dynasties, for Seti I, Ramesses II, Merenptah, and Ramesses III. The palms were generally laid flat in these mummies. However, it seems inconsistent which arm is placed over the other. The left arm was on top of the right for Seti I and Ramesses II, while the right was over the left in the mummies of Merenptah and Ramesses III, as well as in the earlier mummies of Thutmose II and Thutmose III.

Many royal and noble women in the Eighteenth Dynasty, like Thuya (mother of Queen Tiye) and the two fetuses found in the tomb of Tutankhamun, have their arms stretched down the sides of their bodies. Queen Tiye has a different pose, with the left arm crossed over the chest, while the right arm lies at her side.

Arm position could not be assessed in the mutilated mummies of Amenhotep III and Akhenaten.

CT Features of Ancient Egyptian Embalming Materials

Ancient Egyptians primarily used natron, as well as other substances such as resins and spices, for embalming. CT offers a means of suggesting the composition of material, firstly by depicting its morphology and structure, and secondly by measuring the radiological density in HU.[17] Table 25 includes CT densities of material used in mummification, as measured with HU.

Natron

Mummification in ancient Egypt employed tissue preservation via desiccation through the hydrophilic feature of a local salt (natron) found at Wadi al-Natrun, near Cairo. Natron is a naturally occurring mixture of salts composed mainly of sodium carbonates and smaller amounts of sodium bicarbonate (baking soda), sodium sulfate, and sodium chloride (table salt). In addition to its desiccating osmotic action, sodium carbonate is also employed in breaking down protein bonds. This action enhances further the transfer of water out of the body and permits better penetration of liquid reagents into the tissue. There has long been a debate about whether natron was used in mummification in its dry form or as a liquid bath;[18] however, many scholars today adhere to the 'dry natron' concept.[19] Natron salt looks like a white powder in its solid state. Its inclusions may appear as very high densities on CT images.[20]

Resins and similar substances

Resin is a substance that exudes from a tree spontaneously or following incision of the tree. The viscous liquid hardens into brownish globs after being exposed to air. Egyptian embalmers probably obtained their resin from pine trees in Syria or Asia Minor. Beeswax and bitumen from the Dead Sea and Iraq were added as minor components to resin. Embalmers used resin as a heated liquid material on the body following natron desiccation. In addition to its glue effect, hot liquid resin would have had a thermal bactericidal effect. Addition of other substances such as beeswax and bitumen to resin was likely to make the desiccated tissues water-repellent, to prevent moisture absorption and subsequent rehydration.[21] In CT images, resin appears as a structureless substance with homogeneous, moderately high density (70 to 250 HU) that may have a fluid level surface parallel to the dependent body surface (figs. 90a–b).[22]

In CT images, resin and other resin-like[23] materials may be seen in generous quantity in the eviscerated dried body cavities, such as in the mummy of Seti I, as well as within the cranial cavity, as seen in the heads of Amenhotep III, Yuya, and Ramesses II. We identified resin-soaked linen rags as tampons for various body orifices, such as the nose orifices of Thutmose II, Thuya, Merenptah, and Ramesses III; stuffed in the body cavity, as in most of the studied mummies; or between the gaping lips of the abdominal evisceration wound, as found in the mummy of Thuya. In later periods, the body's surface was painted with resin. Resin was also used to attach the initial layer of wrappings to the skin surface to hold them in position, as was the case in the mummified bodies of Seti I and Merenptah. We detected resin mixed with the most superficial wrappings of the mummy of Seti I. Resin-impregnated linen completely surrounded the mummy of Ramesses III, excepting the head; this hindered physical examination of the mummy or obtaining information concerning the treatment of the body before its CT study.[24]

Resin over millennia becomes altered to acquire a black, glistening appearance, which explains the external dark appearance of the mummy of Seti I (see fig. 69 in chapter 9). Foreign travelers to Egypt mistakenly assumed that the blackened, solidified resin covering the mummies was bitumen, the mineral formed from pitch. Since the major source of bitumen was a mountain in Persia (Iran), where the substance was called 'mumia,' these embalmed bodies eventually became known as 'mummies.'[25] Resin also has a surprising ability to penetrate tissues, even reaching the medullary bone spaces and inside the joints, causing the increased densities that we detected in the CT study of the mummy of Seti I. Resin-impregnated linen was also used to wrap viscera placed outside the body within canopic jars.[26]

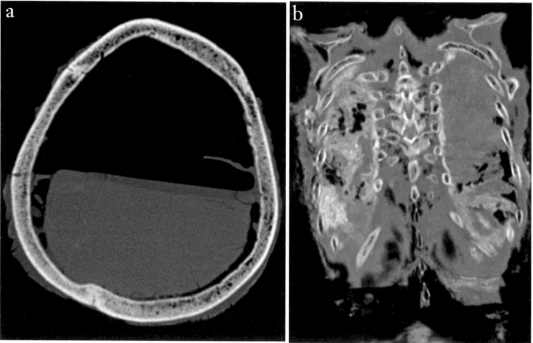

Figs. 90a–b: CT imaging features of resin. Axial CT image (a) of the head of the mummy of Amenhotep III shows intracranial resin, which appears as a structureless substance with homogeneous, moderately high density, and assumes a fluid level parallel to the back of the skull (dependent surface). Coronal CT image (b) of the back of the torso of Seti I shows that the body was immersed in an ample amount of resin. Resin was also mixed with the outer linen wrappings, which may explain the mummy's dark appearance.

Spices and aromatic materials

Materials such as myrrh and frankincense (trees of the *Burseraceae* family) were used in the mummification process for their aromatic properties. Embalmers may have used myrrh as an agent to prevent rehydration or as an antiseptic.[27] Spices such as cinnamon were also employed, though little formal study of their tissue preservation potential has been reported.[28] In a recent study, high-CT-density inclusions (2300 HU) within resin-soaked linen suggested the presence of natron or myrrh.[29] However, the density of an embalming pack must be interpreted with caution, especially at the edges, and the possible presence of beam-hardening artifacts should be considered.[30]

Filling materials

The embalmers used different materials to fill the emptied cranial and body cavities, such as soil, sand, rocks, grains, and sawdust. We suggested that soil may be inside the skull cavity of Seti I's mummy, as we identified an inhomogeneous, low-density material (–150 HU) that included higher densities that could be sand grains and larger stones. Grains and other solid embalming materials could be also identified as variable-sized oval or rounded structures with densities from 430 to 1427 HU, as was seen inserted within the nasal and oral cavities of mummified Ramesses II (fig. 91). CT images also distinguished threadlike, convoluted linen inside the skull of

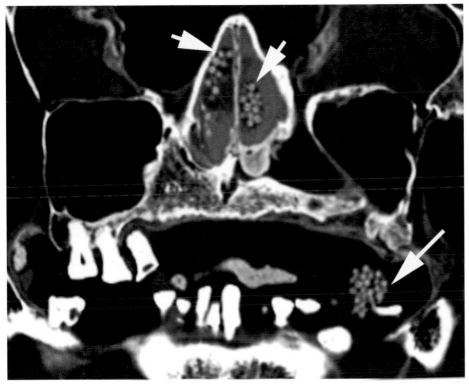

Fig. 91: CT imaging of plant seeds used in mummification. Curved multiplanar reconstructed CT image along the dental arcades of Ramesses II's mummy shows multiple rounded, small, moderately dense structures placed in groups within the cavities of nose (short arrows) and mouth (long arrow).

Merenptah.[31] Semiliquid mud and sawdust were often used to fill the neck region. Fat and soda mixtures filled the faces of some mummies of the Twenty-first Dynasty,[32] though we suggest that this practice may have begun earlier, as discussed below.[33] The literature has also identified different types of abdominal fillers, such as dried lichen in the mummies of Merenptah, Siptah, and Ramesses IV, and sawdust in Ramesses V.[34]

Head Mummification and Excerebration

The ancient Egyptians believed that the 'soul' was associated with the heart, and saw no reason to preserve the brain. Excerebration during mummification became a common practice in the Eighteenth Dynasty, although attempts as early as the Fourth Dynasty have been reported.[35] In a recent study, Andrew D. Wade and colleagues indicated that the peak of excerebration was in the Ptolemaic Period.[36]

The ancient Egyptians removed the brain by inserting a tool into the nose to perforate the thin weak part of the skull base, at the ACF (transnasal craniotomy). According to Herodotus, piecemeal extraction of the brain was expedited by flushing the cranium with "drugs."[37] The body was then turned prone or held in an upright position to allow drainage of the brain. Embalming materials such as resin were sometimes introduced inside the skull.[38] It is worth noting that while excerebration appeared earlier, the introduction of resin into the cranial cavity appeared first in this collection of royal mummies.[39]

MDCT provided the opportunity to examine brain treatment in selected royal mummies from the Eighteenth to the early Twentieth Dynasty. We reported remarkable variations related to brain treatment, skull defects, size of brain removed, and intracranial contents[40] (table 26).

CT of the mummified heads of Thutmose II, Thutmose III, and the mummy that was alleged to be Thutmose I (see chapter 3, "The Discovery of the Mummy of Queen Hatshepsut, and Examination of the Mummies of Her Family"), who have all been dated to the early Eighteenth Dynasty, show intact skull bases with preserved brains and overlying meninges. Reformatted CT images in sagittal planes helped in accurate assessment of the skull base and negated the presence of any defects. The intact desiccated brain appears in CT as a medium-density mass with irregular, undulating border and preserved midline longitudinal fissure; it usually occupies the posterior part of the skull.[41] However, the presence of residual meninges is not an indicator for brain preservation, as they can be found even when the brain has been completely removed. Intactness of the skull and presence of the desiccated brain in CT images indicate that no brain treatment had been performed on those mummies (fig. 92).

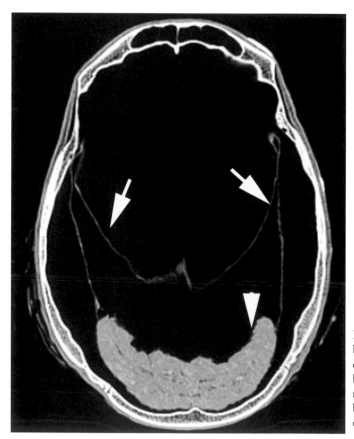

Fig. 92: Intact skull with preserved brain. Axial CT image of the skull of Thutmose II shows shrunken brain at the back of the skull with moderate density and undulating border (arrowhead) as well as the overlying meninges (arrows).

CT study of royal mummies dated later in the Eighteenth Dynasty through the early Twentieth Dynasty shows evidence of transnasal craniotomy; these included Yuya, Thuya, Amenhotep III, Tiye, Seti I, Ramesses II, Merenptah, and Ramesses III.[42] Previous radiographic studies of Eighteenth through Twentieth Dynasty pharaohs also suggested brain removal in Ahmose I, Amenhotep II, Akhenaten,[43] and Tutankhamun.[44]

In transnasal craniotomy, the tool is inserted into one or both nostrils. This approach resulted in damage to the nasal turbinates and the ethmoid bone. Damage to the nasal septum, occasionally detected in mummies, could be due to nasal penetration of the cranium, but could also result from nasal packing alone.[45] In x-ray films, damaged nasal passages could only be hinted at by the absence of obvious contours and interfaces;[46] however, these structures can be clearly visualized on CT scans.[47] Disturbance of the CT anatomy of nasal passages suggests that the right nostril was used in the mummies of Yuya, Amenhotep III, Tiye, and Ramesses II; the left nostril seemed to be utilized in other mummies, such as in Merenptah and Ramesses III. However, in certain occasions with wider destruction of the nasal passages, such as in the mummies of Thuya and Seti I, this distinction was difficult to evaluate, and likely both nostrils were utilized in the procedure.[48]

The study reported variation in the size of a skull defect, a sequela of the transnasal craniotomy, from a small defect in Yuya to a large one in Amenhotep III and Seti I. The average area of ACF bony defects in mummies dated to the Eighteenth Dynasty measured 532 mm², while it was larger (632 mm²) in those dated later, to the Nineteenth to early Twentieth Dynasties. The size of the anatomical

disturbance in the craniotomy passage does not seem to be attributable to carelessness during the procedure, but rather could be related to other technical conditions, such as inflicting a larger defect to enable the introduction of variable intracranial materials (see below).

Removal of the brain by ways other than transnasal has been reported a few times in the literature.[49] Transforaminal craniotomy is removal of the brain by way of the foramen magnum (the large orifice in the base of the skull through which the spinal cord passes to the spine). Transforaminal craniotomy had been described in King Ahmose, the founder of the Eighteenth Dynasty.[50] While the transnasal craniotomy has been linked to the Theban School of mummification, the transforaminal craniotomy has been linked to a different geographic origin: Memphis.[51] It is interesting to note that both embalming approaches (transnasal and transforaminal) have been reported in King Tutankhamun.[52]

In addition to transnasal craniotomy, we reported in Merenptah a right posterior parietal skull defect. The defect has beveled, sharp edges with pointed margins that are longer in the outer than inner skull plate, which indicate that it was inflicted by a sharp, pointed, solid tool. Absence of sclerosis or healing signs suggested that the lesion was likely postmortem and deliberately induced by the embalmers to utilize in brain treatment, rather than being inflicted by tomb robbers[53] (see plate 55).

The size of the brain residues and intracranial contents varied markedly in the mummies with CT evidence of transnasal craniotomies. In Thuya, the embalmers left the skull empty after removal of the brain (see fig. 93). In other mummies, specifically Yuya, Ramesses II, Merenptah, and Ramesses III,

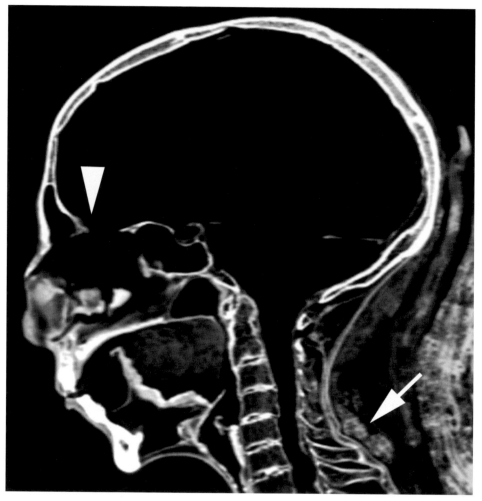

Fig. 93: Removal of brain without introducing an embalming material. Sagittal CT image of the skull of mummified Thuya shows an empty skull. Interruption of the skull base (arrowhead) indicates removal of the brain transnasally. However, the embalmers did not introduce any embalming material intracranially. Note the linen pack that was placed behind the tongue in the mouth cavity. An arrow points to linen packs treated with resin overlying the skin layer and not to be confused with subcutaneous packs. (After Saleem and Hawass, "Variability in Brain Treatment.")

the embalmers filled the cranial cavity after excerebration with variable amounts of different embalming materials such as resin, soil, and linen.[54] CT can also differentiate between desiccated brain residue and intracranial embalming materials. Brain residue is charac-

terized by its low CT density, mottled appearance, and undulating surface.[55] Resin is commonly poured inside the skull; it is identified by its structureless, homogeneous, moderately high-density CT appearance (see fig. 90a).[56] Coexistence of both CT appearances suggests a brain residue impregnated with resin, as in the mummies of Yuya and Seti I. CT images identified the heterogeneous, soil-like material inside the skull of Seti I.[57]

Embalmers used linen as intracranial embalming material in the case of Merenptah. CT identified linen as threadlike, low-density, convoluted structures. Through visual inspection, Elliot Smith previously indicated that Merenptah's skull was stuffed with small pieces of linen and balsam.[58] Unlike CT, plain x-rays cannot detect cranial packing unless it contains radiopaque material such as resin.[59] For this reason, previous plain x-ray studies failed to identify the contents within the skull of Merenptah, but were able to identify the radiopaque resin inside the skulls of Ramesses II and Ramesses III.[60]

When introduced in the nasal cavity as a liquid, resin settles to the most dependent point of the skull and forms a straight level. CT shows that the intracranial contents (brain residue or embalming materials or both) of the royal mummies of Amenhotep III, Tiye, Seti I, Ramesses II, and Ramesses III occupy the dependent posterior aspect of their skulls. This backward position of the contents within the skull indicated that the body was lying supine in a resting position during introduction of this embalming material. Changing the position of the head while introducing the resin may result in multiple fluid levels.[61] In the mummified head of Tutankhamun, the presence of two fluid levels, one along the top of the skull (vertex) and the other backward, suggested that fluid was introduced with the top of the skull lying downwards, and then with the body and head in a resting supine position, although this would seem to be very challenging (fig. 94).[62] CT of the skull of Yuya shows two perpendicular

levels of resin: one at the back and the other parallel to its top (vault). This may suggest that the fluid was introduced inside the skull while the head was first in a resting supine position, then in a sitting position before the resin solidified (see fig. 24a in chapter 4). On the other hand, the CT appearance of multiple resin components inside Ramesses II's skull is likely caused by dural partitions, rather than positioning during mummification.[63]

Brain treatment in the case of Merenptah's mummy was unique, as the embalmers used linen and stuffed it in the front part of the skull. In the other studied mummies, the embalming materials (mostly resin) were placed at the back of the skull. Unlike pouring resin fluid, introducing linen threads using the usual transnasal route would have been a very difficult task for embalmers to do. For this reason, we assumed that in addition to the usual transnasal route, the embalmers inflicted a defect at the back of Merenptah's skull (in the right posterior parietal bone) (see plate 55) to stuff the linen. This assumption is supported by the fact that the bulk of intracranial material is located at the front of the skull, more at the right side with deviation of the interhemispheric dura to the left.[64] Although this hole at the back of Merenptah's skull was noted in previous forensic and radiographic reports, its purpose was not attributed to mummification but rather to an occult reason or a spiritual practice such as providing the spirit with a means of escape.[65]

CT findings emphasized the variability with respect to the style of cranial mummification among these royal mummies. CT documented larger size and more variability in the intracranial embalming materials in mummies dated to the Nineteenth to

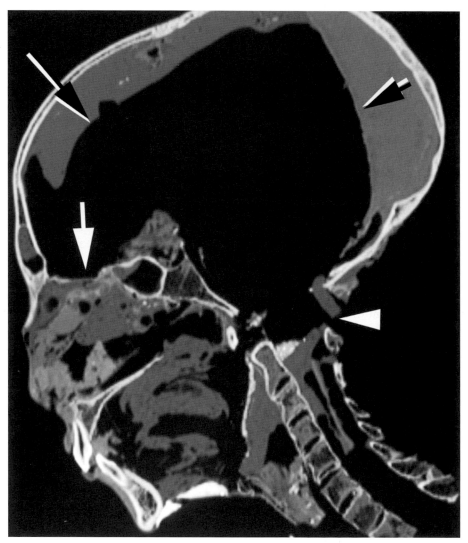

Fig. 94: Sagittal CT image of skull of mummified Tutankhamun. White arrow points to anterior cranial fossa bony defect that the embalmers used for transnasal craniotomy. Short black arrow indicates the resin level at the back of the skull that was introduced in the recumbent position. Long black arrow points to resin lining the vertex that was likely introduced in the skull while the head was tilted backward. White arrowhead shows resin at the opening in the base of the skull (foramen magnum), suggestive of a possible additional (transforaminal) route of cranial mummification.

Twentieth Dynasties (57.5% [SD 5] of the total volume of the skull) in comparison to those dating to the Eighteenth (29% [SD 18.6]). This may explain the relatively larger skull-base defects utilized in transcranial excerebration in Nineteenth to Twentieth

Dynasty mummies when compared with those of the Eighteenth Dynasty, when resin-like fluid was mainly used.

CT documented the variability in brain treatment even over a span of a few years. For example, Thuya's skull had a large skull-base defect, but without CT evidence of cranial packing. This is unlike her husband, Yuya, who had a smaller bony defect and an abundant amount of intracranial resin.[66] This continuous experimentation in brain treatment in royal Egyptian identities was likely for the sake of perfecting the technique of mummification.[67]

The final step in transnasal craniotomy was sealing the nose passages and artificial defects with embalming materials.[68] In CT images, we noted variations in mummification of the nasal passages of the royal mummies in the study (table 27). While there were no significant embalming materials in the nasal passages of the mummies of Amenhotep III, Tiye, and so-called Thutmose I, CT identified different nasal fillings in the mummies of Thutmose II, Thutmose III, Yuya, Thuya, Seti I, Ramesses II, Merenptah, and Ramesses III. Nasal fillings included resin, linen packing, linen tampons impregnated with resin, the bone of a small animal, and plant seeds.[69] CT scanning can identify rolled-linen nasal packs by their characteristic folded appearance. Folded, resin-impregnated nasal linen in Thutmose II appeared as alternating low- and high-density layers, while the likely untreated nasal packs in Thutmose III appeared as heterogeneous low-density structures[70] (fig. 95). Unlike CT, untreated linen packing or low-density nasal tampons are not appreciable on plain x-rays.[71] Nasal passages were sealed with resin in the mummies of Yuya, Seti I, and Ramesses II.[72]

Evisceration: Removal of Viscera and Visceral Packs

The embalmers must have realized early in their practice of mummification that by removing the internal organs, the body would be much less susceptible to putrefaction. Abdominal incisions were inflicted by embalmers to remove viscera. The early evidence of evisceration through an incision in the left flank of the body was dated to the Fourth Dynasty. However, several royal mummies in the Eleventh Dynasty had their viscera removed without evidence of abdominal incisions. In such cases, the viscera could have been dissolved by introducing chemical materials and then extracted through the anus.[73] Before the Eighteenth Dynasty, incisions were vertical on the left flank. Later, incisions extended obliquely from iliac crest to inguinal region. Other reported locations of incisions were the epigastrium and anterior pelvis.

The royal mummies that we studied by CT dated to a time when mummification had developed and achieved its 'classic phase.' At that time, the abdominal incisions were inflicted at the left inguinal region. The incisions were either sealed with resin, stitched, or both (fig. 96).[74] Two- and three-dimensional CT images enabled exact localization and measurements of the extent of the abdominal incisions used in evisceration of the royal mummies (table 28). CT images identified obliquely oriented incisions at the left inguinal region in the mummies of 'Thutmose I,' Thutmose III, Yuya, Ramesses II, and Ramesses III (see plate 64d). The incision was more vertically oriented at the left inguinal region of the mummy of Thuya. Mutilation of and defects in the torsos of the other mummies, likely caused by ancient tomb robbers, prevented the detection of

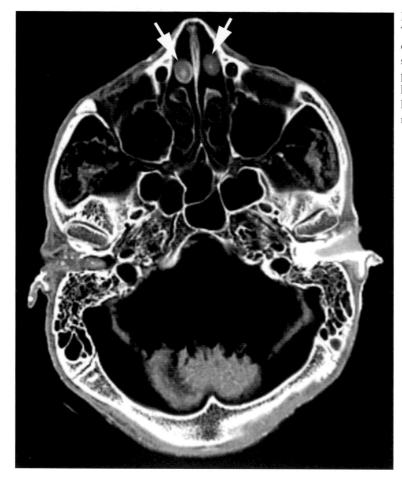

Fig. 95: Nasal packs in Thutmose II. Axial CT image of the skull of Thutmose II shows elaborate rounded nasal packs with alternating low and higher CT densities indicating linen tampons treated with resin (arrows).

abdominal incisions in the mummies of Thutmose II, Amenhotep III, Tiye, the mother of Tutankhamun, Seti I, and Merenptah. A resin-treated pack was detected at the base of the abdominal incision in Thutmose III, Thuya, and Ramesses II (fig. 97). The embalming incision in Tutankhamun is unique in its direction; it extends diagonally from the center of the abdomen (roughly the navel site) toward the left iliac crest. The embalming incisions were not stitched or covered by any metallic plates. However, a small pierced stone (bead) is seen

on the body surface of Thuya, just below the lower edge of the left inguinal incision; this bead could have been placed for wound protection (see plate 64b).

In the New Kingdom, the viscera removed through the incision were generally treated with natron and spices, wrapped, and placed in four canopic jars, each with a lid in either the form of a human head, or a different head of one of the Four Sons of the god Horus who protected the viscera (plate 65). In the latter case, the human-headed (Imesti) jar contained the mummified liver, the baboon-headed

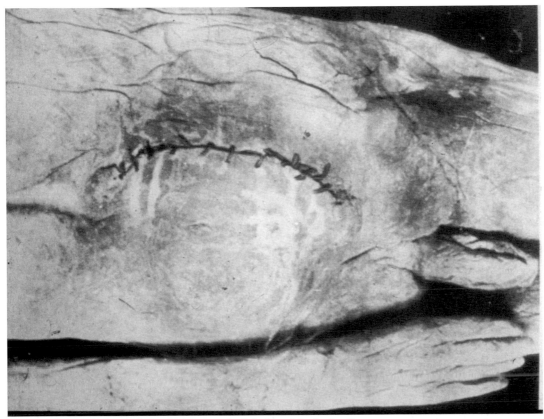

Fig. 96: The stitched embalming incision on the left side of the body of a mummy.

(Hapi) the lungs, the jackal-headed (Duamutef) the stomach, and the falcon-headed (Qebehsenuef) the intestine.[75] The viscera were sometimes inserted into miniature coffins, which were placed in a canopic chest, as was found in the tomb of Tutankhamun (plate 66).

During the process of evisceration, the heart was preserved and kept in place. CT images in coronal plane clearly identified the presence of the heart within the chest of the mummified 'Thutmose I,' Thutmose II, Thutmose III, Thuya, Tiye, the mother of Tutankhamun, Ramesses II, and Ramesses III. Transverse CT images showed that the heart

of Thutmose II was surrounded by a resin-treated pack. A heart amulet likely within heart residue was identified in CT images of the chest of Seti I. No CT evidence of the heart could be identified within the mummies of Yuya, Amenhotep III, Tutankhamun, or Merenptah. Apart from the heart, no other viscera were detected within the torsos of the royal mummies we examined with CT images.

The emptied body cavity would be washed with water and palm wine, then packed with natron for desiccation, spices such as myrrh for scent, resin for disinfection, and linen for absorbing fluids. The body would be covered with natron and allowed to dry. When the

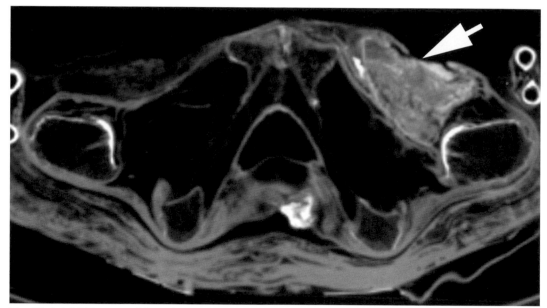

Fig. 97: Axial CT image of the pelvic region of Thuya shows a linen pack within the left inguinal defect that was used for evisceration (arrow).

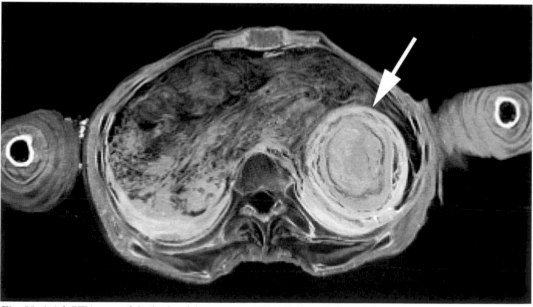

Fig. 98: Axial CT image of the body of the mummy KV60 B identified an elaborate visceral pack of linen impregnated with resin (arrow). The rest of the body cavity is filled with free linen threads partly impregnated with resin. A thin layer of resin is lining the posterior wall.

final wrapping took place, the body cavities would be filled with linen packs soaked in resin to hold their shape and to repel insects (fig. 98).[76] It has been stated that from the Nineteenth Dynasty onward, the body was stuffed very carefully so as not to be squashed by bandages and to preserve its shape.[77] Upon examination of CT images, we found that this applied not only to the Nineteenth and Twentieth Dynasty mummies, but also to royal mummies dated earlier, to the Eighteenth Dynasty. In some of these mummies, namely Thutmose II, Thutmose III, Thuya, and Yuya, we found that the body cavity was almost filled with different embalming materials. However, this could not be assessed in mummies with mutilated torsos (Amenhotep III, Tiye, and the mother of Tutankhamun), due to possible spillage of the cavity contents through the defective wall. The torso cavities of the mummies of Seti I and Ramesses II (Nineteenth Dynasty) as well as Ramesses III (Twentieth Dynasty) were almost filled with embalming materials (fig. 99). This is unlike the mummy of Merenptah (Nineteenth Dynasty), which showed a smaller volume of embalming materials within the torso. The embalmers used different materials to fill the eviscerated torso cavity, such as resin, non-treated linen fibers, linen packs impregnated with resin, soil or sawdust, sand, and stones. CT images showed that the body of Seti I had a distinctive, generous amount of resin that layered its body cavities, extended to the subcutaneous tissues, and partly penetrated the adjacent bones and vertebral bodies. Occasionally, the genital and anal orifices were plugged with linen or dense stone-like materials (as was seen in Thuya), probably to prevent the filler from leaking.

The embalmers stuffed the body of the mummies to retain their shape and to avoid being crushed under the pressure of the bandages;[78] this concurs with the concept of cosmetic care.

Cosmetic Care and Beautification of Mummies

In addition to the elaborate desiccation methods, the embalmers (especially of the royal mummies dated to the New Kingdom) intended to make the corpse look as lifelike as possible. Cosmetic care is identified as efforts involving or relating to treatment intended to restore or improve a subject's appearance.[79]

Cosmetic care of mummies included false hair locks and painted black lines to emphasize eyebrows and hairlines. Occasionally the hair had been hennaed; in the instance of Yuya, the blond hair was likely due to a reaction between henna and the materials used in embalming, or faded henna on white hair.[80]

We studied the CT images of the selected New Kingdom royal mummies and recorded the morphology of the preserved body parts, as well as the presence of embalming materials, filling substances, or packs as evidence of efforts of the embalmers to beautify the corpse. We found that many of these mummies showed signs of cosmetic care lavished on them by the embalmers (tables 26–30).

Eyes

To enhance the face, starting from the latter part of the Eighteenth Dynasty, small pieces of linen were placed over the eyes, to hide sinking, and the eyelids were closed and sealed, usually with glue or other adhesive substance.[81] The embalmers also used onions as artificial eyes, as in the mummy of Ramesses IV (Twentieth Dynasty).[82] The mummies of

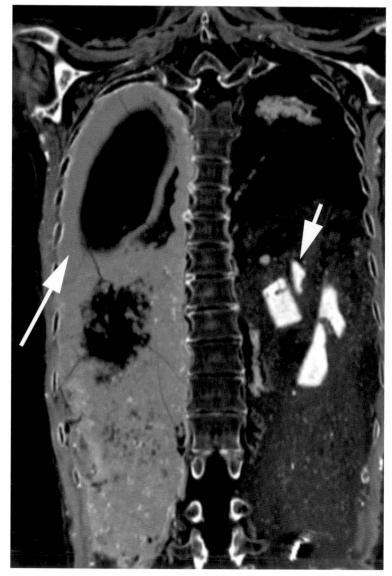

Fig. 99: Coronal reconstructed CT image of the body of Ramesses III shows that it was almost filled with different embalming materials: homogeneous, moderately dense resin (long arrow) and dense amulets (short arrow) buried in a heterogeneous, low-density substance that could be sawdust or soil.

'Thutmose I' and Thutmose II of the early Eighteenth Dynasty showed no embalming materials within their orbits. Desiccated eye globes and other related tissues are seen within the orbits of 'Thutmose I' and Thutmose II, of low CT density except the lens, which has high

CT density (fig. 100). All of the other mummies that we studied from later dates showed inhomogeneous materials inserted within the orbits, likely representing a primitive form of artificial eyes (table 29). The CT densities of the orbital packs varied roughly from –700 to

300 HU; they are likely formed of linen either untreated or treated with resin (fig. 101). Large amounts of resin are exceptionally noted within the orbits of Seti I; the resin had probably been introduced into the orbits in a hot liquid state, as it is seen tracking into the optic canals and smearing the surrounding meninges (fig. 102). We noted dense, small, flat structures (2100 to 2300 HU) in front of both right and left orbital fillings of Seti I; a similar finding was noted at the periphery of the left orbital pack of the mother of Tutankhamun. These dense structures could have been placed by the embalmers for cosmetic reasons or resulted from accidental smearing.

The embalmers usually inserted the orbital packs without removing the eyes, which are sometimes seen displaced by packs. These orbital packs were usually inserted in front of the eye globes. Exceptions are the mummies of Amenhotep III and Seti I, with abundant resin within their orbits. In this situation, the resin likely solidified in the dependent posterior part of the orbit, pushing the eye globe to the front of the pack.

Nose

In addition to their function in plugging the nasal openings to protect the corpse from insects, the nasal packs also seem to have had a cosmetic purpose, to preserve the shape of the nose and make it withstand the pressure of the bandages applied during mummification. The distinctive nose of Ramesses II received special care to preserve its pronounced shape, as it was fully packed with resin, plant seeds, and a small animal bone

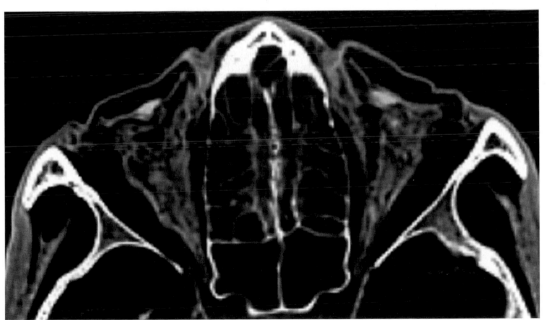

Fig. 100: Axial CT image of the orbits of the mummy of Thutmose II shows desiccated tissues (eye globes, optic nerves, and muscles) with no evidence of any inserted embalming material. Note the concavity of the eyelids, which has resulted in a sunken eye appearance.

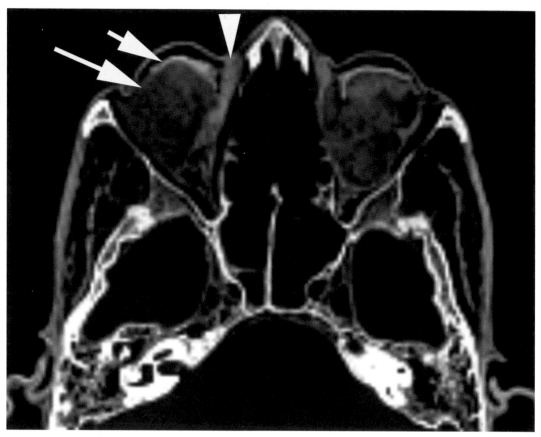

Fig. 101: Axial CT image of the skull of Thuya at the level of the orbits shows low-density linen packs (long arrow) inserted within the orbits. A thin layer of resin was added by the embalmers on the surface of the linen pack (short arrow). The desiccated eye globe or muscles were not usually removed (arrowhead). Note that the orbital pack resulted in a smooth bulge underneath the eyelid, which gives a real-life appearance to the eyes.

(fig. 103). The noses of the other royal mummies in the study contained nontreated or resin-treated linen, were filled with resin, or contained no fillings (see table 27). It seems that the nasal packs preserved well the shapes of the noses of Yuya, Thuya, Tiye, the mother of Tutankhamun, and Seti I. However, despite the presence of nasal packs, the soft parts of the noses of Merenptah and Ramesses III were flattened by the bandages, spoiling the appearance of their faces.

Mouth and throat

Filling the mouth and throat, like packing of the other parts of the body, may have been intended by the embalmers to fill out body areas that otherwise would shrink or collapse. Packing of a mummy's mouth may have helped to mold the face into its proper form,[83] and similar treatment of the throat was meant to maintain a lifelike appearance of the mummy's neck.

Table 30 indicates the different embalming materials detected on CT images in the oral

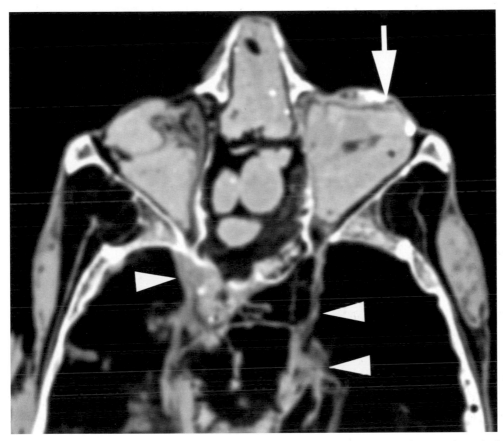

Fig. 102: Axial CT image of the orbits of Seti I: The orbits contain heterogeneous linen packs soaked in large amounts of moderately dense resin. It seems that resin was poured in a hot liquid state, as it is seen tracking into the optic canals and smearing the meninges (arrowheads). The very dense substance on the surface of the orbital pack (arrow) could have been intentionally placed by the embalmers for cosmetic reasons or could be a mere accidental smearing.

cavity and pharynx of the mummies that we studied. No embalming materials were seen within the oral cavity or pharynx of 'Thutmose I.' A linen pack was inserted within the mouth cavity of the mummy of the mother of Tutankhamun. The other examined mummies showed embalming materials inserted in each mouth cavity, as well as in the upper part of the throat (oropharynx) (see fig. 93). The embalming materials inserted within the mouth and pharynx of the royal mummies included resin (Amenhotep III); nontreated linen packs (Yuya, Thuya, and the mother of Tutankhamun); linen impregnated with resin (Tiye and Merenptah); and parcels of grains (Ramesses II). The embalming materials were inserted deeper in the throat (the hypopharynx) of Yuya and Seti I. This, in addition to other maneuvers, namely subcutaneous packing, created a full throat, which likely enhanced the appearance of the neck (figs. 104a–b).[84]

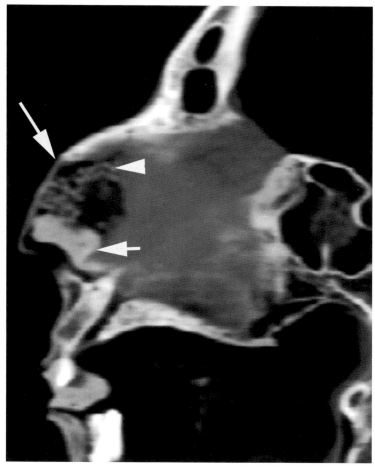

Fig. 103: Sagittal CT image of the head of Ramesses II shows that the embalmers filled the nasal cavity with multiple embalming materials to preserve the distinctive shape of the nose (long arrow). The filling materials include a long bone of a small animal (short arrow), plant seeds (arrowhead), and resin.

Male genitalia (penis and scrotum) (figs. 105a–c)

The ancient Egyptian embalmers were meticulously careful to make all body parts of the mummy look good, including the genital area. The penis of Tutankhamun was mummified as though fully erect, as documented at the time of the unwrapping of the mummy.[85] It was widely thought that the phallus had disappeared since the unwrapping,[86] but it is possible that it can be located in the sand tray on which the mummy now rests.

Physical examinations of the royal mummies by Maspero (1886) and G.E. Smith (1906) identified the external genital organs of some mummies but failed to comment on others, probably due to the presence of wrappings, for example in Seti I and Ramesses III.[87] We examined by CT the external genital regions of the selected New Kingdom mummies[88] (table 31). We noted the presence of the penises of 'Thutmose I,' Thutmose II, Yuya, Merenptah, and Ramesses III. In our CT studies, the mummified penises appeared as cylindrical or flat tubular structures of variable lengths that ranged between 41 and 105 mm. The mummified penile tissues of the kings of

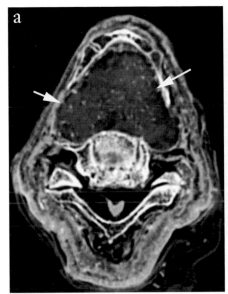

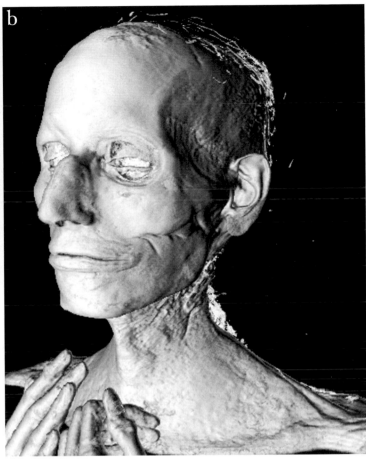

Figs. 104a–b: Embalming material filling the mouth and throat of mummified Yuya. Axial CT image of the neck (a) shows that the embalmers stuffed the throat (hypopharynx) of the mummy with a heterogeneous, low-density material (between arrows). Filling the throat helped to give the neck a full, lifelike appearance, as demonstrated in an oblique frontal 3D CT image of the neck and upper chest region of the mummy of Yuya (b).

the earlier Eighteeenth Dynasty ('Thutmose I' and Thutmose II) have low CT densities (−20 to 40 HU). The mummified penises of later royal family members (Yuya, Merenptah, and Ramesses III) have higher CT densities (200 to 300 HU); this may suggest that resin or other unidentified materials were used to infiltrate and mummify the penile tissues. A central low-density, tube-like structure (−700 to −500 HU) is identified within the higher-density mummified penile tissue (likely representing an air-filled urethra).[89]

We identified a sac of about 5 cm in diameter in the CT images of Yuya, located at the perineum and behind the penis. The sac contains a mixture of high- and low-density materials. The upper part of the sac is in continuity with the body's skin. We suggest that this structure is a scrotum that was opened by the embalmers and filled with embalming materials to give it a lifelike appearance, rather than being a pack that was placed to support the organ. The literature has reported a similar procedure in a mummy dated to the Twenty-first Dynasty: the embalmers filled out the empty scrotum (likely due to a hernia) with mud to make it look better.[90]

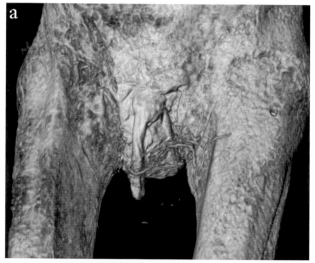

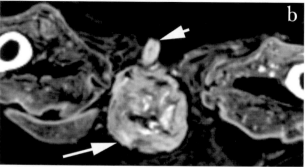

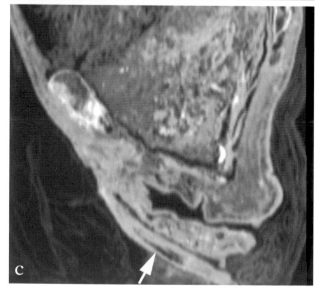

Nonvisualization of the genital organs in the CT images of mummies of Amenhotep III, Seti I, and Ramesses II likely denotes that these organs are missing.[91]

G.E. Smith reported that Merenptah's scrotum was missing. He noted a transverse cut between the base of the penis and anus, and that the area had been coated with resin, indicating that this defect had been inflicted prior to the completion of the embalming process. Our CT studies confirmed the absence of Merenptah's scrotum and most of the penis (except for a stump at the base). Three-dimensional CT images also showed the transverse scar dimple between the penis base and anus (see sidelight in chapter 9, "Questions about Ramesses II and Merenptah").

Subcutaneous packs

With the intention of beautifying the corpse, the embalmers in the Old Kingdom covered the body of some mummies with molded linen and painted their eyes and eyebrows. A famous example is a male mummy from the Fifth Dynasty with his body and face modeled and colored with black for the hair, green for the eyes and eyebrows, and reddish brown for the mouth.[92] However, most mummies of the Middle and New Kingdoms did not involve facial modeling in linen. An exception is an Eleventh Dynasty mummy from Deir al-Barsha, whose face was covered by linen and colored in a manner similar to that of the Old Kingdom.[93]

Figs. 105a–c: CT of the genital organs of Yuya. Three-dimensional reconstructed CT image of the body of Yuya (a) shows a well-preserved male organ and scrotum. Axial CT image (b) shows the scrotum filled with heterogeneous mixed low and high densities (long arrow) and the penis (short arrow). Sagittal CT image along the penis (c) shows a low-density tubular-like structure within (arrow) that could be trapped air within the urethra.

In contrast to Old Kingdom mummification, the trend starting from the Third Intermediate Period was to make the corpse itself look as lifelike as possible. This was done by more elaborate procedures such as making incisions in the skin of the corpse and stuffing packs underneath it (subcutaneously) in order to return it to the shape it had been during life. The locations of these incisions were included in the text of the Rhind Magical Papyrus, which listed seventeen cuts (seven in the head, four in the chest, two in the legs, two in the arms, one in the abdomen, and one in the back). In addition, the face was filled from the mouth (transbuccal) (fig. 106).[94]

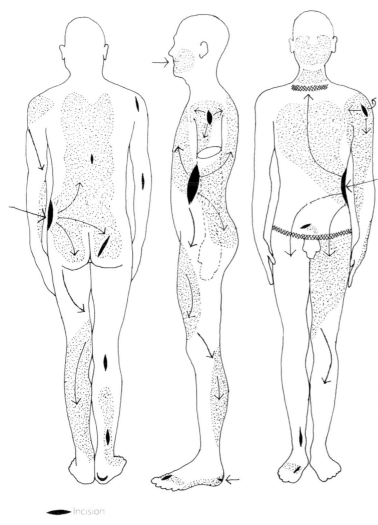

Incision
Stuffing
Linen plugs

Fig. 106: A diagram of the locations of the skin incisions that were used by the embalmers to stuff packs underneath, as included in the text of the Rhind Magical Papyrus. The evisceration cut in the left flank was used to reach the different regions of the body. A space underneath the skin was dissected. The neck was packed, then the torso, followed by the lower back, buttocks, and legs. The packing was stopped up with linen plugs. Additional incisions in the ankles and soles were used to pack the feet. The upper limbs were packed through incisions made in the shoulders, as well as in the elbows and hands. (Diagram courtesy of Salima Ikram; drawing by Nicholas Warner.)

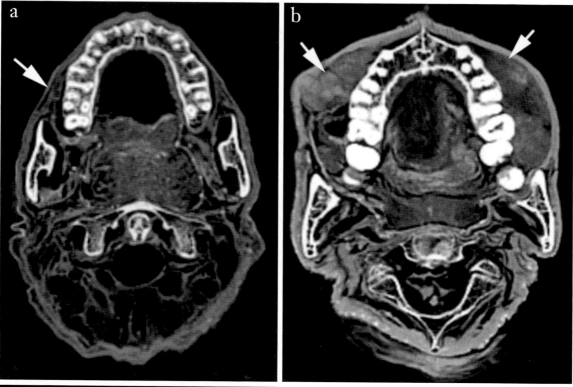

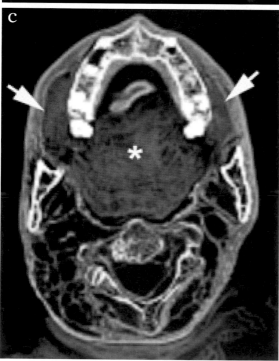

Figs. 107a–f: Subcutaneous packing. Axial CT image of the face of Tiye (a) at the level of the maxillary sinuses shows the thin, desiccated soft tissues of the face (arrow). The mummy was not offered any facial subcutaneous filling. Axial CT image of the face of Thutmose III (b) at the level of the maxilla shows packing beneath the skin on both sides of the face (arrows) with heterogeneous material, likely linen impregnated with resin. Axial CT image of the face of Thuya (c) at the level of the maxilla shows continuation of the subcutaneous low-density material in the face (arrows) with the mouth cavity (asterisk). This proves that the embalmers used the mouth (transbuccal) for packing under the skin of the face. Axial CT image of the right thigh of Tutankhamun (d) shows subcutaneous packing (arrow). Sagittal CT image of the hand of Seti I (e) shows subcutaneous packing of the palm and the first web space (arrow); note also subcutaneous packing of the forearm (arrowhead). Sagittal CT image of the foot and ankle of Seti I (f) shows a thick subcutaneous dense pack (likely resin) at the sole of the foot (arrow).

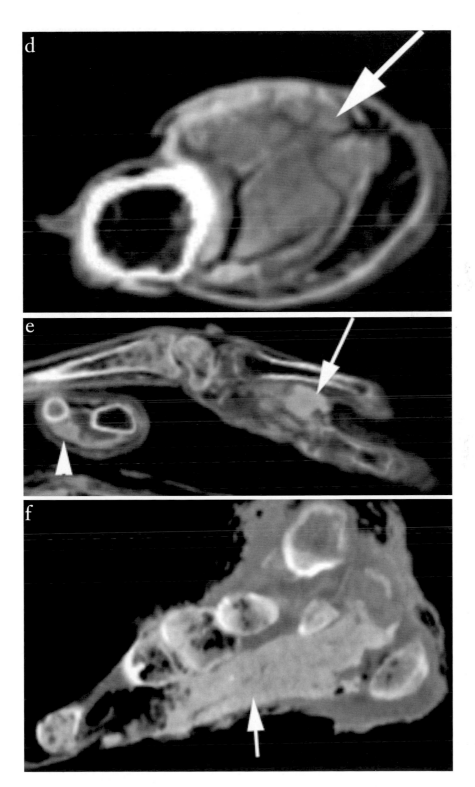

It has been widely disseminated in the archaeological literature that subcutaneous packing was not usually done until the Twenty-first Dynasty, as exemplified in the mummies of Nodjmet, Henttawy, Maetkare, Masaharta, and Nesikhonsu.[95] The only two reports that described the procedure in mummies earlier than the Twenty-first Dynasty were for Amenhotep III by physical inspection, and in a CT study by the authors of a mummified fetus (daughter of Tutankhamun; see chapter 6, "The Two Fetuses Found in the Tomb of Tutankhamun");[96] both were dated to the Eighteenth Dynasty.

The author of this book (SNS) studied the CT scans of thirteen royal mummies dating to the Eighteenth to Twentieth Dynasties to determine if they were stuffed with embalming materials beneath their skin.[97] Our CT studies showed evidence of subcutaneous fillings in twelve mummies, while the mummy of 'Thutmose I' showed no such CT evidence. In each mummy, subcutaneous filling involved one or more of the following regions: face, neck, torso, and limbs. However, the mummies of Tiye (fig. 107a) and Ramesses II showed very limited subcutaneous fillings in the front of the lower neck (suprasternal) in Tiye, and in the medial cheek of Ramesses II.

The subcutaneous packing procedure succeeded in giving a lifelike appearance to the faces of the mummies. The facial packs were comparable in size on both sides and thus had not resulted in significant asymmetry of the mummy's face. The embalmers were meticulously careful to ensure that the procedure did not result in any significant bony or soft-tissue destruction or deformity.[98]

Previous reports of mummies dated to the Twenty-first Dynasty and later indicated variable aesthetic results of the subcutaneous filling of the mummies. In the mummy of Queen Henttawy (Twenty-first Dynasty), the embalmers overfilled her cheeks with a fat and soda mixture that resulted in burst skin and deformed face.[99]

The literature has reported different substances that were used in subcutaneous filling, such as linen tampons, sawdust, sand, semiliquid mud, and mixtures of fat and soda.[100] The chemical nature of the filling substances of the subcutaneous packs was not tested in our studies.

Breasts were left unstuffed in the royal female mummies that we studied by CT. It has been noted, however, that in later times (Third Intermediate Period), females' breasts were also packed beneath the skin.[101]

Multiple Restorations

Some mummies were subjected to several restorations by the embalmers at different times. Although the body of the mummy of Seti I was badly affected by tomb robbers, the head is well preserved and exhibits an excellent mummification job. The mummy was the subject of several later restorations, as the series of linen and coffin dockets associated with his mummy attests. (See details in chapter 9, "The Nineteenth Dynasty.")

Mummification Features as Dating Criteria

There are limitations in the system that scholars have used to date Egyptian mummification, as it was based mainly on observations reported from forensic examinations more than a century ago[102] and later on radiographic studies limited to plain x-rays.[103] One limitation is that some bodies found in the royal caches were placed in antiquity into coffins designed for others; this has resulted in uncertainty regarding the identity of some of the royal mummies.

This CT study of the royal Egyptian mummies is the first to use modern imaging of a large group of royal bodies dated to a limited period of time. The study succeeded in outlining specific features of mummification that are now firmly identified by reliable diagnostic criteria, other than those for the vari-ous periods defined by physical inspection or limited investigations. For example, we proved that the elaborate, unique method of subcutaneous insertion of filling materials, a feature that was long thought to begin in Dynasty Twenty-one, was actually well established in the Eighteenth Dynasty.[104] We also described variability and new routes for brain treatment, stuffing the throat, and preservation of the male organs.[105]

Table 24. Age, stature, preservation status, and position of upper limbs in selected royal mummies, as revealed by MDCT

Name	Royal status	Age	Stature
so-called Thutmose I	Member of the royal family?	About 20 Y	157 cm
Thutmose II	King	30 Y	173 cm
Thutmose III	King	40 Y+	167 cm**
Yuya	Nobleman (father of Queen Tiye)	50–60 Y	165 cm
Thuya	Noblewoman (mother of Queen Tiye)	50–60 Y	145 cm
Amenhotep III	King	50 Y	154 cm**
Tiye	Queen (wife of Amenhotep III)	40–50 Y	146 cm
Akhenaten	King	35–45 Y	160 cm
Mother of Tutankhamun	Queen (wife of Akhenaten)	25–35 Y	158 cm
Tutankhamun	King	19 Y	167 cm
317a	Princess (daughter of Tutankhamun)	Fetus: about 24 weeks (5–6 months)	29.9 cm**
317b	Princess (daughter of Tutankhamun)	Fetus: about 36 weeks (9 months)	45 cm**
Seti I	King	40–50 Y	167 cm
Ramesses II	King	Over 70 Y	170 cm
Merenptah	King	50–60 Y	171 cm
Ramesses III	King	60 Y	163 cm

* Despite injuries to upper limbs inflicted by tomb robbers, the position of the fractured upper limbs was restored in antiquity to the royal crossed-arms position.

Current general preservation status	Upper limb position
Well preserved in general. Both hands are broken and missing; chest injury	Arms are stretched down the side of body and hands are broken off and missing
Fairly preserved. Multiple fractures of upper and lower limbs, thoracic and pelvic girdles. Injury of anterior wall of torso	Arms are crossed over chest, right over left, left hand clenched over the right shoulder, right hand flat over the chest*
Poorly preserved. The head and limbs are detached from the body. Multiple fractures of limbs and pelvis. Injury of soft tissue of the nose	Arms cross over chest, right over left. The right hand is flat. The left hand is flexed with the thumb extended up*
Well preserved. No significant bony or soft-tissue injuries	Flexed elbows, both hands below the chin
Well preserved. No significant bony or soft-tissue injuries	Both upper limbs alongside the body, hands flat
Poorly preserved. Head and limbs are detached from the body. Disrupted pelvis. Missing large amounts of soft tissues of the face and body	Severe mutilation—cannot be assessed
Fairly preserved. A large defect in the anterior wall of the torso and disarticulated feet	Right upper limb alongside body with hand flat over right groin. Left arm crossed over the chest, left hand tightly clenched, with raised thumb (as if holding something)
Poorly preserved. A skeletonized mummy	Cannot be assessed because of severe mutilation
Fairly preserved. Bony and soft-tissue defect of the face and anterior chest wall. Disarticulated fractured right upper limb	Right upper limb is disarticulated at the shoulder joint and placed beside the body; the hand is missing. The left arm extends along the body side with the palm of the hand placed on the upper thigh region
Poor current status with multiple postmortem bony and soft-tissue injures. The head and neck are detached from the body and the limbs are disarticulated	Originally arms were bent at the elbows and the forearms laid, left above right at right angles across his belly, with the elbows jutting out slightly***
Poorly preserved. Multiple bony fractures and soft-tissue mutilations	Arms are alongside the body
Poorly preserved. Multiple bony fractures and soft-tissue mutilations	Arms are alongside the body
Fairly preserved. Head and face are in perfect condition, but the body is separated into three parts at the attachment of neck and body and above the iliac crests	Crossed arms over the chest, left forearm over right, flat hands reach shoulders
Fairly preserved. The neck is fractured at C5-6; body is severed at third–fourth dorsal levels. Both ulnas fractured	Crossed arms over the chest, left forearm over right and at a higher level, fingers mildly flexed
Fairly preserved. Bony fractures of right upper chest wall and right arm. Soft-tissue defects in the torso	Crossed arms over the chest, right forearm over left, flat hands reach shoulders
Well preserved. A cut wound of the neck at C5 to C7	Crossed arms over the chest, right forearm over left, flat

** Measurement is an estimate for mummy's stature; accurate measurement could not be accurately obtained because of mutilated body.

*** Ikram, "Some Thoughts."

Table 25. CT densities of materials related to mummification

Substance	CT morphology feature	CT density (HU)*	Reference
Resin	Homogeneous, feature-less, may show cracks within, straight outer surface (fluid level)	71 SD 23.7	P. Gostner et al., "New Radiological Approach for Analysis and Identification of Foreign Objects in Ancient and Historic Mummies."
Resin-like fluid	Homogeneous, feature-less, may show cracks within, straight outer surface (fluid level)	71	G. Sigmund and M. Minas, "The Trier Mummy Paï-es-tjau-em-aui-nu: Radiological and Histological Findings."
Soil	Heterogeneous, low den-sity, irregular surface, no fluid level. May contain higher densities of sand	−150	K.H. Hübener and W.M. Pahl, "Computertomographische Untersuchungen an altägyptischen Mumien."
Calcite	Dense structures with variable shapes and sizes	2649	Gostner et al., "New Radiological Approach for Analysis and Identification of Foreign Objects in Ancient and Historic Mummies."
Seeds	Rounded or oval dense structures, unified size when in groups	430	P. Soto-Heim, P. Le Floch-Prigent, and M. Laval-Jeantet, "Scanographie d'une momie égypti-enne antique de nourisson et de deux fausses momies de nouveau-nés."
"Son of Horus"	Dense object	1600	Sigmund and Minas, "The Trier Mummy Paï-es-tjau-em-aui-nu: Radiological and Histological Findings."
Heart amulet	Dense object	2410	R.J. Jansen et al., "High Resolution Spiral Computed Tomography with Multiplanar Reformatting, 3D Surface- and Volume Rendering: A Non-Destructive Method to Visualize Ancient Egyptian Mummification Techniques."
Bitumen	Low-density structure	8	Gostner et al., "New Radiological Approach for Analysis and Identification of Foreign Objects in Ancient and Historic Mummies."

*Reference HU values: air, −1000 HU; water, 0 HU; soft tissues, about −100 HU to 100 HU; bone, about 500 HU to 2000 HU.

Table 26. MDCT findings of cranial mummification in selected royal mummies, Eighteenth to Twentieth Dynasties

Name	Skull defects and excerebration route	CT features of intracranial contents
so-called Thutmose I	None	Desiccated brain at post. 1/4 of skull
Thutmose II	None	Desiccated brain at post. 1/4 of skull
Thutmose III	None	Desiccated brain at post. 1/4 of skull
Yuya	Skull-base defect at ACF (129.5 mm²) suggesting transnasal excerebration via R nare	Desiccated brain impregnated with resin and resin-like material Two perpendicular resin levels: at the post. 1/3 parallel to forehead, and at mid 1/3 parallel to the skull vault
Thuya	Skull-base defect at ACF (302 mm²) suggesting transnasal excerebration via both nares	Almost empty skull with minimal dural remains
Amenhotep III	Skull-base defect at ACF (1175 mm²) suggesting transnasal excerebration via R nare	Resin-like at post. 2/5 of skull parallel to the forehead
Tiye	Skull-base defect at ACF (523 mm²) suggesting transnasal excerebration via R nare	Desiccated brain at post. 1/3 of skull
Seti I	Skull-base defect at ACF (1143 mm²), suggesting transnasal excerebration likely via both nares	Desiccated brain with resin, soil and stones, and linen filling the post. 1/2 of skull
Ramesses II	Skull-base defect (ACF) (251 mm²) suggesting transnasal excerebration via R nare	Minimal desiccated brain and resin-like material in post. 2/3 of skull in compartments lined by dura
Merenptah	Skull-base defect (ACF) (703 mm²) suggesting transnasal excerebration via L nare. An additional R post. parietal skull defect (41.6 mm × 30 mm)	Minimal desiccated brain. Linen fibers smeared with resin (–830 HU to +35 HU) at the ant. 2/3 of skull more on the R, likely introduced through the post. skull defect
Ramesses III	Skull-base defect (ACF) (431 mm²) suggesting transnasal excerebration via L nare	Minimal dura and resin-like material at the mid and post. 2/3 of skull

Abbreviations: ACF: anterior cranial fossa; ant: anterior; L: left; post.: posterior; R: right
Source: After Saleem and Hawass, "Variability in Brain Treatment."

Table 27. CT features of embalming of nasal passages in selected royal mummies

Name	CT features of embalming of nasal passages
so-called Thutmose I	No packs
Thutmose II	Linen packs impregnated with resin (70 to 100 HU)
Thutmose III	Untreated linen packs (–240 to –160 HU)
Yuya	Linen (–370 HU) (ant.); resin-like* (–240 HU) (post.)
Thuya	Linen packs impregnated with resin (70 to 100 HU)
Amenhotep III	No nasal packs (minimal resin smears the ethmoids)
Tiye	No nasal packs (minimal resin smears the ethmoids)
Mother of Tutankhamun	Small (resin-like) substance in the right nasal cavity
Seti I	Resin (60 to 100 HU)
Ramesses II	Ant. nasal cavity: a bone of a small animal (transverse 21 mm, length 87 mm) and small dense seeds (4 mm in diameter). Resin fills the post. nasal cavity and ethmoids
Merenptah	Linen packs impregnated with resin (70 to 100 HU)
Ramesses III	Linen packs impregnated with resin (70 to 100 HU)

Abbreviations: ant.: anterior; post.: posterior
* Resin-like: homogeneous appearance but with CT density different than reported with resin

Table 28. CT findings of evisceration and embalming materials in torso cavities of royal mummies

Mummy	Embalming incision	Preserved heart	Torso contents
so-called Thutmose I	L inguinal oblique (77 mm × 44 mm)	Yes	Stuffed with loose linen, linen-resin packs, and resin (resin at R hemithorax and L upper abdomen)
Thutmose II	Cannot be assessed*	Yes	Stuffed with loose linen, linen-resin packs, and resin (resin at post. wall)
Thutmose III	L inguinal oblique (110 mm × 10 mm)	Yes	Stuffed with linen, linen-resin packs, and resin (resin at post. wall)
Yuya	L inguinal oblique (99 mm × 34 mm)	No	Stuffed with loose linen, linen-resin packs, and resin (resin at post. wall and thoracic apices)
Thuya	L inguinal vertical (115 mm × 47 mm) Resin-treated pack at its base	Yes	Stuffed with loose linen, linen-resin packs, and resin (resin at post. wall) A pierced stone bead is seen below the lower edge of the incision.
Amenhotep III	Cannot be assessed*	Cannot be assessed*	Mildly filled* with linen-resin packs and resin
Tiye	Cannot be assessed*	Yes	Mildly filled* with linen, linen-resin packs, and resin (resin at post. wall)
Mother of Tutankhamun	Left inguinal (135 mm × 56 mm)		Moderately filled* with linen and linen-resin
Tutankhamun	Diagonally from the center of the abdomen (navel) to the left iliac crest (149 mm × 90 mm)*§	Yes	Stuffed with linen-resin, and resin at post. wall. N.B.: bilateral symmetrical convexity of the fillings of the upper abdomen (? intact diaphragm)
Seti I	Cannot be assessed	Heart amulet**	Stuffed with loose linen, linen-resin packs, and resin (resin at post. wall)
Ramesses II	L inguinal oblique (165 mm × 55 mm) Resin at its base	Yes	Stuffed with loose linen, linen-resin packs, resin (post. wall & L upper chest cavity), and soil
Merenptah	Cannot be assessed*	No	Mildly filled* with linen, linen-resin, and resin (resin at L upper chest and post. wall)
Ramesses III	L inguinal oblique (149 mm × 56 mm)	Yes	Stuffed with soil or sawdust, linen, and resin (resin at post. wall)

Abbreviations: L: left; R: right; post. wall: torso concavity at the posterior wall of the torso
* Mutilation of the torso is reported
** The heart amulet is wrapped within a linen pack that likely contains heart residue
§ The large gaping wound in the left lower abdomen, packed with a linen pack soaked with resin, was assumed to be the embalming incision

Table 29. Embalming substances in orbits of royal mummies

Mummy	Orbital pack
so-called Thutmose I	No packs *
Thutmose II	No packs*
Thutmose III	Linen impregnated with resin: inhomogeneous (–300 to 20 HU); small amount of resin at the periphery. R: 32 × 36 × 33 mm; L: 31 × 40 × 34 mm. Packs in front of the eye globes.
Yuya	Linen impregnated with resin: inhomogeneous (–600 to 20 HU); small amount of resin at the lower orbit (70 HU). R: 30 × 32 × 16 mm; L: 25 × 32 × 17 mm. Packs in front of the eye globes.
Thuya	Linen impregnated with resin: inhomogeneous (–500 to 45 HU); small amount of resin within and thin layer at the periphery (250 HU). R: 32 × 35 × 35 mm; L: 30 × 31 × 35 mm. Packs in front of the eye globes.
Amenhotep III	Resin and linen impregnated with resin: inhomogeneous (–400 to 100 HU) packs. R: 31 × 39 × 40 mm; L: 30 × 39 × 36 mm. Packs above and behind the eye globes.
Tiye	Linen impregnated with resin: inhomogeneous (–400 to 20 HU); small amount of resin within the pack and at posterior orbit. R: 14 × 14 × 7 mm; L 17 × 17 × 10 mm. Packs in front of the eye globes.
Mother of Tutankhamun	Linen impregnated with resin: inhomogeneous (–500 to –20 HU). R: 35 × 37 × 24 mm; L: 34 × 37 × 25 mm. Packs in front of eye globes. Dense (300 HU) smearing of the periphery of both right and left orbital packs.
Seti I	Linen impregnated with resin: inhomogeneous (–130 HU); large compartments of resin (homogeneous 100 to 250 HU). R: 20 × 28 × 36 mm; L: 33 × 27 × 39 mm. Orbital filling show packs and resin are behind, below, and lateral to eye globes. High densities (2300 HU) at the lower right eyelid and the outer surface of the left.
Ramesses II	Linen impregnated with resin: inhomogeneous (–660 to –300 HU); minimal or no resin. R: 34 × 36 × 35 mm; L: 32 × 34 × 36 mm. Packs are behind and below the eye globes.
Merenptah	Linen impregnated with resin: inhomogeneous (–500 to –200 HU); small amount of resin within the packs. R: 33 × 34 × 34 mm; L: 31 × 35 × 35 mm (less resin). Packs are located behind and lateral to eye globes.
Ramesses III	Linen impregnated with resin: inhomogeneous (–700 to –300 HU); moderate amount of resin (45 HU) within and at the periphery of packs. R: 32 × 32 × 43 mm; L: 37 × 31 × 37 mm. Right orbital pack is below the eye globe; left orbital pack is in front of and below the eye.

Abbreviations: R: right; L: left. * The orbits contain atrophic eye globes
N.B.: Measurements of the packs in transverse, height (craniocaudal), and anteroposterior dimensions, respectively

Table 30. Embalming substances in oral cavity and pharynx of royal mummies

Mummy	Anatomical region	Embalming material
so-called Thutmose I	NA	None
Thutmose II	Oral cavity and orophayrnx	Linen (–600 HU) in ant. oral cavity under the tongue Multiple pellets 10–15 mm in diameter (–350 HU), likely linen balls impregnated with resin (in the post. oral cavity and oropharynx)
Thutmose III	Oral cavity and oropharynx*	Resin-impregnated linen (–300 HU) in ant. oral cavity Solidified resin (100 HU) at floor of mouth, post. oral cavity, and oropharynx
Yuya	Oral cavity, oropharynx, and hypopharynx	Linen (–600 HU) in oral cavity and oropharynx Linen impregnated with resin (–300 HU) in hypopharynx
Thuya	Oral cavity and oropharynx	Linen (–500 HU)
Amenhotep III	Oral cavity and oropharynx*	Resin (70 HU)
Tiye	Oral cavity and oropharynx	Resin-impregnated linen (–200 HU)
Mother of Tutankhamun	Oral cavity	Linen (–600 HU)
Seti I	Oral cavity, oropharynx, and hypopharynx	Resin and linen impregnated with resin (–100 to 30 HU). Solidified resin inside the neck surrounds larynx (200 HU), and prevertebral (400 HU with dense particles)
Ramesses II	Oral cavity and oropharynx	Linen (–600 HU), parcels of seeds (2–4 mm)
Merenptah	Oral cavity and oropharynx	Linen impregnated with resin (–600 to 178 HU). Multiple oblong-shaped linen tampons (about 10 × 30 mm) with central resin-like density (70 HU)**
Ramesses III	Oral cavity and oropharynx	Resin 300 HU, dense spots 1000 HU

* Extent of embalming filling in the lower throat (hypopharynx) in the neck could not be determined due to fracture dislocation of the neck at C4-5 level

** Linen in the mouth cavity is continuous with linen between skin and maxilla/mandible

Table 31. CT findings of external genitalia of male royal mummies

Mummy	CT findings
so-called Thutmose I	Penis appears as a curved cylindrical structure at the base of the perineum measuring 68 mm × 38 mm and –20 to 17 HU; no scrotum detected
Thutmose II	Penis measures 48 mm × 15 mm and 40 HU with higher-density inclusions (500 HU). Thin soft tissue is flattened at the base of perineum (?scrotum)
Thutmose III	Not visualized
Yuya	Penis is a straight tubular structure deviated to the right measuring 105 mm × 14 mm. Its CT density is 300 HU. A spherical structure (about 5 cm in diameter) of mixed densities (–300 to 150 HU) is seen at the base of perineum behind the penis. This could be a scrotum filled with embalming material rather than being a pack placed by the embalmers for protection of the organ.
Amenhotep III	Not visualized
Tutankhamun	Not visualized
Seti I	Not visualized
Ramesses II	Not visualized
Merenptah	Base of penis is preserved (41 mm × 17 mm); its free edge is beveled, denoting that its tip is missing. Penile tissues have moderately high density (240 HU) with a tubular-like central low density seen only in the proximal part. The scrotum is missing. A transverse dimple scar line lies at the perineal region between penis base and anus.
Ramesses III	Penis measures 40 mm in length and 13 mm in width. Its density measures 250 HU with multiple spots of higher densities of 500 HU.

N.B. Dimensions of penis are given as length × transverse

12

Amulets, Funerary Figures, and
Other Objects Found on the Mummies

Introduction

To the ancient Egyptians, the journey to the afterlife was perilous. To aid and protect the deceased, the mummy was often provided with a selection of amulets, funerary figures, and jewelry. Specific amulets and their placement were prescribed by the Book of the Dead, and these were inserted within the wrappings, and sometimes within the body cavities themselves, accompanied by rituals performed by the embalmers.[1]

The use of these funerary objects evolved over time in ancient Egypt. Royal jewelry is known as early as the First Dynasty: four bracelets were found on the arm of a mummy, presumably a queen, in the tomb of Djer at Abydos.[2] There are few remaining mummies from the Old Kingdom that have been unwrapped, and these generally contained only ten to fifteen amulets. The number and variety of amulets increased with time in the Middle and New Kingdoms.[3]

Among the most spectacular jewelry and amulets are those found on relatively intact royal mummies such as the mummy of King Tutankhamun, which had 143 objects scattered throughout the wrappings[4] (plate 67). However, the protective amulets themselves were responsible for the destruction of many mummies, as these valuable objects were the targets of grave robbers over the centuries.[5]

The royal mummies examined by the Egyptian Mummy Project were also provided with a variety of amulets, jewelry, and funerary figures. CT examination enabled noninvasive examination of mummies to determine the presence, precise location, measurements, and identification of foreign objects. CT studies of fifteen royal mummies done by the author (SNS) revealed a total of twenty-five objects distributed among seven of them.[6]

Eleven objects were located within the torso cavities of the mummies, while fourteen were placed within the wrappings or on the surface

Table 32. Foreign objects found in the royal mummies

Name of mummy	Location of object	CT features of object: morphology, dimensions
so-called Thutmose I	Chest cavity	A triangular object (20 mm × 19.8 mm × 19.5 mm) in the right side of chest cavity surrounded by multiple 1–2 mm objects. A rod (7 mm × 18 mm × 10 mm) is at the left lower posterior chest wall (at head of left 11th rib).
Thutmose III	Distal right forearm	A cylinder elliptical in cross section (49.6 mm × 26.6 mm), 50 mm in breadth, and 9 mm thick
	Distal right forearm (distal to the broad bracelet)	A cylinder elliptical in cross section (54 mm × 40 mm); 4.5–9 mm in breadth, and 5 mm thick
Thuya	In front of left upper thigh	Oblong structure (32 mm × 16 mm) with central cavity
	Inside vagina	Irregular spiky structures (27 mm × 15 mm)
	Inside rectum	Oblong object with irregular surface, 49 mm × 15 mm
	Footwear	A rectangular, thin plate with curved sides (R: 70 mm × 174 mm; L: 68 mm × 160 mm) is placed on the plantar surface of each foot (sole). Attached to the back of the sides of each sole plate is a broad band with central constriction that arches on the hindfoot.
Tiye	Torso cavity	Multiple round or oval objects (10–20 mm in width)
Seti I	Right upper chest cavity	Small amulet that looks jar-like with a lid; measures 49 mm × 26 mm × 25 mm
	Within wrappings at back of left arm	Flat plate with processes (projections), measures about 40 mm × 15 mm
	Within wrappings at left side of back opposite 3rd lumbar vertebra	A small amulet (28 mm × 26 mm × 33 mm) with geometric openwork designs
	Within wrappings between both thighs and at medial of lower right thigh	About 11 small barrel-shaped objects (5–6 mm in length)

Source: After Saleem and Hawass, "Multi-detector Computer Tomography."

CT density	Suggested identity of object
3067 HU SD 4	Metallic arrowhead and multiple metallic objects
3060 HU SD 7	Broad metallic bracelet
3067 HU SD 4	Narrow metallic bracelet
2163 HU SD 23	Pierced bead made of stone or faience[7]
1700 HU SD 20	Stone or stopper made of unidentified material
1200 HU SD 23	Stone or stopper made of unidentified material
Sole: 3070 HU; arched band: outer 3070 HU, inner 250 HU	Pair of metallic (likely gold) sandals[8]
1890 HU SD 229	Set of multiple oval or round beads or stones, perhaps faience
2670 HU SD 50	Heart amulet made of stone
3066 HU SD 4	Eye of Horus (wedjat) metallic amulet
3068 HU SD 1	Metallic amulet, likely Eye of Horus
3070 HU SD 3	Multiple barrel-shaped metallic beads or stones

Table 32. Foreign objects found in the royal mummies *(continued)*

Name of mummy	Location of object	CT features of object: morphology, dimensions
Ramesses II	Inside left upper chest cavity	Oblong object (67 mm × 14 mm × 120 mm) with upper and lower processes
Ramesses III	In front of neck at C7 level behind right sternocleido-mastoid muscle	Flat plate with processes, measures about 15 mm × 11 mm × 6 mm
	Inside left lower chest cavity	Four uninscribed or briefly inscribed figures, each measuring approximately 100 mm × 25 mm × 15 mm with heads arranged from front to back: human, falcon, baboon, and jackal
	Left ankle: in front of medial malleolus	Flat plate with processes measuring 41 mm × 20 mm × 2.7 mm
	Left ankle: anteromedial aspect of distal tibia	Flat plate with processes measuring 23.7 mm × 9.8 mm × 2.3 mm
	Left foot: plantar surfaces of distal phalanges of fourth and fifth toes	Two oval-shaped structures that measure 4.7 mm × 4.1 mm × 4 mm, and 4.7 mm × 3 mm × 2.7 mm at the fifth and fourth toes, respectively
	Right ankle: anterolateral aspect of tibia	Thick disc with multiple projections, measures 20 mm × 9.3 mm × 4.1 mm
	Right foot: at tip of distal phalanx of third to fourth toe	A plate with a process, measures 11.9 mm × 9.1 mm × 16.2 mm

of the mummies. Their size varied markedly between 5 mm and 174 mm in length.

The largest number of objects was eleven, in the mummy of Ramesses III, five in Thuya, and four in the mummy of Seti I. The scarcity of objects in these mummies, however, does not seem to be customary in this ancient era, considering their royal status. All of the mummies had been vandalized except for the two female fetuses that were initially found intact in the tomb of their father Tutankhamun. Thus the paucity of amulets and other objects could be attributed to grave robbers, who also caused, at least in part, the mutilation and destruction of the mummies.

In a recent study,[9] measurements of CT density of a foreign object in ancient mummies enabled the identification of its material composition by comparing its value with

CT density	Suggested identity of object
1100 HU SD 30	Oblong figure made of fired clay of unsettled identity (could be crowned Osiris, or unusual presentation of *wedjat* amulet)
2166 HU SD 16	Eye of Horus (*wedjat*) amulet, possibly faience
1034 HU SD 25	Figures of Four Sons of Horus, likely made of fired clay
3069 HU SD 3	Eye of Horus (*wedjat*) metallic amulet
3066 HU SD 4	Eye of Horus (*wedjat*) metallic amulet
3070 HU SD 2	Metallic beads
3070 HU SD 2	Metal amulet, possibly Eye of Horus (*wedjat*)
3069 HU SD 2	Eye of Horus (*wedjat*) metallic amulet

reference data. Metals are identified when an object with a high attenuation value (over 2978 HU) causes a metal streaking artifact in the form of dark streaks along the long axis of the single high-attenuation object, with bright streaks adjacent to the dark streaks. Other substances can be suggested using a range of values; for example, stones (2900 to 2500 HU), quartz substances and possibly faience (1693 to 2317 HU), ivory (around 1260 HU, SD 6.3 HU), and fired clay (1116 HU, SD 54.7). However, because values are in a range of variation, rather than absolute, HU value is not sufficient to unequivocally identify the material composition of an object, but rather to considerably narrow the list of possible substances.

The CT attenuation values of the objects on or in the mummies we studied varied considerably, suggesting that they were made from different materials such as metal, stones, faience, and fired clay. This is consistent with

Table 33. Suggested categories of twenty-five foreign objects found by CT

Suggested category	Number	Mummies
Jewelry	4	Thutmose III, Thuya
Amulets/funerary figures	13	Seti I, Ramesses II, Ramesses III
Stones/beads	2 sets, 3 individual*	Tiye, Seti I, Ramesses III
Other**	3	'Thutmose I,' Thuya

* Set is considered when multiple stones or beads are present in one location as a cluster; these were found in Tiye and on Seti I. Individual beads are those found in separate locations: two were found in Ramesses III's left foot, and one just below the left inguinal region in Thuya.
** 'Other' objects include a metallic arrowhead in 'Thutmose I' and two objects placed in the pelvic orifices of Thuya.

what is known of the various materials used by the ancient Egyptians in the manufacture of their jewelry and amulets.[10]

The reconstructed CT images in multiple planes help in determining the exact location of the objects on the mummies (plates 68a–b), and reconstructed 2D and 3D CT images reveal the morphology of the objects, which helps in determining their identity and purpose. In the case of metal streak artifacts that obscure the CT image and mask the object, processing the image using special software (for example MDT: Metal Deletion Technique) markedly reduces the streak artifacts and allows better delineation of the metallic objects[11] (figs. 108a–b).

We correlated the CT appearance of each object with the archaeological literature and photos of similar objects in world museums to reach a suggested identity for each one. Based on their purpose, we categorized the objects as jewelry, amulets, funerary figures, and stones or beads, as well as a foreign object, possibly a weapon in the form of an arrowhead that might have caused death.

Jewelry

From the Predynastic Period onward, bodies were provided with jewelry constructed of various materials ranging from shells and beads to gold and gemstones. The most common ornaments were necklaces and collars, bracelets, armlets, bands for ankles, earrings, and rings.[12] Two categories of jewelry have been found on ancient Egyptian mummies: jewelry made specifically for the burial, which tended to be of less sturdy manufacture, and jewelry actually used during life. Some of the best-known and most elaborate pieces were found on the intact royal mummy of Tutankhamun.[13] CT images identified two solid metallic bracelets, likely of gold, at the distal right forearm of Thutmose III (plates 69a–b). The bracelets are cylindrical in shape and vary in breadth. A broad bracelet (50 mm in breadth and 9 mm in thickness) is located proximal to a thin bracelet (4.5 to 9 mm in breadth and 5 mm in thickness). This type of solid bracelet was a common adornment of both kings and queens at that time. Metallic, probably gold, footwear seen on the feet of Thuya may also be placed in the category of jewelry (figs. 109a–b).

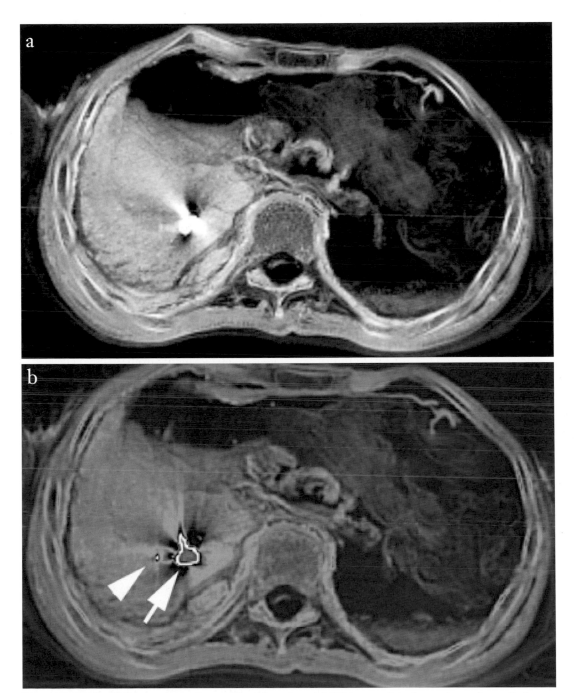

Figs. 108a–b: The CT appearance of a metallic object. An axial CT image of the lower chest of so-called Thutmose I (a) shows a foreign metallic object in the right chest cavity. The object has high attenuation value that measures more than 3000 HU. Metal streak artifacts partially obscure the boundaries of the object. In (b), the metallic artifact is reduced by using CT technology and results in better delineation of the object (arrow) and another adjacent metallic fragment (arrowhead).

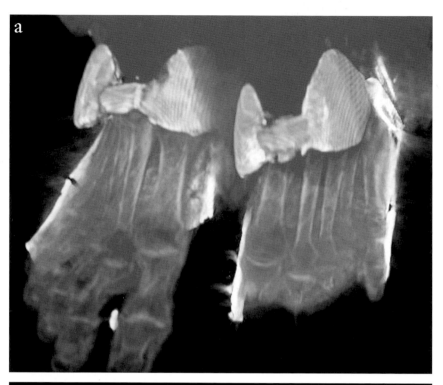

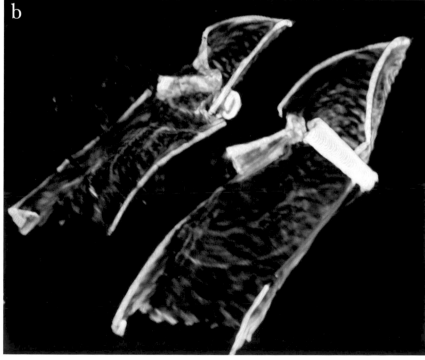

Figs. 109a–b: Three-dimensional CT images of the metallic footwear of Thuya.

Amulets and Funerary Figures

The word 'amulet' comes from the Latin *amuletum*, meaning 'an object that protects a person from trouble.' The ancient Egyptians had several words for amulets, including *sa* and *wedja*, which are related to words for 'protection' and 'well-being.'[14] Amulets were made in a variety of shapes, including deities, parts of the human body, and animals. Each amulet had a specific purpose. The material and color were important elements to enhance its magical properties, though the type of material utilized depended on an individual's wealth.[15]

Small representations of animals appear to have functioned as amulets in the Predynastic Period. In the Old Kingdom, most amulets took animal or human forms. The succeeding Middle Kingdom saw the introduction of the heart scarab, one of the most important funerary amulets, which was inscribed with texts intended to prevent the heart from testifying against the deceased on the Day of Judgment. The New Kingdom showed a further increase in the quantity and forms of amulets, including those of deities, but in the Third Intermediate Period there was a marked proliferation of many different types.[16] In our CT studies of the royal mummies, we observed thirteen amulets or funerary objects. These included a heart amulet, seven Eye of Horus amulets (or most likely so), and figures of the Four Sons of Horus, as well as an oblong-shaped figure of uncertain identity.

Heart amulet

The ancient Egyptians believed that the heart (*ib*) was the source of intelligence, memory, feelings, and passion. Unlike other organs, it was never intentionally removed

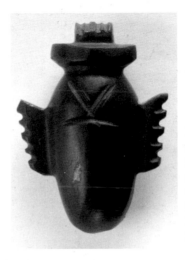

Fig. 110: Obsidian heart amulet. Late Period, 664–332 BC. 1.25 in. x 1.875 in. x 0.5 in. (3.2 cm x 4.8 cm x 1.3 cm). Collected by William A. Shelton, funded by John A. Manget. © Michael C. Carlos Museum, Emory University.

during mummification. The heart amulet stands among the most important items of magical protection in ancient Egypt, as it protected the heart of the deceased and served as a replacement in the event of the original heart's destruction.[17] Several chapters of the Book of the Dead were dedicated to the preservation of the heart, with specific instructions in Chapter 29B for a "heart amulet of *sehert*-stone," or carnelian.[18] Heart amulets were part of the amulet set of the deceased beginning in the New Kingdom and lasting until the end of the Pharaonic Period (fig. 110). They were placed outside or inside the chest cavity above the heart after all of the other organs had been removed. Besides carnelian, the heart amulet was also commonly formed of lapis lazuli, feldspar, and faience. CT images identified a heart amulet within the chest cavity of Seti I's mummy, in the shape of a small jar with a lid; its CT attenuation value suggested that its composition was stone (figs. 111a–b). The amulet is wrapped within a resin-impregnated pack and soft-tissue remnants that could represent cardiac tissue.

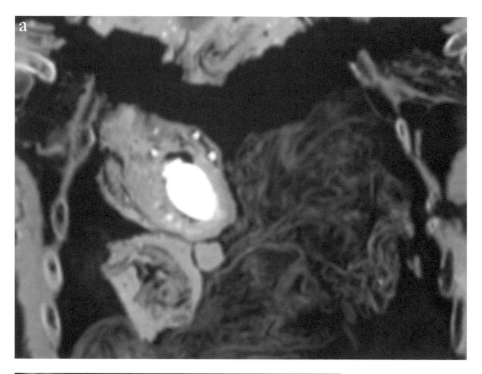

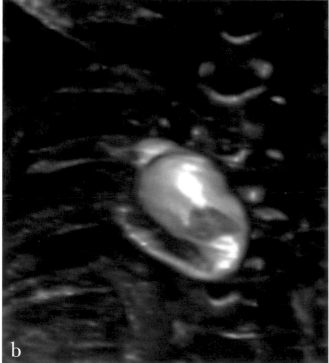

Figs. 111a–b: CT images of the heart amulet in the chest cavity of Seti I. A CT reconstructed image in coronal projection (a) shows a dense amulet within remnants of the heart, surrounded by resin-impregnated linen. Three-dimensional reconstructed CT images (b) show the heart amulet distinctly.

Wedjat Eye of Horus amulets

The *wedjat*[19] is an ancient Egyptian symbol of protection, power, and well-being. The amulet represents a human eye with falcon markings (see plate 67) and is the Eye of Horus, the ancient Egyptian falcon-headed sky god. It protected the wearer against all evils by taking the power of the god. According to the ancient myth, Horus battled his evil uncle Seth to avenge the killing of his father, Osiris. During this fight, Horus's eye was put out and then was healed by the god Thoth. In one version of the myth, Horus offered the eye to his deceased father, Osiris, in order to restore his life. Hence, the Eye of Horus was often used to symbolize sacrifice, healing, restoration, and protection.[20] The *wedjat*-eye amulet was extremely popular with the living and the amulet of choice for the dead for millennia, from the Old Kingdom into the Greco-Roman Period. From the New Kingdom onward, this amulet was placed near the eviscerating incision for protection and healing.[21]

Two- and three-dimensional reconstructed CT images revealed in the mummy of Seti I a fenestrated plate in the shape of the Eye of Horus with its characteristic teardrop marking below (figs. 112a–b). The amulet is located in the wrappings at the back of the left arm. Its orientation has a more backward slope than its traditional vertical position. The attenuation value (3066 HU) of the amulet indicates that it is made of metal, possibly gold.

Another metallic, fenestrated amulet with 3068 HU can be seen within the wrappings of the left side of the back of Seti I's mummy (plates 70a–b). Three-dimensional reconstructed images demonstrate the oval-shaped outline of the amulet, with the characteristic teardrop of the *wedjat* Eye of Horus.

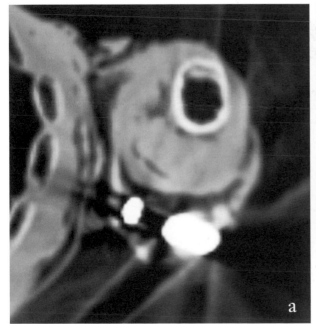

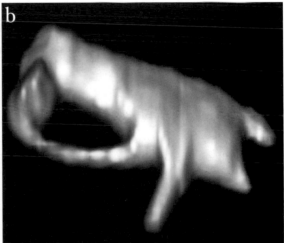

Figs. 112a–b: CT images of the Eye of Horus amulet placed behind the left arm of Seti I. An axial CT image (a) shows a dense structure with a characteristic metal streaking artifact within the wrappings. A 3D CT image (b) shows well the characteristic shape of the Eye of Horus amulet.

We found five *wedjat* amulets on Ramesses III's mummy; one on the neck, opposite his throat injury, and the other four amulets in the region of the ankles and feet, close to the partially chopped left big toe (plates 71a–b). The locations opposite injured body parts confirm the function of the amulet as a symbol of healing. The amulets are solid flat plates with projections that conform with the outline of the Eye of Horus. In Ramesses III, the amulets are small in size and vary in their attenuation values. All of the four amulets at the region of the ankles and feet have high attenuation values (3070 HU) of metal (likely gold). The neck amulet, however, has a lower attenuation value (2166 HU), which indicates that it is made instead from a stone or faience. The different CT morphological appearances of the Eye of Horus in the mummies confirm that variable designs and materials were used in making this particular amulet.[22]

Four Sons of Horus figures

Figures of the Four Sons of the god Horus were sometimes provided to the mummy for the protection and guarding of the organs.[23] The figures have different heads associated with the Four Sons: human-headed Imseti protected the liver; baboon-headed Hapi protected the lungs; jackal-headed Duamutef protected the stomach; and falcon-headed Qebehsenuef protected the intestines.[24] As protectors, the Four Sons of Horus are found from the Old Kingdom through the Greco-Roman era, and they were referenced in both tomb and canopic equipment, as well as in sacred texts. In the Old Kingdom Pyramid Texts, recitation 148 from the tomb of the Sixth Dynasty king Teti tells us: "Hapi, Duamutef, Qebehsenuef, and Imseti shall remove this hunger that is in the belly of Teti and this thirst that is on Teti's lips."[25] In the New Kingdom Book of the Dead, spell 137 states: "O sons of Horus, Imseti, Hapi, Duamutef, Kebehsenuef: as you spread your protection over your father Osiris-Khentimentiu, so spread your protection over (the deceased), as you remove the impediment from Osiris-Khentimentiu, so he might live with the gods and drive Seth from him."[26]

CT images clearly detected four flat, oblong figures of the Sons of Horus within the left side of the chest cavity of Ramesses III's mummy (plates 72a–e). The heads of the Four Sons of Horus are arranged from front to back: human, falcon, baboon, and jackal. The dense objects have an average attenuation value of 1038 HU, suggesting that they were probably made of faience or fired clay. The Four Sons of Horus are common in glazed faience, but more rare in hard stone, gold, silver, bronze, and wax. The presence of low-density patches indicates that the figures are inscribed or have incised decoration. In contrast to Harris and Wente's claim during their x-ray examination of this mummy that there are only three,[27] CT demonstrated the presence of all of the Four Sons. This is believed to be the first time in the Twentieth Dynasty that the Sons of Horus are seen inside a mummy.

An oblong-shaped figure

CT images identified a dense, elongated foreign object (measuring 67 mm x 14 mm x 120 mm in transverse, anteroposterior, and superior-inferior views, respectively) within the left upper chest cavity of the mummy of Ramesses II (plates 73a–c). The attenuation value of the object measures 1100 HU, and it is likely made of fired clay. The oblong-shaped object has two upper and lower hooked processes. Though it cannot be precisely identified, its outline bears some resemblance to a figure of the crowned Osiris carrying scepters, a symbol of the regenerative power of Osiris; or, when viewed from another angle, an unusual presentation of the *wedjat* amulet.

Beads and Stones

There are multiple rounded stones or beads within the torso cavity of Queen Tiye. These objects are seen within the right side of the chest cavity and the left side of the pelvis. The objects measure between 10 mm and 20 mm in length. The CT density of the objects suggests that they are made of quartz. These are likely faience beads placed for spiritual purposes or as part of visceral embalming materials.

A small, oblong-shaped, pierced bead is placed on the surface of the left upper thigh, just below the left inguinal embalming incision.

Multiple (about eleven) small oval and barrel-shaped metallic objects are seen within the wrappings between the mid and lower thighs of the mummy of Seti I.

Two small oval metallic beads are located at the plantar surface of the left fourth and fifth toes of Ramesses III (see fig. 88c in chapter 10). The beads were likely placed by the embalmers for religious or protection purposes.

Other Foreign Objects

CT images show a solid triangular object that measures about 20 mm in its long axis located within the lower right side of the chest cavity of so-called Thutmose I. The metallic object has a high attenuation value (3067 HU) and shows the characteristic streaking artifacts. In 2D reconstructed CT images, the object is triangular in shape, and on 3D images it has

the appearance of an arrowhead with its tip directed upward and to the right side (plates 74a–b). The shape of the arrowhead resembles those used by the ancient Egyptians at that time. The CT findings suggest that an arrow wound to the chest of 'Thutmose I' caused his death.[28] The presence of multiple tiny metallic fragments (1 mm to 2 mm in diameter) surrounding the object supports this assumption. Considering the direction of the arrowhead, the entry point could be at a lower level on the left side of the chest. A metallic fragment (18 mm in long axis) located at the head of the left eleventh rib may be the mark for the entry point of the arrowhead. The right chest wall appears mildly thicker than the left side. Unlike the almost empty left side of the chest cavity, the right side is full of heterogeneous substances surrounding the metallic objects, consisting of a moderately dense material (120 to 275 HU) with a less dense material (–220 HU) at its periphery that could be blood clots resulting from the injury. However, we cannot indicate decisively that it is a blood clot, as the CT appearance of ancient blood residues is not known. An argument against the theory of chest injury in 'Thutmose I' is the fact that the embalmers left the weapon and did not clean the blood clots during the process of evisceration. The substance within the chest cavity thus could have been an atypical embalming material different from resin. The triangular object could have been placed deliberately by the embalmers into the mummy's chest cavity. We could not identify the triangular amulet; the literature does not contain a triangular amulet that matches the shape of the identified object. The presence of smaller metallic objects in the chest cavity in addition to the triangular

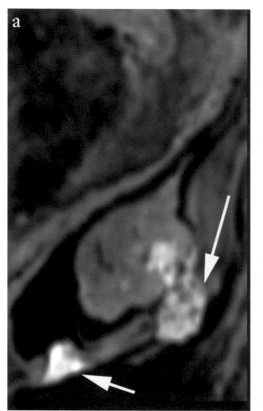

Figs. 113a–d: CT images of objects within the pelvic orifices of Thuya. Localized sagittal oblique reconstructed CT image of the pelvic region (a) shows dense objects plugging the orifices of the vagina (short arrow) and rectum (long arrow). Three-dimensional reconstructed CT image (b) shows the marked irregularity of the objects; short arrow points to the object within the vagina, while the longer arrow points to that in the rectum. Arrows in the axial CT image at the level of the vagina (c), and coronal CT image at the level of the rectum (d), point to the objects that fit well within the corresponding hollow organs.

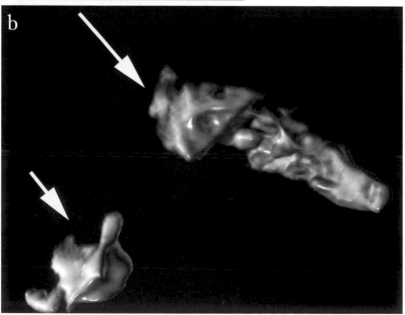

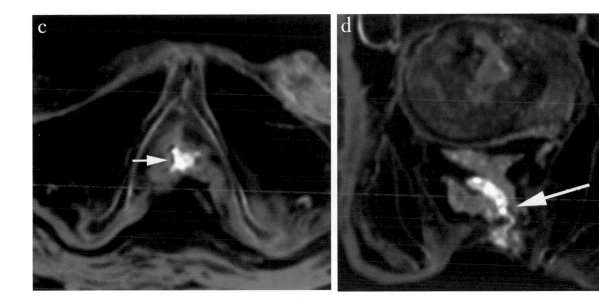

one cannot be justified as part of the mummification process. Accordingly, we conclude that the proposed theory of chest injury is feasible.

Two irregular objects are seen within the pelvic orifices (vagina and rectum) of Thuya (figs. 113a–d). Their high CT densities indicate that they are made of stone or other unidentified substance(s). These objects were likely placed by the embalmers as a stopper to seal the orifices and prevent leakage of the embalming materials within the torso. We noted that the marked irregularities of the surfaces of these objects fit well with the creases of the hollow structures.

In conclusion, MDCT offers detailed, noninvasive analysis of the foreign objects found on or within the royal mummies that helps in protecting human cultural heritage, understanding ancient mortuary practices, and differentiating funerary objects from those that may be related to cause of death.

13

Faces of the Royal Mummies

Introduction

The elaborate process of mummification of the royals in ancient Egypt aimed at preserving the face of the deceased to ensure as lifelike an appearance as possible. Artificial eyes, nasal support, and subcutaneous fillers were occasionally used by the embalmers for this purpose.

Modern computerized tomography using 2D and 3D techniques enabled us not only to look directly into the actual faces of the long-dead Egyptians, but also to discern the elaborate mummification process behind them. CT surface-rendering techniques display the facial features of the mummies, which may reveal data about gender, age, and ethnicity.[1]

CT not only enables detailed nondestructive display of the superficial facial features, but also reveals the bony craniofacial characteristics of the royal mummies. These are inheritable features that may extend from parent to offspring over many generations.[2]

Byron O. Hughes and George R. Moore were among the earliest investigators to subscribe to a multiple-gene concept of inheritance in the craniofacial complex. They observed that craniofacial growth and morphology are under strong hereditary control and expressed this concept in percentages of heritability between parents and siblings.[3]

Ethnicity, or race, and its determination from skeletal remains, is a controversial topic.[4] Egypt was the crossroads for many different cultures, and there is an ongoing debate regarding race in ancient Egypt.[5] There is a great deal of variability in facial features of the ancient Egyptians, with differences in facial shape and contour, skin tone, and hairstyles, findings that may suggest a very cosmopolitan population.[6]

Using 2D and 3D reconstructed CT images, Sahar Saleem described the facial features of selected New Kingdom royal mummies in the Egyptian Museum.

Features of the Faces and Heads of the Royal Mummies in CT Images

So-called Thutmose I (plates 75a–b)

This is the head of a middle-aged man with completely hairless scalp. The skull is a small ovoid with prominent occiput. The face is a narrow ellipsoid. There is prognathism of the maxilla, a weak jaw, and a receding chin. There is no CT evidence of nasal or subcutaneous facial packs. The ear lobules have not been perforated. Physical inspection of the mummy reveals that the face has not been smeared with resin.

Thutmose II (plates 76a–b)

The mummy is a partially bald, middle-aged man with some locks of hair on the temples and the sides of the head. The skull is broad, and the face is ellipsoid. The bridge of the nose is broad and low in position. The nose appears flattened, likely due to the effect of the bandages. Ear openings and nares are distended with linen impregnated with resinous material. The auricles are small, well formed, and the lobules are not perforated. Visual inspection revealed numerous skin eruptions on the face that could not be detected in the CT images.

Thutmose III (plates 77a–b)

The head is separated from the body but is well preserved. The detached head is completely devoid of hair. CT images show a small, narrow, ellipsoid face. The nose is badly damaged, with interruption of the soft tissues surrounding the left nare. Both nares are stuffed with embalming material, likely linen. There is evidence of a marked projection of the upper incisor teeth with pronounced overbite. The auricles are well formed; the lobule of the left auricle is likely perforated. The presence of subcutaneous fillers helped in enhancing the facial contours of the front of the face around the nose and mouth.[7]

Yuya (plates 78a–b)

CT images of the head of Yuya's mummy show a face that must have been handsome in life. Yuya's face is relatively short and elliptical, with a prominent, high-bridged nose and a square chin. Behind the semi-closed lids, the orbits of the shrunken eyes are filled with linen packs. The presence of subcutaneous fillers enhanced the contours of the front of the face around the nose and mouth. Craniofacial features include a sagittal plateau of the skull, narrow triangular nasal openings, square jaw line, and orthognathism. Based on his facial features, some Egyptologists have suggested that Yuya was of foreign origin; however, this is far from certain.[8]

Thuya (plates 79a–b)

CT images of the head of Thuya show a well-preserved elderly female mummy with ovoid face and high cheekbones. The opened eyelids show that the orbits were stuffed with amorphous embalming materials. The intranasal embalming materials did not distort the delicate nose of Thuya. The facial contours around the mouth are enhanced by subcutaneous packing.[9] There are multiple piercings of both ear pinnas: one in the right lobule, two in the left lobule, as well as multiple piercings in the upper auricles of both ears, a common practice at that time. There is a rise near the top of the skull, a receding chin, inclined mandible with downward slope from the jaw to the chin, and mild prognathism. In fact, the physical characteristics of Thuya's face are similar to many Egyptian women of today.

Amenhotep III (plates 80a–b)

The poorly preserved mummy of Amenhotep III displays a skeletonized head with scarce facial flesh. The bones of the skull and face of the mummy have suffered from multiple postmortem fractures. Most of the soft tissues of the face are missing. The remnant of soft tissues of the lower face and neck shows packs of resin and linen bits. The orbits are filled with an embalming material.

There is a rise near the top of the skull with mildly projected glabella, rectangular sloping orbits, prominent nasal septum, and steepled nasals. The chin is long and pointed downward with straight lines (receding). The mandible shows a steep slope from the jaw to the chin, likely with mild maxillary and mandibular prognathism. Occipital buns are present in the form of a flattened lambdoid region with upper and lower eminences causing sharp angles.

Tiye (plates 81a–b)

CT images of the head of Queen Tiye display an elderly woman with long locks of hair overlying the head and falling onto both shoulders. Queen Tiye had a narrow face with narrow nose and pointed chin. There are orbital packs behind the semi-closed eyelids. A lack of facial subcutaneous packing explains the striking hollow cheeks and drawn appearance of the facial contours. There are multiple piercings of the lobe of the left ear auricle. There is a high skull vault, sagittal plateau, occipital buns, sharply receding chin, inclined mandible, and mild maxillary prognathism.

Akhenaten (see figs. 6a–b in chapter 1)

The head of the poorly preserved mummy of Akhenaten is skeletonized, with almost no facial flesh. The CT features of the face indicate moderate length, unlike the drawings and statues of the king. The elongated appearance of Akhenaten's face in artistic representations of the Amarna Period could be thus attributed to an imaginative expression of the pharaoh's image characteristic of the Amarna Period, rather than being a real-life appearance. The head of Akhenaten has a rise near its top, rectangular sloping orbit, and prominent nasal septum with steepled nasals. The chin is long and pointed downward with straight lines. The mandible has a downward slope from the jaw to the chin with incisor protrusion and mild prognathism. There are occipital buns with sharp angles caused by a flattened lambdoid region with upper and lower eminences.

The mother of Tutankhamun (plate 82; see also plates 29a–b)

This is a shaved head of a young female. The skull is moderately elongated, with a mild rise near the top. The skull base is intact, but there is a frontal rounded defect (33 mm in diameter) with nonsclerotic sharp beveled edges. The face is oval; the nose descends unbroken from the brow and the angle of the orbits. The mandible is smooth, with an obtuse angle. The right ear auricle is partly missing. The left auricle (not shown) has two piercings in its lobe. The presence of subcutaneous fillers enhances the contours of the right cheek and adjacent jaw area.

The significant injury of the left side of the face and jaw has been described above (see chapter 4, "CT Examination of Selected Mid- to Late Eighteenth Dynasty Mummies").

Seti I (plates 83a–b)

The mummy of King Seti I has the most lifelike and attractive face of the many Egyptian mummies, royal and commoner, that have survived down to the present time. CT images display an ovoid face with narrow nose, big jaw, and wide chin. Orbital packs are behind the semi-closed eyelids. The elaborate subcutaneous packing in Seti I enhanced the facial contours smoothly and almost symmetrically, combating the hollow, depressed appearance characteristic of mummified tissues.[10]

The skull shows a sagittal plateau; the forehead is sloping, the glabella is arched, and there is a forward projection of the zygomatic arches. The incisors are very straight, and the mandible is moderately steep with a broad ramus. The chin is receding. The stronger build of the face of Seti I presents a marked contrast to the features of the Eighteenth Dynasty mummies, as is to be expected from a new ruling dynasty. This does not necessarily imply that Seti I was less Egyptian, ethnically or physically.

Ramesses II (plates 84a–b; see also fig. 4g)
Three-dimensional CT images of King Ramesses II reveal a large, narrow face with very prominent hooked nose. The characteristic shape of the nose was preserved by stuffing different embalming materials within the nasal cavity (a small animal bone and plant seeds). The lack of subcutaneous packing (see chapter 11, "CT Findings on the Mummification Process of Royal Ancient Egyptians") explains the hollow cheeks and depressed facial contours of the mummy. The lobes of the ears have been pierced, as was the fashion at that time. The skull shows a rounded forehead, roundish glabella, and a sagittal plateau. There is a forward projection of the zygomatic arch, receding chin, and inclined mandible.

Merenptah (plates 85a–b)
Three-dimensional CT images of the mummy of King Merenptah show an elderly male with a wide face and a wide sloping forehead. The eyelids are semi-closed; orbital packs are placed to combat sunken areas characteristic of mummified tissues. Despite the presence of nasal packs, the soft parts of the nose have become flattened, spoiling the appearance of the face; this was presumably caused by the pressure of the bandages. There is a forward projection of the zygomatic arch and receding chin. Merenptah has a strong, mildly inclined mandible with slight overbite. The jaw is strong. Subcutaneous packs symmetrically enhanced the contour of the mid face around the nose and mouth. Both ear auricles are preserved. The lobe of the right ear shows a large piercing, while the lobe of the left ear is missing.

Ramesses III (plates 86a–b)
The head of Ramesses III reveals an impressive face, as displayed in three-dimensional surface-rendering images. The skull shows a sagittal plateau. The orbits are filled with heterogeneous embalming material. The deformed, flattened nose is likely caused by pressure from bandages, despite being stuffed with embalming materials (mostly soft and resinous). The nasal openings are narrow and triangular. Symmetrical enhancement of the facial contours is the result of the skillful insertion of packs underneath the skin of the face. The chin is rounded, not receding. The mandible shows a square line and orthognathism.

CT Craniofacial Features
Wendell L. Wylie was the first to quantify the inheritance of craniofacial features by means of measurements on x-ray images (cephalograms).[11] The measurements include several lines, angles, ratios, and so on, related to conventional anatomic or anthropologic landmarks on lateral cephalometric x-rays.[12]

James E. Harris and his colleagues used an approach of cephalometric x-ray tracings with a statistical technique called cluster analysis to study a small sample of kings and queens of the royal mummy collection at the Egyptian Museum in Cairo. Using this sophisticated technique, the investigators compared similarities and dissimilarities between superimposed cephalometric tracings of the mummies and inferred data related to their position in the genealogical sequence.[13] In his notes, Edward F. Wente claimed that these superimposed cephalometric tracings illustrate dissimilarity between Amenhotep III and Tutankhamun and between Amenhotep III and Thutmose IV. He further stated that several mummies were found to be anomalous in terms of their position within the genealogical sequences.[14] However, this study has faced some criticism.

Two-dimensional and 3D CT images can be used to obtain reliable bony and soft-tissue craniofacial measurements. In a previous study, M.G. Cavalcanti and colleagues investigated the precision and accuracy of bony and soft-tissue anthropometric measurements using 2D and 3D reconstructed CT imaging of thirteen cadaver heads, performed by two radiologists. They found no statistically significant differences between interobserver and intraobserver measurements or between CT imaging and physical measurements.[15] The process of measuring the heads and faces of the royal mummies using 2D and 3D CT images is in progress.

Facial Reconstruction

More details may be obtained by facial reconstruction to render the likely facial appearance of these ancient mummies.[16] Variability in the phenotypes of faces reconstructed for ancient Egyptian mummies can come from a variety of sources, as reviewed by Victoria Lywood and Andrew Nelson.[17] Reconstruction techniques recognized in the literature include the Russian School, the American School, and the UK School.[18] The Russian School used the muscle markings on the skull as the basis of a detailed anatomical method of rebuilding the face muscle by muscle, arguing that the muscles determine the face's contours, while the skull determines the essential shape of the face.[19] The American School relies on specific tables of average facial tissue thickness, where pegs of appropriate lengths are placed at specific anatomical landmarks and strips of clay are used to build out from the skull to the end of the pegs.[20] The UK Manchester School uses the Russian muscle-based approach, but is guided by the tissue-thickness tables used by the American School.[21] Recently a variety of computerized methods of facial reconstruction have been developed, such as warping transformations, virtual sculpting techniques, and facial averaging.[22] Following 3D CT images of the head of a mummy, a resin or plastic model of the skull is built using a selective laser sintering system or stereolithography. The facial anatomy is then built using strips of plasticine or clay laid according to wooden pegs to construct the face.[23] The proper tissue-depth data is determined by race, gender, and age. Eye color, hair color, and lips are independent of bony structure. The different approaches to facial reconstruction have the potential to produce quite different results,[24] as do the anthropological assumptions that underlie the undertaking. The recent development of computerized techniques has introduced new variables in methodology, such as three-dimensional printing. There is considerable scholarly and popular interest in this matter, and facial reconstructions play an important role in shaping perceptions, as demonstrated by the controversy that surrounded the King Tutankhamun reconstruction.[25]

The Facial Reconstruction of Tutankhamun (plates 87, 88a–c)

A project to reconstruct the face of Tutankhamun was undertaken in 2005 by the Egyptian Supreme Council of Antiquities and National Geographic. Three teams were chosen, each representing a different country and headed by the following individuals:

- Egyptian: Khaled el-Said, biomedical engineer and team leader
- French: Jean-Noël Vignal, forensic expert, Institute de recherche criminelle de la gendarmerie nationale, Paris
- American: Susan Antón, physical anthropologist, New York University, and Michael Anderson, forensic sculptor, Peabody Museum, Yale University

The French and American participants were chosen and sponsored by National Geographic, and the Egyptian member was selected by the Supreme Council of Antiquities. The teams worked independently of each other; the French and Egyptian members were told that the subject was Tutankhamun, but this was not disclosed to the Americans, who worked 'blind.'

All three teams started with the CT data. The American and French teams were given a plastic model of the skull produced in Paris. The Egyptian team made their own model directly from the data. Based on this skull, the American and French teams both concluded that the subject was Caucasoid (the human type usually found, for example, in North Africa, Europe, and the Middle East). The American team, working blind, correctly identified the subject as North African.

Using the plastic model as a guide, the teams added clay to sculpt the features, based on the racial type. The French and Egyptian sculptors also were able to consult ancient images of Tutankhamun, and the Egyptian team did the work with the assistance of a detective from Boston. When the French team's model was complete, their sculptor created a silicone cast and, based on the archaeological information, added glass eyes, hair, and color to the skin and lips. The results of the three teams' work were identical or very similar in the proportions of the skull, the basic shape of the face, and the size and setting of the eyes. Variations occurred in the shape of the end of the nose and the ears. The noses are all different, though those of the French and the American versions resemble each other more closely than that of the Egyptian. The jaw and chin of the Egyptian reconstruction are stronger than those of the American and French, which are more similar to each other. In all, the Egyptian reconstruction looks the most Egyptian, and the French and American versions have more unique personalities.

The skull and facial shapes bear a remarkable resemblance to those on a famous image of the king found in his tomb, where he is depicted as the sun god rising from a lotus at dawn, in the guise of a child. This confirms the usefulness of the science and techniques of forensic reconstruction for recreating images of people who lived long ago.

Conclusion

Both the Egyptological and radiological results of the project confirm the Egyptian origins of the royal family. Though some scholars theorize a foreign origin for some of the pharaohs, this was contradicted by the Egyptian Mummy Project's analyses.

Appendix: List of the Royal Mummies in the Egyptian Museum, Cairo

In the first mummy room (P56), located on the east side of the museum, the following mummies are exhibited:

Seqenenre Tao II	CG 61051, JE 26209(b), SR 1/ 10192
Amenhotep I	CG 61058, JE 26211(b), SR 1/ 10194
Queen Meritamun	JE 55150, SR 1/ 10215
Unknown man, labeled 'Thutmose I'	CG 61065, JE 26217(c), SR 1/ 10195
Thutmose II	CG 61066, JE 26212(b), SR 1/ 10196
Thutmose III	CG 61068, JE 26203(b), SR 1/ 10197
Amenhotep II	CG 61069, SR 1/ 10198
Thutmose IV	CG 61073, JE 34559(b), SR 1/ 10199
Seti I	CG 61077, JE 26213(b), SR 1/ 10202
Ramesses II	CG 61078, JE 26214(b), SR 1/ 10203
Merenptah	CG 61079, JE 34562(b), SR 1/ 10204
Seti II	CG 61081, JE 34561(b), SR 1/ 10206
Sitre-In	TR 24.12.161, SR 7/23510(b), SR 1/
14437(b) Hatshepsut	JE 99575, SR 1/ 15143
Box of Hatshepsut containing liver	JE 26250
Hair samples of Ramesses II	JE 26214(b).1, CG 61078.1, SR 1/ 10203.1

On the west side of the Egyptian Museum, the second mummy room (P52) contains the following mummies:

Ramesses III	CG 61083, JE 26208a(d), SR 1/ 10207
Ramesses IV	CG 61084, JE 34567(b), SR 1/ 10208
Ramesses V	CG 61085, JE 34564(b), SR 1/ 10209
Ramesses IX	SR 1/10211
Queen Nodjmet	CG 61087, JE 26215(c), SR 1/ 10216
Henttawy	CG 61090, JE 26204(c), SR 1/ 10218
Maetkare + baboon	CG 61088, JE 26200(d), SR 1/ 10217(a); CG 61089, JE26200(e), SR 1/ 10217(b)
Pinudjem II	CG 61094, JE 26197(d), SR 7/ 19396(b), SR 1/ 10327(b)
Isetemkheb D	CG 61093, JE 26198(d), SR 1/ 10219
Nesikhonsu	CG 61095, JE 26199, SR 7/ 19394(c), SR 1/ 10325(c)
Djedptahiufankh	CG 61097, JE 26201(d), SR 7/ 19418(d), SR 1/ 10349(d)

At the entrance of this room are exhibited the mummies of Akhenaten (CG 61075, TR 16/9/15/1, SR 1/10201), the mother of Tutankhamun (CG 61072), and Queen Tiye (CG 61070). It is planned that the royal mummies (kings only) will be exhibited at the National Museum of Egyptian Civilization in Fustat, Old Cairo, when it is completed. The mummy of Tutankhamun remains in his tomb in the Valley of the Kings.

Glossary

Amduat: The New Kingdom Egyptian royal funerary text, "That Which Is in the Underworld." It describes the voyage of the sun god through the twelve hours of the night and is for the use of the pharaoh to overcome obstacles in the afterworld.

ankylosing spondylitis: A chronic inflammatory disease of the axial skeleton with variable involvement of peripheral joints.

ankylosis: Fusion of the joints.

axial images: Two-dimensional cross sections.

beam hardening artifact: Falsification of the structure of the imaged object due to sudden change in tissue density from a relatively low density (as in brain) to relatively high density (as skull).

Book of Gates: New Kingdom funerary text that chronicles the journey of the sun through the underworld during the twelve hours of the night. It corresponds to the journey of the dead into the afterlife, passing through a series of gates, each associated with a different deity.

Book of the Celestial Cow: New Kingdom mythological text first found in the tomb of Tutankhamun. It recounts mankind's rebellion against the sun god Re, and punishment by the goddess Hathor. Though Re prevented the total destruction of humans, he withdrew to the sky on the back of the celestial cow (the goddess Nut), and due to this separation, suffering and death were said to come into the world.

canopic jars: Four jars that held the mummified viscera of the deceased. Each jar was under the protection of one of the Four Sons of the god Horus, and in the New Kingdom, the lids often took the forms of the human-headed Imseti (liver), baboon-headed Hapi (lungs), falcon-headed Qebehsenuef (intestines), and jackal-headed Duamutef (stomach).

cine view: Sequential images are displayed on a monitor rapidly in a dynamic movie display format.

coronal plane: A vertical plane that divides the body into ventral (front) and dorsal (rear) sections.

diffuse idiopathic skeletal hyperostosis (DISH): Calcification or bony hardening of the ligaments in areas where they attach to the spine.

dorsal kyphosis: Hunchback.

ectocranial: Outside the skull.

ectocranial sutures: The sutures at the outer surface of the skull.

enthesopathy: Abnormal calcification of the tendons or joints.

epigastrium: The part of the upper abdomen immediately over the stomach.

hallux valgus complex: A deformity in which the big toe of the foot (hallux) deviates inward (valgus) in the direction of the little toe.

Hounsfield scale (measured in Hounsfield Units [HU]): A quantitative scale for describing the density in CT images that is calibrated with reference to water (0) and a scale from –1000 (air) to +1000 (bone).

hydrophilic: Having a tendency to mix with, dissolve in, or be wetted by water.

hyperostosis: Excessive bone growth.

iliac crest: The thick curved upper border of the ilium, the most prominent bone on the pelvis.

inguinal region: The lowest lateral region of the abdomen.

intra vitam: During life.

in vivo: Occurring in a living body.

lipping: Osteophytic lipping is the buildup of bone spurs, usually as the result of some form of arthritis.

Litany of Re: New Kingdom funerary text that invokes the sun god Re in seventy-five different forms, and contains a series of prayers associating the king with the sun god.

magic bricks: A set of four mud bricks sometimes placed at the cardinal points of a tomb chamber. They were intended to protect the deceased from evil. Each brick was inscribed with a text from the Book of the Dead and was provided with an amulet.

malocclusion: A problem in the way the upper and lower teeth fit together in biting or chewing. The word literally means 'bad bite,' and usually refers to crossbite or overbite.

metal streaking artifact: Dark streaks along the long axis of a single high-attenuation object, with bright streaks adjacent to the dark streaks.

midsagittal image: An image at the midline of the sagittal plane.

multiplanar reconstruction (or reformatting) (MPR): A post-processing technique to create new images from a stack of images in planes defined by the user. The use of thin slices increases the spatial resolution.

oblique plane: Inclined in direction.

occipital bun: A prominent bulge or projection of the occipital bone at the back of the skull.

occlusal wear: Loss of substance on the chewing surface of a tooth from use or other destructive factors.

orthopantomographic-like images: Panorama for teeth.

osteophyte: Small, abnormal bony outgrowth.

perimortem: Shortly before or after death.

popliteal fossa: A shallow depression at the back of the knee joint.

prognathism: A protruding jaw; the positional relationship of the mandible and/or maxilla to the skeletal base where either of the jaws protrudes beyond a predetermined imaginary line in the coronal plan of the skull.

pubic symphyseal face: The surface of the pubis where one pubis joins the other at the pubic symphysis.

sagittal plane: A vertical plane that passes from front to rear, dividing the body into right and left halves.

scoliosis: Lateral (sideways) curvature of the spine.

scout view or image: A preliminary image obtained prior to performing a major study.

sequela: An aftereffect or pathological condition resulting from a disease.

shawabti: A funerary figure intended to work as a stand-in for the deceased in the afterlife when called upon to perform agricultural labor in the fields.

spinal dysraphism: A congenital disorder in which some vertebrae overlying the spinal cord are not fully formed and remain unfused and open.

Sprengel's deformity (or high scapula): A rare congenital skeletal abnormality in which one shoulder blade (scapula) sits higher on the back than the other.

suture: The place where skull bones join and fuse later in life.

talatat: Small sandstone blocks used during Akhenaten's reign for the rapid construction of buildings and temples at Karnak and Amarna. These structures were dismantled and used as rubble in later buildings, enhancing their preservation.

trabecular bone: Anastomosing bony spicules in cancellous bone that form a meshwork of intercommunicating spaces that are filled with bone marrow.

volume data sets: Data in three dimensions.

voxel: The smallest distinguishable box-shaped part of a three-dimensional image.

wab-priest: Lower-level priest who assisted in cultic and maintenance activities in the temple.

window level: Determines the center CT number value displayed by the grayscale range.

window width: Determines the range of CT numbers displayed by the grayscale. CT numbers above the range are displayed as white and CT numbers below the range are displayed as black.

Illustration Credits

All CT images are from the Egyptian Mummy Project. The reconstructed CT images are the work of Sahar Saleem.

All other images are from the photo archive of Zahi Hawass, with the exception of the following:

Fig. 106. Courtesy of Salima Ikram, drawing by Nicholas Warner.

Fig. 110. © Michael C. Carlos Museum, Emory University. Photograph by Peter Harholdt.

Abbreviations

Acta Anat	*Acta Anatomica*
AJNR	*American Journal of Neuroradiology*
AJPA	*American Journal of Physical Anthropology*
AJR	*American Journal of Roentgenology*
Amarna Letters	*Amarna Letters*: Essays on Ancient Egypt series, ed. D. Forbes (San Francisco: KMT Communications)
Am J Anat	*American Journal of Anatomy*
Am J Med Genet	*American Journal of Medical Genetics*
Am J Orthod Dentofacial Orthop	*American Journal of Orthodontics and Dentofacial Orthopedics*
Anc Biomol	*Ancient Biomolecules*
Ann Hum Biol	*Annals of Human Biology*
Ann Méd Légale	*Annales de Médicine Légale*
Ann Rheum Dis	*Annals of the Rheumatic Diseases*
ASAE	*Annales du Service des Antiquités de l'Égypte*
BEM	*Bulletin of the Egyptian Museum*
BIE	*Bulletin de l'Institut Égyptien*
BIFAO	*Bulletin de l'Institut Français d'Archéologie Orientale*
BMJ	*British Medical Journal*
Br J Radiol	*British Journal of Radiology*
BSEG	*Bulletin de la Société d'égyptologie de Genève*
Bull Mém Soc Anthrop Paris	*Bulletins et Mémoires de la Société d'anthropologie de Paris*

Can Assoc Radiol J	*Canadian Association of Radiologists Journal*
CAPA	*Canadian Association for Physical Anthropology*
Clin Rheum Dis	*Clinics in Rheumatic Diseases*
Coll Antropol	*Collegium Antropologicum*
Comput Med Imaging Graph	*Computerized Medical Imaging and Graphics*
CSEG	*Cahiers de la Sociéte d'Égyptologie*
DE	*Discussions in Egyptology*
Dent Clin North Am	*Dental Clinics of North America*
Dentomaxillofac Radiol	*Dentomaxillofacial Radiology*
Eur Radiol	*European Radiology*
Fortschr Geb Röntgenstr Nuklearmed	*Fortschritte auf dem Gebiete der Röntgenstrahlen und der Nuklearmedizin*
GM	*Göttinger Miszellen*
Hum Evol	*Human Evolution*
IFAO	*Institut Français d'Archéologie Orientale*
Int J Legal Med	*International Journal of Legal Medicine*
Int J Osteoarchaeol	*International Journal of Osteoarchaeology*
JADA	*Journal of the American Dental Association*
JAMA	*Journal of the American Medical Association*
JARCE	*Journal of the American Research Center in Egypt*
J Arch Sci	*Journal of Archaeological Science*
JCAT	*Journal of Computer Assisted Tomography*
JEA	*Journal of Egyptian Archaeology*
JMFA	*Journal of the Museum of Fine Arts, Boston*
JNES	*Journal of Near Eastern Studies*
J Rheumatol	*Journal of Rheumatology*
JSSEA	*Journal of the Society for the Study of Egyptian Antiquities*
LÄ	*Lexikon der Ägyptologie*, ed. W. Helck, E. Otto, and W. Westendorf, 7 vols., 1972–92
Leg Med	*Legal Medicine*
MDAIK	*Mitteilungen des deutschen archäologischen Instituts, Abt. Kairo*
MMAF	Mémoires publiés par les membres de la Mission Archéologique Française au Caire
Pediatr Radiol	*Pediatric Radiology*
Rheumatol Int	*Rheumatology International*
SAOC	Studies in Ancient Oriental Civilization
Skeletal Radiol	*Skeletal Radiology*
Theo Med Bioeth	*Theoretical Medicine and Bioethics*
World J Surg	*World Journal of Surgery*
ZÄS	*Zeitschrift für Ägyptische Sprache und Altertumskunde*

Notes

Notes to Chronology

1   Dates through the Late Period are approximate. There are a number of new findings or interpretations of existing evidence that may change the lengths of some of these reigns (including Horemheb, Tawosret, Sethnakht, Ramesses VIII, and Ramesses X); these are not incorporated into this chronology.

Notes to Introduction

1   For the CT scanning of this mummy and additional information about Ramesses I, see "Ramesses I: The Search for the Lost Pharaoh," www.carlos.emory.edu/RAMESSES/index.html, and H. Hoffman and S. D'Auria, "Mummies and Modern Medical Imaging," in *The Realm of Osiris: Mummies, Coffins, and Ancient Egyptian Funerary Art in the Michael C. Carlos Museum*, ed. P. Lacovara and B.T. Trope (Atlanta: Michael C. Carlos Museum, Emory University, 2001), 38–39.

Notes to Chapter 1

1   F. Cesarani et al., "Whole-Body Three-Dimensional Multidetector CT of 13 Egyptian Human Mummies," *AJR* 180:3 (2003): 601.

2   T. Böni, F.J. Rühli, and R.K. Chhem, "History of Paleoradiology: Early Published Literature, 1896–1921," *Can Assoc Radiol J* 55:4 (October 2004): 203–10.

3   W. Seipel, "Research on Mummies in Egyptology: An Overview," in *Human Mummies: A Global Survey of Their Status and the Techniques of Their Conservation*, ed. K. Spindler et al. (Vienna: Springer, 1996), 42–44.

4   R.K. Chhem and D.R. Brothwell, *Paleoradiology: Imaging Mummies and Fossils* (Berlin and Heidelberg: Springer, 2010), 2.

5   Z. Hawass et al. "Ancestry and Pathology in King Tutankhamun's Family," *JAMA* 303:7 (2010): 638–47.

6   G.E. Smith, *The Royal Mummies*, Catalogue général des antiquités égyptiennes du Musée du Caire (Cairo: IFAO, 1912, repr. London: Duckworth, 2000), 45.

7   D.E. Derry, "An X-ray Examination of the Mummy of King Amenophis I," *ASAE* 34 (1934): 47–48.

8   Seipel, "Research," 42.

9   J.E. Harris and K.R. Weeks, *X-Raying the Pharaohs* (New York: Charles Scribner's Sons, 1973).

10 J.E. Harris and E.F. Wente, *An X-Ray Atlas of the Royal Mummies* (Chicago: University of Chicago Press, 1980).

11 Seipel, "Research," 42–44.

12 E.M. Braunstein et al., "Paleoradiologic Evaluation of the Egyptian Royal Mummies," *Skeletal Radiol* 17 (1988): 348–52.

13 Chhem and Brothwell, *Paleoradiology*, 26.

14 Hawass et al., "Ancestry and Pathology."

15 W. Recheis et al., "New Methods and Techniques in Anthropology," *Coll Antropol* 23:2 (1999): 495–509.

16 A motorized table moves the mummy through a circular opening in the CT machine. As the mummy passes through the machine, a source of x-rays rotates around the circular opening, producing a narrow beam to irradiate a thin section of the mummy's body to be received by opposing detectors. The detectors send the data to a computer to create a cross-sectional image of the body.

17 Recheis et al., "New Methods."

18 Somatom Emotion 6; Siemens Medical Solutions, Malvern, Pennsylvania.

19 Lightspeed; GE.

20 Hawass et al., "Ancestry and Pathology."

21 Leonardo Workstation, Siemens Medical Solution.

22 ORS-Visual (Object Research Systems, available at http://www.theobjects.com/en/; ImageJ (available at http://rsb.info.nih.giv/ij); and InVesalius 3.0 (available at http://www.cti.gov.br/invesalius)

23 F.E. Boas and D. Fleischmann, "Evaluation of Two Iterative Techniques for Reducing Metal Artifacts in Computed Tomography," *Radiology* 259:3 (2011): 894–902.

24 G. Luccichenti et al., "3D Reconstruction Techniques Made Easy: Know-how and Pictures," *Eur Radiol* 15:10 (October 2005): 2146–56.

25 In SSD, the pixel's value of the final picture corresponds to the value of the point that is closest to the screen and above a selected threshold. A depth-encoded shading scale makes the closer voxel appear brighter, enhancing the depth perception.

26 Cesarani et al., "Whole-Body."

27 Cesarani et al., "Whole-Body."

28 S.N. Saleem and Z. Hawass, "Multi Detector CT of Royal Ancient Egyptian Mummies: An Approach to Study" (presentation, Radiological Society of North America (RSNA), Chicago, November 25–30, 2012).

29 Smith, *Royal Mummies*, passim; S. Ikram and A. Dodson, *The Mummy in Ancient Egypt* (Cairo: American University in Cairo Press; London: Thames & Hudson Limited, 1998), 320–30.

30 Z. Hawass and S.N. Saleem, "Mummified Daughters of King Tutankhamun: Archeologic and CT Studies," *AJR* 197:5 (November 2011): W829–36.

31 S. Grabherr et al., "Estimation of Sex and Age of 'Virtual Skeletons': A Feasibility Study," *Eur Radiol* 19:2 (February 2009): 419–29.

32 S. Brooks, "Skeletal Age at Death: The Reliability of Cranial and Pubic Age Indicators," *AJPA* 13 (1955): 567–97; C.O. Lovejoy et al., "Multifactoral Determination of Skeletal Age at Death: A Method and

Blind Tests of Its Accuracy," *AJPA* 68:1
(1985): 1–14; D. Franklin, "Forensic Age
Estimation in Human Skeletal Remains:
Current Concepts and Future Directions,"
Leg Med 12:1 (January 2010): 1–7; Grabherr et
al., "Estimation."

33   Franklin, "Forensic Age."

34   Grabherr et al., "Estimation."

35   R.H. Biggerstaff, "Forensic Dentistry and the
Human Dentition in Individual Age
Estimation," *Dent Clin North Am* 21:1 (1977):
167–74.

36   L. Scheuer and S. Black, *Developmental
Juvenile Osteology* (San Diego: Academic Press,
2000), 12.

37   I. Schour and M. Massler, "The Development
of the Human Dentition," *JADA* 28 (1941):
1153–60.

38   Franklin, "Forensic Age."

39   Hawass et al., "Ancestry and Pathology";
Hawass et al., "Computed Tomographic
Evaluation of Pharaoh Tutankhamun, ca. 1300
BC," *ASAE* 81 (2007): 159–74.

40   R.S. Meindl and C.O. Lovejoy, "Ectocranial
Suture Closure: A Revised Method for the
Determination of Skeletal Age at Death Based
on the Lateral-Anterior Sutures," *AJPA* 68:1
(1985): 57–66.

41   Grabherr et al., "Estimation."

42   S. Brooks and J.M. Suchey, "Skeletal Age
Determination Based on the Os Pubis: A
Comparison of the Acsádi-Nemeskéri and
Suchey-Brooks Methods," *Hum Evol* 5:3
(1990): 227–38.

43   Grabherr et al., "Estimation."

44   Franklin, "Forensic Age."

45   Grabherr et al., "Estimation."

46   Franklin, "Forensic Age."

47   Grabherr et al., "Estimation."

48   G. Fully and H. Pineau, "Détermination de la
stature au moyen du squelette," *Ann Méd
Légale* 40 (1960): 145–54; B.R. Kate and R.D.

Mujumdar, "Stature Estimation from Femur
and Humerus by Regression and Autometry,"
Acta Anat 94:2 (1976): 311–20.

49   M.H. Raxter et al., "Stature Estimation in
Ancient Egyptians: A New Technique Based
on Anatomical Reconstruction of Stature,"
AJPA 136:2 (June 2008): 147–55.

50   Ikram and Dodson, *Mummy*, chapter 3.

Notes to Chapter 2

1   For the caches, see D.C. Forbes, *Tombs,
Treasures, Mummies: Seven Great Discoveries of
Egyptian Archaeology* (Sebastopol, CA: KMT
Communications, Inc., 1998), 17–55; S.
Ikram and A. Dodson, *The Mummy in
Ancient Egypt* (Cairo: American University in
Cairo Press, 1998), 316–30; V. Loret, "Le
tombeau d'Aménophis II et la cachette
royale de Biban el-Molouk," *BIE* (3rd series)
9 (1899): 98–112; D. Fouquet, *Le momies
royales de Deir el-Bahari: Rapport addressé à M.
Le Directeur Général des fouilles en Egypt*
(Cairo: IFAO, 1890); N. Reeves and R.H.
Wilkinson, *The Complete Valley of the Kings:
Tombs and Treasures of Egypt's Greatest
Pharaohs* (London: Thames & Hudson,
1996), 194–207; G.A. Belova, "TT320 and
the History of the Royal Cache during the
Twenty-first Dynasty," in *Egyptology at the
Dawn of the Twenty-first Century 1:
Archaeology*, ed. Z. Hawass and L.P. Brock
(Cairo: American University in Cairo Press,
2004), 73–80.

2   For the tomb robberies, see British Museum,
"The Abbott Papyrus," http://www.british-
museum.org/explore/highlights/highlight_obj
ects/aes/t/the_abbott_papyrus.aspx; J. Capart,
A.H. Gardiner, and B. van de Walle, "New
Light on the Ramesside Tomb Robberies,"
JEA 22:2 (1936): 169–93; A.J. Peden, *Egyptian
Historical Inscriptions of the Twentieth Dynasty*
(Jonsered, Sweden: Paul Åströms Förlag,

1994), xviii ff, 259 ff; T.E. Peet, *The Great Tomb Robberies of the Twentieth Egyptian Dynasty* (Oxford: Clarendon Press, 1930).

3   For discussion, see N. Reeves, *Valley of the Kings: The Decline of a Royal Necropolis* (London: Kegan Paul, 1990), 276–78; Reeves and Wilkinson, *Complete Valley*, 204–207.

4   Forbes, *Tombs*, 17–49. See also A. Edwards, "Lying in State in Cairo," *Harper's New Monthly Magazine* 65 (July 1882): 185–204.

5   G. Maspero, *Les Momies Royales de Déir el-Baharî*, MMAF 3 (Paris: Leroux, 1889), 518.

6   'Pasha' was a title given to important people by the king, before 1952.

7   Maspero, *Momies Royales*, 518.

8   An Arabic expression indicating that honesty is like a weapon that can be carried.

9   E. Wilson, "Finding Pharaoh," *Century Magazine* 34:1 (May 1887): 3–10.

10 Wilson, "Finding Pharaoh," 7–8; Edwards, "Lying in State," 190.

11 Forbes, *Tombs*, 26–27. See also G.E. Smith, *The Royal Mummies*, Catalogue général des antiquités égyptiennes du Musée du Caire (Cairo: IFAO, 1912, repr. London: Duckworth, 2000), 107; Maspero, *Momies Royales*, 520–24.

12 Maspero, *Momies Royales*, 513–14.

13 S. Hassan, *Misr al-qadima* (Cairo: Maktabat al-Usra, 2000), 8:676.

14 A. Fakhry, *Misr al-far'uniya*, 2nd ed. (Cairo: Maktabat al-Anglu, 1960), 391.

15 Ikram and Dodson, *Mummy*, 78.

16 Forbes, *Tombs*, 21.

17 In 2005, I excavated the tunnel until I came to its end, and nothing was found. See Z. Hawass and T. El Awady, "The Tunnel Inside the Tomb of Seti I (KV17): Secrets Revealed," *ASAE*, forthcoming.

18 Forbes, *Tombs*, 59.

19 Forbes, *Tombs*, 60–61.

20 Smith, *Royal Mummies*, 38–39.

21 Loret, "Tombeau d'Aménophis II," 104.

22 Loret, "Tombeau d'Aménophis II," 107–108.

23 See, for example, Reeves and Wilkinson, *Complete Valley*, 157.

24 Smith, *Royal Mummies*, 84.

25 P. Piacentini, ed., *Victor Loret in Egypt (1881–1899): From the Archives of the Milan University to the Egyptian Museum in Cairo* (Cairo: Supreme Council of Antiquities, 2008), 22–23. Some sources, such as Forbes, *Tombs*, 78, indicate that Loret did not sail with the cargo, but it is clear from Loret's notes that he did begin the journey to Cairo.

26 Forbes, *Tombs*, 78–81; Piacentini, *Victor Loret*, 8.

27 However, Loret's archives were acquired by the University of Milan in 2002; see P. Piacentini, *La Valle de Re riscoperta: I giornali di scavo di Victor Loret (1898–1899) e altri inediti* (Milan: University of Milan, 2004) and Piacentini, *Victor Loret*.

28 Forbes, *Tombs*, 78–81.

Notes to Chapter 3

1   For Hatshepsut's reign, see A.H. Gardiner, *Egypt of the Pharaohs* (Oxford: Oxford University Press, 1961), 181–88; W.C. Hayes, "Egypt: Internal Affairs from Thutmosis I to the Death of Amenophis III," in *Cambridge Ancient History*, 3rd ed., vol. 2, part 1, ch. 9, ed. I.E.S. Edwards, C.J. Gadd, N.G.L. Hammond, and E. Sollberger (Cambridge: Cambridge University Press, 1973); Z. Hawass, *Silent Images: Women in Pharaonic Egypt* (Cairo: American University in Cairo Press, 2008), 33–35; C.H. Roehrig, R. Dreyfus, and C.H. Keller, eds., *Hatshepsut: From Queen to Pharaoh* (New York: Metropolitan Museum of Art, 2005); J. Tyldesley, *Hatchepsut: The Female Pharaoh* (New York: Viking, 1996).

2   Roehrig et al., *Hatshepsut*, fig. 41.

3   D. O'Connor, "Thutmose III: An Enigmatic Pharaoh," in *Thutmose III: A New Biography*, ed. E. Cline and D. O'Connor (Ann Arbor: University of Michigan Press, 2009), 26.

4   P. Dorman, *The Monuments of Senenmut: Problems in Historical Methodology* (London and New York: Kegan Paul International, 1988), 78–79.

5   P. Lacau, *Stèles du Nouvel Empire*, vol. 1, Catalogue général des antiquités égyptiennes du Musée du Caire 45 (Cairo: IFAO, 1909), 21–22.

6   E. Naville, *The Temple of Deir el Bahari* (London: Egypt Exploration Fund, 1894–1908), vol. 5, pls. 141, 143; K. Kitchen, "A Long-Lost Portrait of Princess Neferurēʿ from Deir el-Baḥri," *JEA* 49 (1963): 38–39, pl. 7.

7   R. Pirelli, *The Queens of Ancient Egypt* (Cairo: American University in Cairo Press, 2008), 168.

8   Pirelli, *Queens*, 166.

9   For the career of Senenmut, see Dorman, *Monuments*.

10 H. Carter, "A Tomb Prepared for Queen Hatshepsut Discovered by the Earl of Carnarvon (October 1916)," *ASAE* 16 (1916): 79–82.

11 T. Davis, E. Naville, and H. Carter, *The Tomb of Hâtshopsîtû* (London: Constable, 1906).

12 L. Gabolde, "La montagne thébaine garde encore des secrets," *Dossiers d'Archéologie*, 149–50 (1990): 56–59; J. Romer, "Tuthmosis I and the Bibân el-Molûk: Some Problems of Attribution," *JEA* 60 (1974): 119–33.

13 Reeves and Wilkinson, *Complete Valley*, 91–94.

14 Davis, Naville, and Carter, *Tomb of Hâtshopsîtû*, xiv.

15 JE 47032.

16 MFA 04.278.

17 For a discussion of the two sarcophagi, see P. Der Manuelian and C. Loeben, "From Daughter to Father: The Recarved Egyptian Sarcophagus of Queen Hatshepsut and King Thutmose I," *JMFA* 5 (1993): 24–61.

18 Davis, Naville, and Carter, *Tomb of Hâtshopsîtû*, 77–112; H. Carter, "Report of Work Done in Egypt, 1903–1904," *ASAE* 6 (1905): 112–19; L. Gabolde, "Les tombes d'Hatchepsout," *Egypte: Afrique et Orient* 17 (2000): 51–56.

19 CG 61056 in the Egyptian Museum.

20 Egyptian Museum CG 61052.

21 G.E. Smith, *The Royal Mummies*, Catalogue général des antiquités égyptiennes du Musée du Caire (Cairo: IFAO, 1912, repr. London: Duckworth, 2000), 7.

22 Z. Hawass, "The Discovery of the Mummy of Queen Hatshepsut," in Ola El-Aguizy Festschrift, *BIFAO*, forthcoming.

23 Z. Hawass, "Quest for the Mummy of Hatshepsut," *KMT* 17:2 (Summer 2006): 40–43.

24 G. Maspero, *Les Mummies Royales de Déir el-Baharî*, MMAF 3 (Paris: Leroux, 1889), 581–82; Maspero, *The Struggle of the Nations* (London: Society for Promoting Christian Knowledge, 1896), 242, n2.

25 Smith, *Royal Mummies*, 25–28; see also D.C. Forbes, *Tombs, Treasures, Mummies: Seven Great Discoveries of Egyptian Archaeology* (Sebastopol, CA: KMT Communications, Inc., 1998), 621–25.

26 See Hawass, "Discovery"; see also M. Luban, "Is the Mummy 'Tuthmosis I' Really Hatshepsut?" *DE* 42 (1998).

27 S.N. Saleem and Z. Hawass, "Variability in Cranial Mummification of Royal Ancient Egyptians (18th–20th Dynasties): A Multi-detector Computed Tomography Study," lecture presented at the Eighth World Congress on Mummies Studies, Rio de Janeiro, Brazil, August 8, 2013.

28 S.N. Saleem and Z. Hawass, "Multi-Detector Computed Tomography Study of Amulets, Jewelry, and Other Foreign Objects in Royal Egyptian Mummies Dated to the 18th to 20th Dynasties," *JCAT* 38:2 (2013): 153–58.

29 Z. Hawass, "Discovery."

30 J.E Harris and E.F. Wente, *An X-Ray Atlas of the Royal Mummies* (Chicago: University of Chicago Press, 1980), 206.

31 T. Davis, G. Maspero, E. Ayrton, and G. Daressy, *The Tomb of Siphtah; The Monkey Tomb and the Gold Tomb* (London: Constable, 1908), 18.

32 E. Thomas, *The Royal Necropoleis of Thebes* (Princeton: privately published, 1966), 161.

33 Email from Donald Ryan to Zahi Hawass, November 13, 2009.

34 See D.C. Forbes, "Akheperenre Djehutymes: The All-But-Forgotten Second Thutmose," *KMT* 11:2 (Summer 2000): 62–75; see also Forbes, *Tombs*, 626–29; L. Gabolde, "La montagne thébaine."

35 Hawass, "Discovery."

36 See D. Laboury, "A propos de l'authenticité de la momie attribuée à Thoutmosis III (CG 61068)," *GM* 156 (1997): 73–79; Gabolde, "La montagne thébaine"; G. Gibson, "How Tall Was Thutmose III? An Investigation into the Nature of Information," *KMT* 11:1 (Spring 2000): 60–65.

37 Smith, *Royal Mummies*, 32; Maspero, *Momies Royales*, 547–48; Forbes, *Tombs*, 43–47, 631.

38 Hawass, "Discovery."

39 Forbes, *Tombs*, 32, 48.

40 JE 26250.

41 H. Carter, "Report of Work Done in Upper Egypt (1902–1903)," *ASAE* 4 (1903): 176–77.

42 Z. Hawass, "Quest for the Mummy of Queen Hatshepsut," *KMT* 17:2 (Summer 2006): 41; Thomas, *Royal Necropoleis*, 137; D.P. Ryan, "Who is Buried in KV60?" *KMT* 1 (1990): 34–39. See also Z. Hawass, "The Scientific Search for Hatshepsut's Mummy," *KMT* 18:3 (Fall 2007): 20–25.

43 It was registered as TR 24.12.16.1 in 1916.

44 Email from Donald Ryan to Zahi Hawass, 2010.

45 Thomas, *Royal Necropoleis*, 138.

46 Ryan, "Who is Buried?"

47 JE 56264.

48 According to the examination of both the mummy and the CT scans by Ashraf Selim and other Egyptian and foreign consultants.

49 Email from Paul Gostner to Zahi Hawass, 2009.

50 Hawass, "Discovery."

51 Hawass, "Quest."

52 Hawass, "Discovery."

53 J. Guevara-Aquirre and A.L. Rosenbloom, "Obesity, Diabetes and Cancer: Insight into the Relationship from a Cohort with Growth Hormone Receptor Deficiency," *Diabetologia* 58:1 (Jan. 2015): 37–42, doi: 10.1007/s00125-014-3397-3, Epub 2014 Oct 15.

54 Pirelli, *Queens*, 54.

55 For further discussion of this concept, see Hawass, *Silent Images*, 28–30.

Notes to Chapter 4

1 Z. Hawass, *The Golden King: The World of Tutankhamun* (Cairo: American University in Cairo Press, 2006), 23–24.

2 Hawass, *Golden King*, 27–28.

3 H. Sourouzian, "Beyond Memnon: Buried More than 3,300 Years, Remnants of Amenhotep III's Extraordinary Mortuary Temple at Kom el-Hettan Rise from Beneath the Earth," *ICON Magazine* (Summer 2004): 10–17.

4 Z. Hawass and A.G. Wagdy, "Excavations North-West of Amenhotep III Temple: Season 2010–11," *MDAIK* 70/71 (2014/2015), forthcoming; Z. Hawass, A.G. Wagdy, and M.A. Badea, "The Discovery of the Missing Pieces

of the Statue of Amenhotep III and Queen Tiye at the Egyptian Museum," *ASAE* 85 (2011): 165–76.

5   J. Quibell, *Tomb of Yuaa and Thuiu*, Catalogue général des antiquités égyptiennes du Musée du Caire (Cairo: IFAO, 1908). See also D.C. Forbes, *Tombs, Treasures, Mummies: Seven Great Discoveries of Egyptian Archaeology* (Sebastopol, CA: KMT Communications, Inc., 1998), 116–85.

6   N. Reeves and R.H. Wilkinson, *The Complete Valley of the Kings: Tombs and Treasures of Egypt's Greatest Pharaohs* (London: Thames & Hudson, 1996), 176–77.

7   Hawass, *Golden King*, 27–28. See also W.R. Johnson, "Monuments and Monumental Art under Amenhotep III," in *Amenhotep III: Perspectives on His Reign*, ed. D. O'Connor and E.H. Cline (Ann Arbor: University of Michigan Press, 1998), 90.

8   Johnson, "Monuments," 90.

9   A. Dodson and D. Hilton, *The Complete Royal Families of Ancient Egypt* (London: Thames & Hudson, 2004), 157.

10   For the coregency, see the following recent articles in *KMT* 35:2 (Summer 2014): A. Dodson, "The Coregency Conundrum," 28–35; F.M. Valentin and T. Bedman, "Proof of a 'Long Coregency' between Amenhotep III and Amenhotep IV Found in the Chapel of Vizier Amenhotep-Huy (Asasif Tomb 28), West Luxor," 17–27; and D. Forbes, "Circumstantial Evidence for an Amenhotep III/Amenhotep IV Coregency," 36–49.

11   For the reign of Akhenaten and the city of Akhetaten, see C. Aldred, *Akhenaten and Nefertiti* (New York: The Brooklyn Museum, 1973); J. Allen, "Akhenaten's 'Mystery' Coregent and Successor," *Amarna Letters* 1 (1991): 74–85; J.D.S. Pendlebury, *The City of Akhenaten* 3 (London: Egypt Exploration Society, 1951); E. Hornung, *Echnaton: die Religion des Lichtes* (Zurich: Artemis and Winkler, 1995); C. Aldred, "The Horizon of the Aten," *JEA* 62 (1976): 184; R.E. Freed, Y.J. Markowitz, and S.H. D'Auria, eds., *Pharaohs of the Sun: Akhenaten, Nefertiti, Tutankhamun* (Boston: Museum of Fine Arts, 1999); and B. Kemp, *The City of Akhenaten and Nefertiti: Amarna and Its People* (London: Thames & Hudson, 2012).

12   N. Reeves, *The Complete Tutankhamun: The King, the Tomb, the Royal Treasure* (London: Thames & Hudson, 1990), 24.

13   N. de G. Davies, *The Rock Tombs of El Amarna, Part 2: The Tombs of Panehesy and Meryra II* (London: Egypt Exploration Society, 1905), 38–43, pls. 37–40, 47.

14   For a discussion of Neferneferuaten and Smenkhkare, see J. Allen, "The Amarna Succession," in *Causing His Name to Live: Studies in Epigraphy and History in Memory of William Murnane*, ed. P. Brand and L. Cooper, Culture and History of the Ancient Near East 37 (Leiden: Brill, 2009), 9–20.

15   A. van der Perre, "The Year 16 Graffito of Akhenaten in Dayr Abu Hinnis: A Contribution to the Study of the Later Years of Nefertiti," *Journal of Egyptian History* 7:1 (2014): 67–108; Van der Perre, "Nefertiti's Last Documented Reference (for Now)," in *In the Light of Amarna: One Hundred Years of the Nefertiti Discovery*, ed. F. Seyfried (Berlin: Ägyptisches Museum und Papyrussammlung, Staatliche Museen zu Berlin), 195–97; T.L. Gertzen, "New Evidence for Nefertiti in Akhenaten's Regnal Year 16," *KMT* 24:1 (Spring 2013): 34.

16   For discussion, see Reeves and Wilkinson, *Complete Valley*, 117–21; T. Davis, *The Tomb of Queen Tiye*, 2nd ed. (San Francisco: KMT Communications, 1990).

17   Quibell, *Tomb*, 68–73.

18 S.N. Saleem and Z. Hawass, "Variability in Brain Treatment during Mummification of Royal Ancient Egyptians Dated to the 18th–20th Dynasties: MDCT Findings Correlated with the Archaeologic Literature," *AJR* 200:4 (April 2013): W336–44.

19 S. Saleem and Z. Hawass, "Multi Detector CT of Royal Ancient Egyptian Mummies: An Approach to Study," presentation at the Radiological Society of North America (RSNA), Chicago, November 25–30, 2012.

20 T. Davis et al., *The Tomb of Iouiyu and Touiyou* (London: Constable, 1907), xxix.

21 S.N. Saleem and Z. Hawass, "Subcutaneous Packing in Royal Egyptian Mummies Dated from the 18th to 20th Dynasties," *JCAT* (in press).

22 Saleem and Hawass, "Multi Detector CT."

23 Saleem and Hawass, "Variability in Brain Treatment."

24 Z. Hawass et al., "Ancestry and Pathology in King Tutankhamun's Family," *JAMA* 303:7 (2010): 638–47.

25 D. O'Connor and E. Cline, *Amenhotep III: Perspectives on His Reign* (Ann Arbor: University of Michigan Press, 1998), 3; G.E. Smith, *The Royal Mummies*, Catalogue général des antiquités égyptiennes du Musée du Caire (Cairo: IFAO, 1912, repr. London: Duckworth, 2000), 46–51.

26 Forbes, *Tombs*, 676–77.

27 Smith, *Royal Mummies*, 50–51.

28 Saleem and Hawass, "Variability in Brain Treatment."

29 Saleem and Hawass, "Subcutaneous Packing."

30 Griffith Institute, Carter 320e, http:www.griffith.ox.ac.uk/gri/carter3203.html

31 J.E. Harris et al., "The Identification of the Elder Lady in the Tomb of Amenhotep II as Queen Tiye," *Delaware Medical Journal* 51:2 (1979): 89–93.

32 Hawass et al., "Ancestry and Pathology."

33 Smith, *Royal Mummies*, 38. See also G.E. Smith, "On the Mummies in the Tomb of Amenhotep II," BIE 51, series 1 (1907), 224–25.

34 Harris et al., "Identification."

35 Report submitted by the team to the SCA in 2003.

36 E.F. Wente, "Age at Death of Pharaohs of the New Kingdom Determined from Historical Sources," in *An X-Ray Atlas of the Royal Mummies*, ed. J.E. Harris and E.F. Wente (Chicago: University of Chicago Press, 1980), 256–57.

37 Saleem and Hawass, "Variability in Brain Treatment."

38 S. Ikram and A. Dodson, *The Mummy in Ancient Egypt* (Cairo: American University in Cairo Press, 1998), 124.

39 Saleem and Hawass, "Subcutaneous Packing."

40 Hawass et al., "Ancestry and Pathology."

41 Saleem and Hawass, "Subcutaneous Packing."

42 Smith, *Royal Mummies*, 41.

43 Reeves and Wilkinson, *Complete Valley*, 121.

44 M. Gabolde, "Under a Deep Blue Starry Sky," in *Causing His Name to Live: Studies in Egyptian Epigraphy and History in Memory of William Murnane*, ed. P. Brand and L. Cooper (Leiden: Brill, 2009), http://cassian.memphis.edu/history/murnane/M_Gabolde.pdf, 8 ff.

45 Smith, *Royal Mummies*, 54.

46 F. Hussein and J.E. Harris, "The Skeletal Remains from Tomb No. 55," in *Fifth International Congress of Egyptology, October 29–November 3, Cairo, 1988, Abstracts of Papers* (Cairo: International Association of Egyptologists), 140–41.

47 R.C. Connolly, R.G. Harrison, and S. Ahmed, "Serological Evidence for the Parentage of Tut'ankhamūn and Smenkharē'," *JEA* 62 (1976): 184–86; Forbes, *Tombs*, 317; D.B. Redford, *Akhenaten: The Heretic King*

(Princeton: Princeton University Press, 1984), 190–91; R.G. Harrison et al., "Kinship of Smenkhkare and Tutankhamun Affirmed by Serological Micromethod: Kinship of Smenkhkare and Tutankhamen Demonstrated Serologically," *Nature* 224 (1969): 325–26; Reeves and Wilkinson, *Complete Valley*, 120–21.

48 Hussein and Harris, "Skeletal Remains."

49 J. Filer, "Anatomy of a Mummy," *Archaeology* 55:2 (March/April 2002): 26–29.

50 Hawass et al., "Ancestry and Pathology."

Notes to Chapter 5

1 See Z. Hawass, *Discovering Tutankhamun: From Howard Carter to DNA* (Cairo: American University in Cairo Press, 2013), chapter 1.

2 For the origins of Tutankhamun, see N. Reeves, *The Complete Tutankhamun: The King, the Tomb, the Royal Treasure* (London: Thames & Hudson, 1990), 24.

3 For the name, see G. Roeder, *Amarna-Reliefs aus Hermopolis* (Hildesheim: Gerstenberg, 1969), pl. 106, no. 831/VIIIC; see also Z. Hawass, "Newly Discovered Scenes of Tutankhamun from Memphis and Rediscovered Blocks from Heliopolis," in *The Art and Culture of Ancient Egypt: Studies in Honor of Dorothea Arnold*, ed. O. Goelet and A. Oppenheim, *BES* 19 (2012), forthcoming.

4 For Tutankhamun at Memphis, see J. van Dijk and M. Eaton-Krauss, "Tutankhamun and Memphis," *MDAIK* 42 (1986): 35–41.

5 Hawass, "Newly Discovered Scenes."

6 To be published in the upcoming Festschrift for Betsy Bryan: R. Jasnow and K.M. Cooney, eds., *Joyful in Thebes: Egyptological Studies in Honor of Betsy M. Bryan* (Atlanta: Lockwood Press, 2015).

7 Hawass, *Discovering Tutankhamun*, 154–57. See also S. Holm, "The Privacy of Tutankhamen–Utilising the Genetic Information in Stored Tissue Samples," *Theo Med Bioeth* 22 (2001): 437–49.

8 Z. Hawass, *Discovering Tutankhamun*, chapter 1.

9 Griffith Institute, Diaries 4th Season, "Tutankhamun: Anatomy of an Excavation. Howard Carter's Diaries. The Fourth Excavation Season in the Tomb of Tutankhamun, September 23, 1925 to May 21, 1926," http://www.griffith.ox.ac.uk/gri/4sea4not.html

10 H. Carter and A.C. Mace, *The Tomb of Tut-Ankh-Amen* (London: Cassell & Co., 1927, repr. New York: Cooper Square Publishers, 1963), 2:106–61.

11 D.C. Forbes, *Tombs, Treasures, Mummies: Seven Great Discoveries of Egyptian Archaeology* (Sebastopol, CA: KMT Communications, Inc., 1998), 704–10; The Griffith Institute, "Tutankhamun: The Anatomy of an Excavation," photo p. 1566, http//www.griffith.ox.ac.uk/gri/4tut.html

12 F.F. Leek, *The Human Remains from the Tomb of Tutankhamun* (Oxford: Griffith Institute, 1972).

13 Leek, *Human Remains*, 7, 9, 13, 19.

14 R.G. Harrison and A.B. Abdalla, "The Remains of Tutankhamun," *Antiquity* 46 (1972): 9.

15 Harrison and Abdalla, "Remains," 11.

16 Forbes, *Tombs*, 712; B. Brier, *The Murder of Tutankhamun* (Berkeley: Berkeley Publishing Group, 1999); M.R. King, G.M. Cooper, and D. DeNevi, *Who Killed King Tut? Using Modern Forensics to Solve a 3300-Year-Old Mystery* (Amherst, NY: Prometheus Books, 2004).

17 Harrison and Abdalla, "Remains," 11, 13; F.F. Leek, "How Old was Tutankhamun?" *JEA* 63 (1977): 112–15.

18 See Forbes, *Tombs*, 711.

19 Z. Hawass, "New Evidence for the Cause of Tutankhamun's Death," *Bibliotheca Alexandrina*, http://www.bibalex.org/archeology/attachments/lectures/201201221342049314.pdf. See also Z. Hawass, *Tutankhamun and the Golden Age of the Pharaohs* (Washington, D.C.: National Geographic, 2005) 263–70.

20 Z. Hawass et al., "Computed Tomographic Evaluation of Pharaoh Tutankhamun, ca. 1300 BC," *ASAE* 81 (2007): 159–74.

21 Cf. Harrison and Abdalla, "Remains," 9.

22 It is impossible to tell exactly when the ribs, which seem to be visible in the photographs taken by Harry Burton, were removed from the body. There are various theories current, including the idea that the king was killed by the kick of a horse, and the crushed ribs were removed by the embalmers (W.B. Harer, Jr., "An Explanation of King Tutankhamun's Death," *BEM* 3 (2006): 83–88); or that the king was killed by a hippopotamus (Harer, "New Evidence for King Tutankhamun's Death: His Bizarre Embalming," *JEA* 97 (2011): 228–232; "Was Tutankhamun Killed by a Hippo?" *Ancient Egypt* 72 (2012): 50–54); or that the ribs were removed sometime between 1926 and 1968 in order to steal the now-missing jewelry that Carter left on the body (D.C. Forbes, S. Ikram, and J. Kamrin, "Tutankhamun's Ribs: A Proposed Solution to the Problem," *KMT* 18:1 (Spring 2007): 50–56). I personally (Z.H.) believe that the ribs were removed by Carter himself.

23 Cf. Leek, "How Old?" 115.

24 Hawass et al., "Ancestry and Pathology in King Tutankhamun's Family," *JAMA* 303:7 (2010): 638–47.

25 R.G. Harrison, "Postmortem on Two Pharaohs: Was Tutankhamun's Skull Fractured?" *Buried History* 4 (1971): 114–29.

26 J.D. Swales, "Tutankhamun's Breasts," *The Lancet* 301:7796 (27 January 1973): 201.

27 M.E. Müller et al., *Manual der Osteosynthese* (Berlin: Springer, 1971).

28 Carter and Mace, *Tomb of Tut-Ankh-Amen*, 2:156, pl. XXXV, B.

29 N. Reeves, *The Complete Tutankhamun: The King, The Tomb, The Royal Treasure* (London: Thames & Hudson, 1990), 178.

30 Griffith Institute, http://www.griffith.ox.ac.uk/gri/carter/229.html; Reeves, *Complete Tutankhamun*, 178.

31 *Ägyptisches Museum, Staatliche Museen Preußischer Kulturbesitz* (Stuttgart: Belser, 1980), no. 35, 84.

32 R. Vergnieux, "Recherches sur les monuments Thébains d'Amenhotep IV à l'aide d'outils informatiques: Methodes et résultats," *CSEG* 4 (1999): pls. 22, 31b, 35, 37b.

33 M. Saleh and H. Sourouzian, *Official Catalogue of the Egyptian Museum, Cairo* (Mainz: Philipp von Zabern, 1987), Carter 540, Carter 551, cat. no. 188, also Carter 108, cat. no. 178.

34 Hawass, "Newly Discovered Scenes."

35 N.M. Davies, *Ancient Egyptian Paintings* (Chicago: University of Chicago Press, 1936), pl. 7.

36 N. de G. Davies, *The Tomb of Ken-Amūn at Thebes* (New York: Metropolitan Museum of Art, repr. 1973), pl. 53.

37 According to W. Raymond Johnson, a scene exists of Akhenaten seated while using a bow and arrow to hunt fish and fowl. However, the context is different from the depiction of Tutankhamun, which takes place in the desert at Memphis, where the king hunts wild animals, something that could not easily be done from a seated position.

38 R.S. Boyer et al., "The Skull and Cervical Spine Radiographs of Tutankhamen: A Critical Appraisal," *AJNR* 24:61 (2003): 1142–47.

39 Egyptian Museum, JE 26210/CG61057. G.E. Smith, *The Royal Mummies*, Catalogue général des antiquités égyptiennes du Musée du Caire (Cairo: IFAO, 1912, repr. London: Duckworth, 2000), 10–17; S. Ikram and A. Dodson, *The Mummy in Ancient Egypt* (Cairo: American University in Cairo Press, 1998), 118, 122–23, 322, ill. 125.

40 Hawass et al., "Computed Tomographic," 162.

41 For a discussion of malaria in the royal family, see Z. Hawass, *Discovering Tutankhamun*, 158.

42 There are no details in the medical papyri about the recurrent fevers and chills associated with malaria (J.F. Nunn, "Disease," in *The Oxford Encyclopedia of Ancient Egypt* 1, ed. D. Redford (Cairo: American University in Cairo Press, 2001), 398). There are also no real details given by the ancient Egyptians, although Herodotus notes that Lower Egypt was infested with gnats, and people slept under nets to avoid the mosquitos (Herodotus, *The Histories*, Book 2, translated by A. de Sélincourt, rev. A.R. Burns. (Harmondsworth: Penguin, 1972), 94). This is sometimes taken as evidence of malaria. The Ebers Papyrus mentions rigors, fever, and enlargement of the spleen for one medical problem, which could be a reference to malaria symptoms (A.J. McMichael, *Human Frontiers, Environments and Disease: Past Patterns, Uncertain Futures* (Cambridge: Cambridge University Press, 2001), 80). However, Nunn states that there is no evidence of periodic fevers in the medical papyri (J.F. Nunn, *Ancient Egyptian Medicine* (London: British Museum, 1996), 73). Generally, malaria is not referenced in the medical papyri.

43 R. Bianucci et al., "Immunological Evidence of *Plasmodium falciparum* Infection in an Egyptian Child Mummy from the Early Dynastic Period," *J Arch Sci* 35:7 (2008): 1880–85.

44 Hawass et al., "Ancestry and Pathology."

Notes to Chapter 6

1 H. Carter and A.C. Mace, *The Tomb of Tut-Ankh-Amen* 3 (London: Cassell & Co., 1927, repr. New York: Cooper Square Publishers, 1963), 88–89, 167–69. See also N. Reeves, *The Complete Tutankhamun: The King, the Tomb, the Royal Treasure* (London: Thames & Hudson, 1990), 123–25; and D.C. Forbes, *Tombs, Treasures, Mummies: Seven Great Discoveries of Egyptian Archaeology* (Sebastopol, CA: KMT Communications, Inc., 1998), 450–54.

2 Griffith Institute, "Tutankhamun: Anatomy of an Excavation. The Howard Carter Archives," database entries for fetus mummies: http://www.griffith.ox.ac.uk/gri/carter/300-349.html.

3 D.E. Derry, "Report upon the Two Human Fetuses Discovered in the Tomb of Tut-Ankh-Amen," in *The Tomb of Tut-Ankh-Amen* 2, ed. H. Carter and A.C. Mace (London: Cassell and Company, 1933), 167–69.

4 Derry, "Report."

5 R.G. Harrison et al., "A Mummified Foetus from the Tomb of Tutankhamun," *Antiquity* 53:207 (1979): 19–21.

6 C.A. Hellier and R.C. Connolly, "A Reassessment of the Larger Fetus Found in Tutankhamen's Tomb," *Antiquity* 83:319 (2009): 165–73.

7 Ahmed Sameh Farid was convinced that the fetuses should be transported to the Egyptian Museum because of their poor preservation at Kasr Al-Ainy. However, we were unable to make this transfer because of the revolution that began in January 2011.

8 Z. Hawass and S.N. Saleem, "Mummified Daughters of King Tutankhamun: Archeologic and CT Studies," *AJR* 197:5 (November 2011): W829–36.

9   G. Olivier and H. Pineau, "Nouvelle détermination de la taille foetale d'après les longueurs diaphysaires des os longs," *Ann Méd Légale* 40 (1960): 141–44.

10 J.L. Scheuer et al., "The Estimation of Late Fetal and Perinatal Age from Limb Bone Length by Linear and Logarithmic Regression," *Ann Hum Biol* 7:3 (1980): 257–65.

11 E. Gilbert-Barness and D. Debich-Spicer, *Embryo and Fetal Pathology: Color Atlas with Ultrasound Correlation* (Cambridge, UK: Cambridge University Press, 2004), 1–22.

12 Derry, "Report."

13 Z. Hawass and S.N. Saleem, "Reply," *AJR* 198:6 (2012): W630.

14 Hawass and Saleem, "Mummified Daughters," W830.

15 N. Stempflé et al., "Fetal Bone Age Revisited: Proposal of a New Radiographic Score," *Pediatr Radiol* 25:7 (1995): 551–55.

16 Ø.E. Olsen et al., "Ossification Sequence in Infants Who Die during the Perinatal Period: Population-based References," *Radiology* 225:1 (2002): 240–44.

17 Hawass and Saleem, "Mummified Daughters," W831.

18 Harrison et al., "Mummified Foetus," 19.

19 Harrison et al., "Mummified Foetus," 20.

20 S.N. Saleem and Z. Hawass, "Mummification of Fetuses in Ancient Egypt: Anthropology and Multi-detector Computed Tomography Study (MDCT)," presented at American Anthropology Association (AAA) annual meeting, Chicago, November 22, 2013.

21 Saleem and Hawass, "Mummification of Fetuses."

Notes to Chapter 7

1   J. Allen, "The Amarna Succession," in *Causing His Name to Live: Studies in Epigraphy and History in Memory of William Murnane*, ed. P. Brand and L. Cooper, Culture and History of the Ancient Near East 37 (Leiden: Brill, 2009), http://cassian.memphis.edu/history/murnane/Allen.pdf

2   W.J. Murnane, *Texts from the Amarna Period in Egypt*, Writings from the Ancient World 5 (Atlanta: Society of Biblical Literature, 1995), 207–208.

3   A. Dodson, *Amarna Sunset: Nefertiti, Tutankhamun, Ay, Horemheb, and the Egyptian Counter-Reformation* (Cairo: American University in Cairo Press, 2009), 45; A. Dodson, "Were Nefertiti and Tutankhaten Coregents?" *KMT* 20:3 (Fall 2009): 49.

4   During her tenure as a queen, Nefertiti also bore the name Neferneferuaten.

5   See Allen, "Amarna Succession," and Dodson, *Amarna Sunset*, 40.

6   See N. Reeves, *Akhenaten: Egypt's False Prophet* (London: Thames & Hudson, 2005), 172–73.

7   Dodson, "Nefertiti and Tutankhaten?," 47; P. Clayton, *The Complete Pharaohs* (Cairo: American University in Cairo Press, 2006), 126; A. Dodson and D. Hilton, *The Complete Royal Families of Ancient Egypt* (London: Thames & Hudson, 2004), 150. See also the discussion in Dodson, *Amarna Sunset*, 29–39.

8   Z. Hawass, *Tutankhamun and the Golden Age of the Pharaohs* (Washington, D.C.: National Geographic, 2005), 89–90; M. Eaton-Krauss, "Tutankhamun," *LÄ* 6, col. 816.

9   Z. Hawass, "Newly Discovered Scenes of Tutankhamun from Memphis and Rediscovered Blocks from Heliopolis," in *The Art and Culture of Ancient Egypt: Studies in Honor of Dorothea Arnold*, ed. O. Goelet and A. Oppenheim, *BES* 19 (2012), forthcoming. The text also refers to the "King's Daughter, Ankhesenpaaten."

10 G. Roeder, *Amarna-Reliefs aus Hermopolis* (Hildesheim: Gerstenberg, 1969), pl. 106, no. 831/VIII C; W. Helck, "Kije," *MDAIK* 40 (1984): 166; J. Allen, "Akhenaten's 'Mystery' Coregent and Successor," *Amarna Letters* 1 (1991): 74–85; Hawass, "Newly Discovered."

11 See the discussions in J. Harris and E.F. Wente, *An X-Ray Atlas of the Royal Mummies* (Chicago: University of Chicago Press, 1980), 136, 352; Helck, "Kije," 166; R.C. Connolly, R.G. Harrison, and S. Ahmed, "Serological Evidence for the Parentage of Tut'ankhamūn and Smenkharē," *JEA* 62 (1976): 184–86; D.P. Silverman, J. Wegner, and J.H. Wegner, *Akhenaten and Tutankhamun: Revolution and Restoration* (Philadelphia: University of Pennsylvania Museum of Archaeology and Anthropology, 2006), 141–44.

12 W.J. Murnane, "The Return to Orthodoxy," in *Pharaohs of the Sun: Akhenaten, Nefertiti, Tutankhamun*, ed. R. Freed, Y. Markowitz, and S. D'Auria (Boston: Museum of Fine Arts, 1999), 177–78.

13 D. Franke, "Verwandschaftsbezeichnungen," *LÄ* 6, col. 1033; Hawass, "Newly Discovered"; Allen, "Akhenaten's 'Mystery'," 85.

14 Allen, "Amarna Succession," 6.

15 Harris and Wente, *X-Ray Atlas*, 140; Helck, "Kije,"166; N. Reeves, *Valley of the Kings: The Decline of a Royal Necropolis* (London: Kegan Paul, 1990), 49; N. Reeves and R.H. Wilkinson, *The Complete Valley of the Kings: Tombs and Treasures of Egypt's Greatest Pharaohs* (London: Thames & Hudson, 1996), 122; Allen, "Akhenaten's 'Mystery'," 85; A. Kozloff, B. Bryan, and L. Berman, *Egypt's Dazzling Sun: Amenhotep III and His World* (Cleveland: Cleveland Museum of Art, 1992), 44; J. van Dijk, "Kiya Revisited," in *Seventh International Congress of Egyptologists, Cambridge, 3–9 September 1995, Abstracts of Papers*, ed. C. Eyre (Oxford: Oxford Books, 1995), 50; N. Reeves, "The Royal Family," in *Pharaohs of the Sun: Akhenaten, Nefertiti, Tutankhamun*, ed. R. Freed, Y. Markowitz, and S. D'Auria (Boston: Museum of Fine Arts, 1999), 91; Murnane, "Return," 177–78.

16 Allen, "Akhenaten's 'Mystery'," 85; N. Reeves, "Tuthmosis IV as 'Great-grandfather' of Tut'ankhamūn," *GM* 56 (1982): 65–69.

17 M. Bell, "An Armchair Excavation of KV55," *JARCE* 27 (1990): 135; Reeves and Wilkinson, *Complete Valley*, 121.

18 Reeves and Wilkinson, *Complete Valley*, 121.

19 G. Martin, *The Royal Tomb at El-Amarna*, 2 (London: Egypt Exploration Society, 1974), 38–40, fig. 7, pls. 58, 59f, 60–61.

20 Martin, *Royal Tomb*, 40; van Dijk, "Kiya Revisited," 3, 5; Silverman et al., *Akhenaten and Tutankhamun*, 101–102.

21 van Dijk, "Kiya Revisited," 6, 7, 9.

22 Silverman et al., *Akhenaten and Tutankhamun*, 141, 144, 161.

23 D. Forbes, *Tombs*, 304.

24 R.G. Harrison, R.C. Connolly, and A. Abdalla, "Kinship of Smenkhkare and Tutankhamun Affirmed by Serological Micromethod: Kinship of Smenkhkare and Tutankhamen Demonstrated Serologically," *Nature* 224 (1969): 325–26.

25 Connolly et al., "Serological Evidence," 184–85; Kozloff et al., *Egypt's Dazzling Sun*, 26; Silverman et al., *Akhenaten and Tutankhamun*, 144.

26 S. Ikram and A. Dodson, *The Mummy in Ancient Egypt* (Cairo: American University in Cairo Press, 1998), 324.

27 J.E. Harris and E.F. Wente, "Mummy of the 'Elder Lady' in the Tomb of Amenhotep II: Egyptian Museum Catalog Number 61070," *Science* (9 June 1978): 1149–51.

28 Harris and Wente, *X-Ray Atlas*, 140; Helck, "Kije," 166; Reeves, *Complete Tutankhamun*, 21; Kozloff et al., *Egypt's Dazzling Sun*, 44; D. Arnold, *The Royal Women of Amarna: Images of Beauty from Ancient Egypt* (New York: Metropolitan Museum of Art, 1996), 14–15; Reeves and Wilkinson, *Complete Valley*, 122; Reeves, "Royal Family," 91; A.J.

Thomas, "The Other Woman at Akhetaten, Royal Wife Kiya," *Amarna Letters* 3 (1994): 81; Silverman et al., *Akhenaten and Tutankhamun*, 141, 144.

29 Martin, *Royal Tomb*, 40.

30 See van Dijk, "Kiya Revisited"; Silverman et al., *Akhenaten and Tutankhamun*, 144.

31 Helck, "Kije," 166.

32 Dodson and Hilton, *Complete Royal Families*, 155.

33 Forbes, *Tombs*, 511; Silverman et al., *Akhenaten and Tutankhamun*, 144; van Dijk, "The Death of Meketaten," in *Causing His Name to Live: Studies in Egyptian Epigraphy and History in Memory of William J. Murnane*, ed. P. Brand and L. Cooper, http://www.jacobus-vandijk.nl/docs/Meketaten.pdf, 65–82.

34 M. Gabolde, "Baketaten fille de Kiya?" *BSEG* 16 (1992): 39.

35 Carter and Mace, *Tomb*, vol. 3, 88.

36 Z. Hawass, *King Tutankhamun: The Treasures of the Tomb* (New York: Thames & Hudson, 2007), 232; Forbes, *Tombs*, 452–53.

37 A total of sixteen mummies were included in the study. Two of these mummies, from KV21, will be discussed in chapter 8, and there was a morphological and genetic control group of five Eighteenth Dynasty mummies from DB320 and KV60. See Hawass et al., "Ancestry and Pathology," table 1.

38 Reeves and Wilkinson, *Complete Valley*, 176–77.

39 Reeves and Wilkinson, *Complete Valley*, 110–13.

40 Forbes, *Tombs*, 694.

41 Z. Hawass, "King Tut's Family Secrets," *National Geographic Magazine*, September 2010, 34–59, http://ngm.nationalgeographic.com/print/2010/09/tut-dna/hawass-text

42 Hawass et al., "Ancestry and Pathology," 640–41.

43 Hawass et al., "Ancestry and Pathology."

44 R.K. Beals and L. Mason, "The Marfan Skull," *Radiology* 140:3 (1981): 723–25.

45 A. De Paepe et al., "Revised Criteria for the Marfan Syndrome," *Am J Med Genet* 62:4 (1996): 417–26.

46 D. Magid, R.E. Pyeritz, and E.K. Fishman, "Musculoskeletal Manifestations of the Marfan Syndrome: Radiologic Features," *AJR* 155:1 (1990): 99–104.

47 See Beals and Mason, "The Marfan Skull"; De Paepe et al., "Revised Criteria for the Marfan Syndrome"; and Magid, Pyeritz, and Fishman, "Musculoskeletal Manifestations of the Marfan Syndrome: Radiologic Features."

48 This applies to patients with no known family history of Marfan's Disease. We assume that this can be applied to an ancient mummy with no known medical history. See A. De Paepe et al., "Revised Criteria for the Marfan Syndrome."

49 A wrist sign is positive when the terminal bones of the first and fifth fingers of one hand overlap when wrapping the opposite wrist. A thumb sign is positive when the thumb, clenched in the hand, projects beyond the fingers.

50 The skull index, the ratio between its breadth and length, determines the shape of the skull. A normal skull (mesocranic) has an index of 75–79.9; an elongated skull (dolichocephalic) has an index of less than 75.

51 Hawass et al., "Ancestry and Pathology," table 2.

Notes to Chapter 8

1 See, for example, W.M.F. Petrie, *Tell el Amarna* (London: Methuen and Co., 1894), 38. For additional discussion, see J. Tyldesley, *Nefertiti: Egypt's Sun Queen* (New York: Penguin, 1998), 41–46.

2 N. de G. Davies, *The Rock Tombs of El Amarna, Part 2: The Tombs of Panehesy and Meryra II* (London: Egypt Exploration Society, 1905), 38–43 , pls. 37–40, 47; D.P. Silverman, J. Wegner, and J.H. Wegner, *Akhenaten and Tutankhamun: Revolution and Restoration* (Philadelphia: University of Pennsylvania Museum of Archaeology and Anthropology, 2006), 98–101.

3 J. Allen, "The Amarna Succession," in *Causing His Name to Live: Studies in Epigraphy and History in Memory of William Murnane*, ed. P. Brand and L. Cooper, Culture and History of the Ancient Near East 37 (Leiden: Brill, 2009), http://cassian.memphis.edu/history/murnane/Allen.pdf, 1.

4 N. Reeves, "The Royal Family," in *Pharaohs of the Sun: Akhenaten, Nefertiti, Tutankhamun*, ed. R. Freed, Y. Markowitz, and S. D'Auria (Boston: Museum of Fine Arts, 1999), 88; Reeves, *Akhenaten: Egypt's False Prophet* (London: Thames & Hudson, 2005), 172–73.

5 N. Reeves, *The Complete Tutankhamun: The King, the Tomb, the Royal Treasure* (London: Thames & Hudson, 1990), 22–23.

6 On a stela in Berlin (17813) belonging to Pase, a soldier; illustrated in Reeves, *Complete Tutankhamun*, 22.

7 Reeves, "Royal Family," fig. 59, p. 88; cat. no. 110, p. 238.

8 R.W. Smith and D. Redford, *The Akhenaten Temple Project 1: Initial Discoveries* (Warminster: Aris & Phillips, 1976), 81, pl. 23:2.

9 Reeves, *Akhenaten*, 175.

10 For the tomb, see http://www.kv-63.com/publications.html

11 E. Ertman, "The Eyes of Nefertiti," *Archaeology* 61:2 (March/April 2008): 28–32.

12 J. Fletcher, *The Search for Nefertiti* (New York: Harper Collins, 2004), 370–71.

13 Fletcher, *Search*, 374.

14 According to a report submitted to the SCA by Ashraf Selim. The mummy was also examined by G. Elliot Smith in 1907 (Smith, *The Royal Mummies*, Catalogue général des antiquités égyptiennes du Musée du Caire (Cairo: IFAO, 1912, repr. London: Duckworth, 2000), 40–42) and by Harris and Wente in 1980 (J.E. Harris and E.F. Wente, *An X-Ray Atlas of the Royal Mummies* (Chicago: University of Chicago Press, 1980)).

15 Fletcher, *Search*, 116.

16 Fletcher, *Search*, 351.

17 A. Dodson and D. Hilton, *The Complete Royal Families of Ancient Egypt* (London: Thames & Hudson, 2004), 146, n103.

18 Z. Hawass, "Newly Discovered Scenes of Tutankhamun from Memphis and Rediscovered Blocks from Heliopolis," in *The Art and Culture of Ancient Egypt: Studies in Honor of Dorothea Arnold*, ed. O. Goelet and A. Oppenheim, *BES* 19 (2012), forthcoming.

19 Sitamun, Iset, Henuttaneb, Nebetiah, Beketaten. Amenhotep III is shown with eight unnamed daughters in the tomb of Kheruef.

20 D.C. Forbes, *Tombs, Treasures, Mummies: Seven Great Discoveries of Egyptian Archaeology* (Sebastopol, CA: KMT Communications, Inc., 1998), 694.

21 G.B. Belzoni, *Narrative of the Operations and Recent Discoveries in Egypt and Nubia* (London: John Murray, 1820), 228.

22 Email from D. Ryan to Z. Hawass, December 9, 2007. For the tomb, see Ryan, "Who Is Buried in KV60? A Field Report," *KMT* 1 (1990): 35–39; "Return to Wadi Biban el Moluk: The Second (1990) Season of the Valley of the Kings Project," *KMT* 2:1 (Spring 1991): 29–30; and N. Reeves and R.H. Wilkinson, *The Complete Valley of the Kings: Tombs and Treasures of Egypt's Greatest Pharaohs* (London: Thames & Hudson, 1996), 115.

23 This violation as reported by Ryan took place during the nineteenth century, sometime after 1826.

24 Female stature: 2.340 x femur length + 56.99 = stature ± 2.517 cm. See M.H. Raxter et al., "Stature Estimation in Ancient Egyptians: A New Technique Based on Anatomical Reconstruction of Stature," *AJPA* 136:2 (June 2008): 147–55.

25 Femoral head diameter is an example of a measurement that is greater in males than females, often enough that it can make an adequate estimation of sex. See W.M. Bass, *Human Osteology: A Laboratory and Field Manual*, 5th ed. (Columbia: Missouri Archaeological Society, 2005), 26, 231.

26 M.H. Raxter et al., "Stature Estimation."

27 G. Martin, *The Memphite Tomb of Horemheb, Commander-in-Chief of Tut'ankhamūn* 1 (London: Egypt Exploration Society, 1990).

28 E. Strouhal, "Queen Mutnodjmet at Memphis: Anthropological and Paleopathological Evidence," in *L'Égyptologie en 1979: Axes prioritaires de recherches* 2 (Paris: Éditions du Centre national de la recherche scientifique, 1982), 317–22.

Notes to Chapter 9

1 For the reign of Horemheb, see A. Dodson, *Amarna Sunset: Nefertiti, Tutankhamun, Ay, Horemheb, and the Egyptian Counter-Reformation* (Cairo: American University in Cairo Press, 2009), 109–34.

2 H.D. Schneider, "Horemheb," in *The Oxford Encyclopedia of Ancient Egypt* 2, ed. D. Redford (Cairo: American University in Cairo Press, 2001), 114.

3 G. Martin, *The Memphite Tomb of Horemheb, Commander-in-Chief of Tut'ankhamūn* 1 (London: Egypt Exploration Society, 1990).

4 For Mutnodjmet, see G. Martin, *Memphite Tomb*; Dodson, *Amarna Sunset*, 114–17;

W.M.F. Petrie, *A History of Egypt*, part 2 (London: Methuen and Co., 1896, repr. Michael S. Sanders, 1991), 256.

5 J. van Dijk, "New Evidence on the Length of the Reign of Horemheb," *JARCE* 44 (2008): 193–200.

6 Dodson, *Amarna Sunset*, 128–32.

7 T. Davis, G. Maspero, and G. Daressy, *The Tombs of Harmhabi and Touatânkhamanou* (London: Constable, 1912); E. Hornung, *Das Grab des Haremhab im Tal der Könige* (Bern: Francke Verlag, 1971); N. Reeves and R.H. Wilkinson, *The Complete Valley of the Kings: Tombs and Treasures of Egypt's Greatest Pharaohs* (London: Thames & Hudson, 1996), 130–33.

8 Reeves and Wilkinson, *Complete Valley*, 204.

9 P. Clayton, *The Complete Pharaohs* (Cairo: American University in Cairo Press, 2006) 140–41.

10 G.B. Belzoni, *Narrative of the Operations and Recent Discoveries in Egypt and Nubia* (London: John Murray, 1820), 229–30; A. Piankoff, "La tombe de Ramsès 1er," *BIFAO* 56 (1957): 189–200; Reeves and Wilkinson, *Complete Valley*, 134–35.

11 Clayton, *Complete Pharaohs*, 141–45.

12 For the monuments of Seti I, see P.J. Brand, *The Monuments of Seti I: Epigraphic, Historical, and Art Historical Analysis*, Probleme der Ägyptologie 16 (Leiden: Brill, 2000).

13 J. van Dijk, "The Amarna Period and the Later New Kingdom," in *The Oxford History of Ancient Egypt*, ed. I. Shaw (Oxford: Oxford University Press, 2000), 288.

14 Brand, *Monuments*, 308.

15 Belzoni, *Narrative*, 230–37; E. Hornung, *The Tomb of Pharaoh Seti I* (Zurich and Munich: Artemis Verlag, 1971); Reeves and Wilkinson, *Complete Valley*, 136–39.

16 For further details, see Z. Hawass, *Discovering Tutankhamun: From Howard Carter to DNA* (Cairo: American University in Cairo Press, 2013), 186–89.

17 K.A. Kitchen, *Pharaoh Triumphant: The Life and Times of Ramesses II* (Warminster: Aris and Phillips, 1982), 27; for further discussion, see Brand, *Monuments*, 312–32.

18 For the family of Ramesses II, see A. Dodson and D. Hilton, *The Complete Royal Families of Ancient Egypt* (London: Thames & Hudson, 2004), 164–75.

19 Dodson and Hilton, *Complete Royal Families*, 166.

20 K.R. Weeks, ed., *KV5: A Preliminary Report on the Excavation of the Tomb of the Sons of Ramesses II in the Valley of the Kings*, rev. ed. (Cairo: American University in Cairo Press, 2006), http://www.thebanmapping-project.com/sites/browse_tomb_819.html

21 For further details, see Hawass, *Discovering Tutankhamun*, 175–80.

22 C. Leblanc, "The Tomb of Ramesses II and Remains of His Funerary Treasure," *Egyptian Archaeology* 10 (1997): 11–13; C. Maystre, "Le tombeau de Ramsès II," *BIFAO* 38 (1939): 183–90; Reeves and Wilkinson, *Complete Valley*, 140–43.

23 Kitchen, *Pharaoh Triumphant*, 112, 206.

24 Dodson and Hilton, *Complete Royal Families*, 176–83.

25 R.H. Wilkinson, *Tausret: Forgotten Queen and Pharaoh of Egypt* (Oxford: Oxford University Press, 2012).

26 See M. Görg, "Exodus," in *The Oxford Encyclopedia of Ancient Egypt* 1, ed. D. Redford, (Cairo: American University in Cairo Press, 2001), 489–90.

27 C. De Wit, *The Date and Route of the Exodus* (London: Tyndale Press, 1960), 20.

28 C. Desroches-Noblecourt, *Ramses II: An Illustrated Biography* (Paris: Flammarion, 2007), 134.

29 M. Bietak, "Comments on the 'Exodus,'" in *Egypt, Israel, Sinai: Archaeological and Historical Relationships in the Biblical Period*, ed. A.F. Rainey (Tel Aviv: Tel Aviv University, 1987), 163–71; D. Redford, "An Egyptological Perspective on the Exodus," in *Egypt, Israel, Sinai: Archaeological and Historical Relationships in the Biblical Period*, ed. A.F. Rainey (Tel Aviv: Tel Aviv University, 1987), 137–61.

30 J. van Dijk, "Amarna Period," 294; A. Weigall, *Histoire de l'Égypte ancienne* (Paris: Payot, 1949), 163. However, Ramadan Abdou does not agree that the word "Jezreel" (an alternative reading) is "Israel" because the text did not mention Palestine, and the kingdom of Israel did not exist at that time. See R. Abdou, *Tarikh Misr al-qadima* (Cairo: al-Majlis al-A'la li-l-Athar, 1993), 2:175–85.

31 Abdou, *Tarikh Misr al-qadima*, 175–85.

32 Exod. 2:23.

33 M. Bucaille, *Mummies of the Pharaohs: Modern Medical Investigations* (New York: St. Martin's Press, 1990), 60.

34 S.N. Saleem and Z. Hawass, "Variability in Brain Treatment during Mummification of Royal Egyptians Dated to the 18th–20th Dynasties: MDCT Findings Correlated with the Archaeologic Literature," *AJR* 200:4 (April 2013): W336–44 (doi: 10.2214/AJR.12.9405).

35 G.E. Smith, *The Royal Mummies*, Catalogue général des antiquités égyptiennes du Musée du Caire (Cairo: IFAO, 1912, repr. London: Duckworth, 2000), 57; S. Ikram and A. Dodson, *The Mummy in Ancient Egypt* (Cairo: American University in Cairo Press, 1998), 325.

36 Saleem and Hawass, "Variability in Brain Treatment."

37 S.N. Saleem and Z. Hawass. "Multi-detector Computerized Tomography (MDCT) Study of Cosmetic Care and Beautification of Royal

Ancient Egyptian Mummies Related to the 18th to 20th Dynasties," presentation at the Eighth World Congress on Mummies Studies, Rio de Janeiro, Brazil, August 8, 2013.

38 S.N. Saleem and Z. Hawass, "Subcutaneous Packing in Royal Egyptian Mummies Dated from the 18th to 20th Dynasties," *JCAT* (in press).

39 N. Reeves, *Valley of the Kings: The Decline of a Royal Necropolis* (London: Kegan Paul, 1990), 92–94.

40 Ikram and Dodson, *Mummy*, 122.

41 Ikram and Dodson, *Mummy*, 129.

42 Saleem and Hawass, "Variability in Brain Treatment," W343.

43 Saleem and Hawass, "Multi-detector Computerized Tomography."

44 Saleem and Hawass, "Subcutaneous Packing."

45 S.N. Saleem and Z. Hawass, "Multi-detector Computed Tomography Study of Amulets, Jewelry, and Other Foreign Objects in Royal Egyptian Mummies Dated to the 18th to 20th Dynasties," *JCAT* 38:2 (2013): 153–58.

46 Smith, *Royal Mummies*, 59.

47 S.N. Saleem and Z. Hawass, "Multi Detector CT of Royal Ancient Egyptian Mummies: An Approach to Study," presentation at the Radiological Society of North America (RSNA), Chicago, November 25–30, 2012.

48 E.F. Wente, "Age at Death of Pharaohs of the New Kingdom, Determined from Historical Sources," in *An X-Ray Atlas of the Royal Mummies*, ed. J.E. Harris and E.F. Wente (Chicago: University of Chicago Press, 1980), 259–60.

49 Saleem and Hawass, "Variability in Brain Treatment."

50 With the presence of hunchback, the position of the head would have been raised above the body during recumbency in the king's old age. During mummification, and in order to rest the position of the head at the same level of the body during recumbency, the embalmers might have snapped the neck of the mummy between the fifth and sixth vertebrae. Saleem and Hawass, "Multi-detector Computerized Tomography."

51 There is mild sclerosis and narrowing of the articulating surfaces of both sacroiliac joints, predominantly left. Changes involve the nonsynovial part of the joint as well as the synovial part. In absence of fusion or significant erosions, findings are considered age-related degenerative changes rather than inflammatory.

52 Saleem and Hawass, "Multi-detector Computed Tomography."

53 Saleem and Hawass, "Multi-detector Computerized Tomography."

54 Saleem and Hawass, "Subcutaneous Packing."

55 D. Resnick and G. Niwayama, "Entheses and Enthesopathy: Anatomical Pathological and Radiological Correlation," *Radiology* 146 (1983): 1–9.

56 Saleem and Hawass, "Variability in Brain Treatment," W343.

57 Saleem and Hawass, "Multi-detector Computerized Tomography."

58 Saleem and Hawass, "Multi-detector Computerized Tomography."

59 Saleem and Hawass, "Multi-detector Computerized Tomography."

60 E. Feldtkeller, E.M. Lemmel, and A.S. Russell, "Ankylosing Spondylitis in the Pharaohs of Ancient Egypt," *Rheumatol Int* 23 (2003): 1–5; W.M. Whitehouse, "Radiologic Findings in the Royal Mummies," in *An X-Ray Atlas of the Royal Mummies*, ed. J.E. Harris and E.F. Wente (Chicago: University of Chicago Press,

1980), 286–97; C. Massare, "Anatomo-radiologie et vérité historique: à propos du bilan xéroradiographique de Ramsès II," *Bruxelles Medical* 59:3 (1979): 163–70.

61 R.K. Chhem, P. Schmit, and C. Fauré, "Did Ramesses II Really Have Ankylosing Spondylitis? A Reappraisal," *Can Assoc Radiol J* 55:4 (October 2004): 211–17.

62 Chhem et al., "Did Ramesses II?"

63 D. Resnick and G. Niwayama, "Radiographic and Pathologic Features of Spinal Involvement in Diffuse Idiopathic Skeletal Hyperostosis (DISH)," *Radiology* 119 (1976): 559–68.

64 S.N. Saleem and Z. Hawass, "Ankylosing Spondylitis or Diffuse Idiopathic Skeletal Hyperostosis (DISH) in Royal Egyptian Mummies of the 18th–20th Dynasties? CT and Archaeology Studies," *Arthritis and Rheumatology* 66:12 (December 2014), published online October 20, 2014 (doi:10.1002/art.38864).

65 P.D. Utsinger, "Diffuse Idiopathic Skeletal Hyperostosis," *Clin Rheum Dis* 11 (1985): 325–51.

66 Resnick and Niwayama, "Radiographic."

67 J. Rogers, I. Watt, and P. Dieppe, "Palaeopathology of Spinal Osteophytosis, Vertebral Ankylosis, Ankylosing Spondylitis, and Vertebral Hyperostosis," *Ann Rheum Dis* 44:2 (February 1985): 113–20; C. Kiss et al., "Risk Factors for Diffuse Idiopathic Skeletal Hyperostosis: A Case-Control Study," *Rheumatology* 41 (2002): 27–30.

68 Wente, "Age at Death," 260–62.

69 Smith, *Royal Mummies*, 68–69.

70 Whitehouse, "Radiologic Findings," 291.

71 Smith, *Royal Mummies*, 68–69.

72 Saleem and Hawass, "Variability in Brain Treatment," W343.

73 Smith, *Royal Mummies*, 67.

74 Ikram and Dodson, *Mummy*, 326.

75 M.A. Ruffer, *Studies in the Palaeopathology of Egypt* (Chicago: University of Chicago Press, 1921), 172.

76 N. Dorairajan, "Inguinal Hernia—Yesterday, Today and Tomorrow," *Indian Journal of Surgery* 66:3 (June 2004): 137.

77 N.S. Papavramidou and H. Christopoulou-Aletras, "Treatment of 'Hernia' in the Writings of Celsus (First Century AD)," *World J Surg* 29 (2005): 1343–47.

Notes to Chapter 10

1 For the reign of Ramesses III, see E. Cline and D. O'Connor, eds., *Ramesses III: The Life and Times of Egypt's Last Hero* (Ann Arbor: University of Michigan Press, 2012).

2 P. Clayton, *The Complete Pharaohs* (Cairo: American University in Cairo Press, 2006), 160.

3 J. Grist, "The Identity of the Ramesside Queen Tyti," *JEA* 71 (1985): 71–81; Clayton, *Complete Pharaohs*, 164.

4 For discussion, see S. Redford, *The Harem Conspiracy: The Murder of Ramesses III* (Dekalb, IL: Northern Illinois University Press, 2008), 37–38; A. Dodson and D. Hilton, *The Complete Royal Families of Ancient Egypt* (London: Thames & Hudson, 2004), 188–89.

5 W. Erichsen, *Papyrus Harris I: Hieroglyphische Transkription* (Brussels: Édition de la Fondation égyptologique Reine Élisabeth, 1933); P. Grandet, *Le Papyrus Harris I, BM 9999* (Cairo: IFAO, 1994–99).

6 Epigraphic Survey, University of Chicago, *Medinet Habu*, 9 vols. (Chicago: University of Chicago Press, 1930–2009; Architectural Survey, University of Chicago, Oriental Institute, *The Excavation of Medinet Habu*, 5 vols. (Chicago: University of Chicago Press, 1934–54).

7 A. Erman, *Zur Erklärung des Papyrus Harris* (Berlin: Akademie der Wissenschaften, 1903), 456–74.

8 For the Libyans, see A.M. Leahy, "The Libyan Period in Egypt: An Essay in Interpretation," *Libyan Studies* 16 (1985): 51–65; A.M. Leahy, ed., *Libya and Egypt c. 1300–750 BC* (London: SOAS Centre of Near and Middle Eastern Studies and the Society for Libyan Studies, 1990); and A. Spalinger, "Some Notes on the Libyans of the Old Kingdom and Later Historical Reflexes," *JSSEA* 9 (1979): 125–60.

9 N.K. Sandars, *The Sea Peoples: Warriors of the Eastern Mediterranean* (London: Thames & Hudson, 1978), 114–19.

10 Redford, *Harem Conspiracy*, 32–33, 73–74.

11 J.H. Breasted, *Ancient Records of Egypt*, (Chicago: University of Chicago Press, 1906), vol. 4, §§192–94, p. 115.

12 J. Černy, *A Community of Workmen at Thebes in the Ramesside Period* (Cairo: IFAO, 1973), 112.

13 P.J. Frandsen, "Editing Reality: The Turin Strike Papyrus," in *Studies in Egyptology Presented to Miriam Lichtheim* 1, ed. S. Israelit-Groll (Jerusalem: Magness Press, Hebrew University, 1990), 166–99.

14 A.H. Gardiner, *Egypt of the Pharaohs* (Oxford: Oxford University Press, 1961), 293.

15 W. Edgerton, "The Strikes in Ramses III's Twenty-ninth Year," *JNES* 10 (1951): 137–45; C.J. Eyre, "A Strike Text from the Theban Necropolis," in *Glimpses of Ancient Egypt: Studies in Honor of H.W. Fairman*, ed. J. Ruffle, G.A. Gaballa, and K. Kitchen (Warminster: Aris and Phillips, 1979), 80–91. See also A. Gardiner, *Ramesside Administrative Documents* (Oxford: Griffith Institute, 1948).

16 See K.A. Kitchen, *Ramesside Inscriptions: Historical and Biographical*, vol. 5, no. 148, (Oxford: Wiley-Blackwell, 1968–93), 350–60; translation in A. de Buck, "The Judicial Papyrus of Turin," *JEA* 23:2 (1937): 152–66; J.H. Breasted, *Ancient Records of Egypt* (Chicago: University of Chicago Press, 1906–1907), vol. 4, §416–53.

17 For discussion of the harem in ancient Egypt, see E. Haslauer, "Harem," in *The Oxford Encyclopedia of Ancient Egypt* 2, ed. D. Redford (Cairo: American University in Cairo Press, 2001), esp. p. 80; E. Reiser, *Der königliche Harim im alten Ägypten und seine Verwaltung*, reviewed by B.J. Kemp in *JEA* 62 (1976), 191–92; B. Kemp, "The Harim Palace at Medinet el-Ghurab," *ZÄS* 105 (1978): 122–23.

18 J.H. Breasted, *Ancient Records*, vol. 4, §423–56; de Buck, "Judicial Papyrus," 152–66.

19 P. Rifaud is preserved only in hand copies; see Redford, *Harem Conspiracy*, 5.

20 Redford, *Harem Conspiracy*, 8.

21 Redford, *Harem Conspiracy*, 72.

22 H. Goedicke, "Was Magic Used in the Harem Conspiracy against Ramesses III?" *JEA* 49 (1963): 71–92; R.K. Ritner, *The Mechanics of Ancient Egyptian Magical Practice*, SAOC 54 (Chicago: Oriental Institute of the University of Chicago, 1993), 192–98.

23 Breasted, *Ancient Records*, vol. 4, §427.

24 Breasted, *Ancient Records*, vol. 4, §§419, 541.

25 Breasted, *Ancient Records*, vol. 4, §420.

26 Redford, *Harem Conspiracy*, 105.

27 Breasted, *Ancient Records*, vol. 4, §418.

28 Redford, *Harem Conspiracy*, 133.

29 Redford, *Harem Conspiracy*, 9.

30 The CT study of the neck was done by a group of authors (see note 33 below), while the CT study of the rest of the body of this mummy was done by Sahar Saleem.

31 Maspero's text is quoted in full, with further references, in G.E. Smith, *The Royal Mummies*, Catalogue général des antiquités égyptiennes du Musée du Caire (Cairo: IFAO, 1912, repr. London: Duckworth, 2000), 84–86.

32 Smith, *Royal Mummies*, 87; D.C. Forbes, *Tombs, Treasures, Mummies: Seven Great Discoveries of Egyptian Archaeology* (Sebastopol, CA: KMT Communications, Inc., 1998), 643, 645.

33 Z. Hawass et al., "Revisiting the Harem Conspiracy and Death of Ramesses III: Anthropological, Forensic, Radiological, and Genetic Study," *BMJ* 2012; 345: e8268; S.N. Saleem and Z. Hawass, "Multi-detector Computed Tomography Study of Amulets, Jewelry, and Other Foreign Objects in Royal Egyptian Mummies Dated to the 18th to 20th Dynasties," *JCAT* 38:2 (2013): 153–58.

34 D. Resnick and G. Niwayama, "Entheses and Enthesopathy: Anatomical Pathological and Radiological Correlation," *Radiology* 146 (1983): 1–9.

35 J. Haller et al., "Diffuse Idiopathic Skeletal Hyperostosis: Diagnostic Significance of Radiographic Abnormalities of the Pelvis," *Radiology* 172 (1989): 835–39.

36 J. Rogers, I. Watt, and P. Dieppe, "Palaeopathology of Spinal Osteophytosis, Vertebral Ankylosis, Ankylosing Spondylitis, and Vertebral Hyperostosis," *Ann Rheum Dis* 44:2 (February 1985): 113–30; I. Olivieri et al., "Diffuse Idiopathic Skeletal Hyperostosis May Give the Typical Postural Abnormalities of Advanced Ankylosing Spondylitis," *Rheumatology* (Oxford) 46 (2007): 1709–11.

37 Hawass et al., "Revisiting."

38 Redford, *Harem Conspiracy*, 112.

39 I. Shaw and P. Nicholson, *The Dictionary of Ancient Egypt* (London: British Museum, 1995), 133–34.

40 R.H. Wilkinson, *Reading Egyptian Art: A Hieroglyphic Guide to Ancient Egyptian Painting and Sculpture* (New York: Thames & Hudson, 1992), 42–43.

41 Smith, *Royal Mummies*, 114–16; Forbes, *Tombs*, 612–13; B. Brier, "The Mystery of Unknown Man E," *Archaeology* 59 (2006): 36–42, and "The Mummy of Unknown Man E: A Preliminary Re-examination," *Bulletin of the Egyptian Museum* 3 (2006): 23–32.

42 W.K. Simpson, ed., *The Literature of Ancient Egypt* (New Haven: Yale University Press, 1972), 68.

43 Smith, *Royal Mummies*, 115.

44 Smith, *Royal Mummies*, 115.

45 Brier, " Mummy of Unknown Man E," 23–32.

46 See Brier, "Mystery," 38.

47 For full results, see Hawass et al., "Revisiting the Harem Conspiracy."

48 See Hawass et al., "Revisiting the Harem Conspiracy."

49 Redford, *Harem Conspiracy*, 16.

50 Applied Biosystems, Poster City, California.

51 Hawass et al., "Revisiting the Harem Conspiracy."

Notes to Chapter 11

1 A.T. Sandison and E. Tapp, "Disease in Ancient Egypt," in *Mummies, Disease, and Ancient Cultures*, 2nd ed., ed. A. Cockburn, E. Cockburn, and T.A. Reyman (Cambridge, UK: Cambridge University Press, 1998), 38–58.

2 S. Ikram and A. Dodson, *The Mummy in Ancient Egypt* (Cairo: American University in Cairo Press, 1998), 103.

3 Herodotus, *The Histories*, trans. A. de Sélincourt, rev. A.R. Burns (Harmondsworth: Penguin, 1972), 160–61.

4 Herodotus, *Histories*, 160–61.

5 A.C. Aufderheide, *The Scientific Study of Mummies* (Cambridge: Cambridge University Press, 2003), 418–98.

6 Ikram and Dodson, *Mummy*, 118.

7   G.E. Smith, *The Royal Mummies*, Catalogue général des antiquités égyptiennes du Musée du Caire (Cairo: IFAO, 1912, repr. London: Duckworth, 2000).

8   Smith, *Royal Mummies*, 87.

9   J.E. Harris and E.F. Wente, *An X-Ray Atlas of the Royal Mummies* (Chicago: University of Chicago Press, 1980), 169.

10 Harris and Wente, *X-Ray Atlas*, 287.

11 F. Cesarani et al., "Whole-Body Three-Dimensional Multidetector CT of 13 Egyptian Human Mummies," *AJR* 180:3 (2003): 597–606; E.M. Braunstein et al., "Paleoradiologic Evaluation of the Egyptian Royal Mummies," *Skeletal Radiol* 17 (1988): 348–52; A.D. Wade, A.J. Nelson, and G.J. Garvin, "A Synthetic Radiological Study of Brain Treatment in Ancient Egyptian Mummies," *HOMO—Journal of Comparative Human Biology* 62:4 (2011): 248–69.

12 S.N. Saleem and Z. Hawass, "Multi-detector Computerized Tomography (MDCT) Study of Cosmetic Care and Beautification of Royal Ancient Egyptian Mummies Related to the 18th to 20th Dynasties," presentation at the Eighth World Congress on Mummies Studies, Rio de Janeiro, Brazil, August 8, 2013; S.N. Saleem and Z. Hawass, "Variability in Brain Treatment During Mummification of Royal Egyptians Dated to the 18th–20th Dynasties: MDCT Findings Correlated with the Archaeologic Literature," *AJR* 200:4 (April 2013): W336–44.

13 S.N. Saleem and Z. Hawass, "Multi Detector CT of Royal Ancient Egyptian Mummies: An Approach to Study," presentation at the Radiological Society of North America (RSNA), Chicago, November 25–30, 2012.

14 Ikram and Dodson, *Mummy*, 109.

15 Ikram and Dodson, *Mummy*, chapter 3.

16 S. Ikram, "Some Thoughts on the Mummification of King Tutankhamun," in *Institut des Cultures Méditerranéennes et Orientales de l'Académie Polonaise des Sciences, Études et Travaux* 26 (2013) (Cairo: American University in Cairo Press; London: Thames & Hudson Limited, 1998), 293–94.

17 F.J. Rühli, R.K. Chhem, and T. Böni, "Diagnostic Paleoradiology of Mummified Tissue: Interpretation and Pitfalls," *Can Assoc Radiol J* 55:4 (2004): 218–27.

18 R. David, "Mummification," in *Ancient Egyptian Materials and Technology*, ed. P.T. Nicholson and I. Shaw (Cambridge: Cambridge University Press, 2000), 383–84.

19 Aufderheide, *Scientific Study*, 255.

20 A.D. Wade et al., "Scenes from the Past: Multidetector CT of Egyptian Mummies of the Redpath Museum," *Radiographics* 32:4 (2012): 1235–50.

21 For properties of resin, see M. Serpico and R. White, "Resins, Amber and Bitumen," in *Ancient Egyptian Materials and Technology*, ed. P.T. Nicholson and I. Shaw (Cambridge: Cambridge University Press, 2000), 430–51; Aufderheide, *Scientific Study*, 253.

22 Rühli, Chhem, and Böni, "Diagnostic Paleoradiology."

23 In our experience, we noted substances with CT appearance similar to resin (homogeneous texture, and may show fluid level) but with lower CT densities than what has been reported in the literature. As we do not have the chemical analysis of these substances yet, we may refer to them as "resin-like."

24 Smith, *Royal Mummies*, 87.

25 Ikram and Dodson, *Mummy*, 64.

26 Aufderheide, *Scientific Study*, 237.

27 Aufderheide, *Scientific Study*, 252.

28 Aufderheide, *Scientific Study*, 55.

29 Wade et al., "Scenes from the Past."

30 Rühli, Chhem, and Böni, "Diagnostic Paleoradiology."

31 Saleem and Hawass, "Variability in Brain Treatment."

32 Ikram and Dodson, *Mummy*, 124–26.

33 Saleem and Hawass, "Multi-detector Computerized Tomography."

34 Ikram and Dodson, *Mummy*, 121.

35 Ikram and Dodson, *Mummy*, 129.

36 A.D. Wade et al., "Synthetic Radiological Study."

37 Herodotus, *Histories*, 160.

38 Ikram and Dodson, *Mummy*, 106, 118.

39 A.D. Wade and A.J. Nelson, "Evisceration and Excerebration in the Egyptian Mummification Tradition," *JAS* 40:12 (2013): 4198–4206.

40 Saleem and Hawass, "Variability in Brain Treatment."

41 Wade et al., "Synthetic Radiological Study."

42 Saleem and Hawass, "Variability in Brain Treatment."

43 Harris and Wente, *X-Ray Atlas*, 168–69.

44 Z. Hawass et al., "Computed Tomographic Evaluation of Pharaoh Tutankhamun, ca. 1300 BC," *ASAE* 81 (2007): 159–74.

45 Harris and Wente, *X-Ray Atlas*, 168.

46 Harris and Wente, *X-Ray Atlas*, 168.

47 Wade et al., "Synthetic Radiological Study."

48 Saleem and Hawass, "Variability in Brain Treatment."

49 Wade et al., "Synthetic Radiological Study."

50 Smith, *Royal Mummies*, 17.

51 Wade et al., "Synthetic Radiological Study," 250–51.

52 Z. Iskander, "Mummification in Ancient Egypt: Development, History and Techniques," in *An X-Ray Atlas of the Royal Mummies*, ed. J.E. Harris and E.F. Wente (Chicago: University of Chicago Press, 1980), 19; M. Shafik et al., "Computed Tomography of King Tut-Ankh-Amen," *The Ambassadors Online Magazine* 11:23 (2008): Selected Study 3, http://ambassadors.net/archives/issue23/selectedstudy3.htm

53 Saleem and Hawass, "Variability in Brain Treatment."

54 Saleem and Hawass, "Variability in Brain Treatment."

55 Wade et al., "Synthetic Radiological Study"; Saleem and Hawass, "Variability in Brain Treatment."

56 Wade et al., "Synthetic Radiological Study."

57 Saleem and Hawass, "Variability in Brain Treatment."

58 Smith, *Royal Mummies*, 67.

59 Harris and Wente, *X-Ray Atlas*, 169.

60 Harris and Wente, *X-Ray Atlas*, 170.

61 Z. Hawass et al., "Ancestry and Pathology in King Tutankhamun's Family," *JAMA* 303:7 (2010): 643–47; R.S. Boyer et al., "The Skull and Cervical Spine Radiographs of Tutankhamen: A Critical Appraisal," *AJNR* 24:61 (2003), referencing R.G. Harrison and A.B. Abdalla, "The Remains of Tutankhamun," *Antiquity* 46 (1972): 8–14.

62 R.S. Boyer et al., " Skull and Cervical Spine," referencing Harrison and Abdalla, "The Remains of Tutankhamun."

63 Saleem and Hawass, "Variability in Brain Treatment."

64 Saleem and Hawass, "Variability in Brain Treatment."

65 Smith, *Royal Mummies*, 68–69.

66 Saleem and Hawass, "Variability in Brain Treatment."

67 Harris and Wente, *X-Ray Atlas*, 169–70.

68 Harris and Wente, *X-Ray Atlas*, 168; Wade et al., "Synthetic Radiological Study," 250.

69 Saleem and Hawass, "Variability in Brain Treatment."

70 Saleem and Hawass, "Variability in Brain Treatment."

71 Wade et al., "Synthetic Radiological Study."

72 Saleem and Hawass, "Variability in Brain Treatment."

73 Ikram and Dodson, *Mummy*, 114.

74 Ikram and Dodson, *Mummy*, 118–19; Aufderheide, *Scientific Study*, 240–41.

75 Ikram and Dodson, *Mummy*, 278; Aufderheide, *Scientific Study*, 237.

76 Ikram and Dodson, *Mummy*, 121.

77 Ikram and Dodson, *Mummy*, 121.

78 Ikram and Dodson, *Mummy*, 121.

79 *The American Heritage Medical Dictionary*, "Cosmetic," http://medical-dictionary. thefreedictionary.com/cosmetic

80 Ikram and Dodson, *Mummy*, 121.

81 Ikram and Dodson, *Mummy*, 121.

82 Ikram and Dodson, *Mummy*, 121.

83 Ikram and Dodson, *Mummy*, 324.

84 S.N. Saleem and Z. Hawass, "Subcutaneous Packing in Royal Egyptian Mummies Dated from the 18th to 20th Dynasties," *JCAT* (in press).

85 Ikram, "Some Thoughts," 299. Ikram theorizes that the unique mummified, erect penis of Tutankhamun was deliberately done by the embalmers in an attempt to make the king appear as Osiris, the god of the underworld, in as literal a way as possible.

86 Ikram and Dodson, *Mummy*, 121–22.

87 Smith, *Royal Mummies*, 27.

88 Saleem and Hawass, "Multi-detector Computerized Tomography."

89 We noted the very prominent low central density within the mummified penis of Yuya. We first assumed that this was an embalming prosthesis (a reed or a similar tube) that had been inserted by the embalmers for support. However, we noted a similar central low density with penises of other mummies (royal and nonroyal). We became more cautious about our conclusions concerning this appearance, which may be a normal variation of mummification caused by an innate air-filled urethra in contrast with the higher-density penile tissue (which has possibly been treated with a resin-like substance).

90 Ikram and Dodson, *Mummy*, 126.

91 Saleem and Hawass, "Multi-detector Computerized Tomography."

92 Ikram and Dodson, *Mummy*, 110.

93 P.H. Chapman and R. Gupta, "The Mummified Head of Tomb 10A," in *The Secrets of Tomb 10A: Egypt 2000 BC*, ed. R.E. Freed, L.M. Berman, D.M. Doxey, and N.S. Picardo (Boston: Museum of Fine Arts, 2009), 180–82.

94 Ikram and Dodson, *Mummy*, 125.

95 Ikram and Dodson, *Mummy*, 329–30.

96 Z. Hawass and S.N. Saleem, "Mummified Daughters of King Tutankhamun: Archeologic and CT Studies," *AJR* 197:5 (November 2011): W829–36.

97 Saleem and Hawass, "Multi-detector Computerized Tomography."

98 Saleem and Hawass, "Subcutaneous Packing."

99 Ikram and Dodson, *Mummy*, 126.

100 Ikram and Dodson, *Mummy*, 124.

101 Ikram and Dodson, *Mummy*, 126.

102 Smith, *Royal Mummies*.

103 Harris and Wente, *X-Ray Atlas*.

104 Saleem and Hawass, "Subcutaneous Packing."

105 Saleem and Hawass, "Variability in Brain Treatment."

Notes to Chapter 12

1   S. Ikram and A. Dodson, *The Mummy in Ancient Egypt* (Cairo: American University in Cairo Press, 1998), 137–38; C. Andrews, *Amulets of Ancient Egypt* (London: British Museum Press, 1994), 6–8.

2   Now in the Egyptian Museum, JE 35054;

see W.M.F. Petrie, *A History of Egypt* 1 (London: Methuen and Co., 1896, repr. Michael S. Sanders, 1991), 17; Petrie, *The Royal Tombs of the Earliest Dynasties, 1901*, Part 2 (London: Egypt Exploration Fund, 1901), 17–19 and frontispiece.

3 Ikram and Dodson, *Mummy*, 138.

4 Ikram and Dodson, *Mummy*, 138; H. Carter and A.C. Mace, *The Tomb of Tut-Ankh-Amen*, vol. 2 (London: Cassell & Co., 1927, repr. New York: Cooper Square Publishers, 1963), 106–40.

5 Ikram and Dodson, *Mummy*, 137.

6 S.N. Saleem and Z. Hawass, "Multi-detector Computed Tomography Study of Amulets, Jewelry, and Other Foreign Objects in Royal Egyptian Mummies Dated to the 18th to 20th Dynasties," *JCAT* 38:2 (2013): 153–58.

7 The CT density of original ancient Egyptian faience has not yet been measured and presently is unknown. It is expected that the radiological density of ancient Egyptian faience may differ from modern ceramics due to potential pigment additions. See P. Gostner et al., "New Radiological Approach for Analysis and Identification of Foreign Objects in Ancient and Historic Mummies," *J Arch Sci* 40:2 (2013): 1003–11.

8 D.C. Forbes, *Tombs, Treasures, Mummies: Seven Great Discoveries of Egyptian Archaeology* (Sebastopol, CA: KMT Communications, Inc., 1998), 173.

9 Gostner et al., "New Radiological Approach."

10 Ikram and Dodson, *Mummy*, 137–52.

11 F.E. Boas and D. Fleischmann, "Evaluation of Two Iterative Techniques for Reducing Metal Artifacts in Computed Tomography," *Radiology* 259:3 (2011): 894–902.

12 Ikram and Dodson, *Mummy*, 147–48.

13 Ikram and Dodson, *Mummy*, 147–49; Carter and Mace, *Tomb*, vol. 2, 106–40.

14 Andrews, *Amulets*, 6.

15 Ikram and Dodson, *Mummy*, 137; Andrews, *Amulets*, 100–106.

16 Ikram and Dodson, *Mummy*, 138–44; Andrews, *Amulets*, 8–12.

17 For the heart amulet, see R. Sousa, "The Heart Amulet in Ancient Egypt: A Typological Study," in *Proceedings of the Ninth International Congress of Egyptologists* 1, ed. J.-C. Goyon and C. Cardin (Dudley, MA: Peeters, 2007), 713–21 and "The Meaning of the Heart Amulets in Egyptian Art," *JARCE* 43 (2007): 59–70.

18 Andrews, *Amulets*, 72–73; Ikram and Dodson, *Mummy*, 142.

19 Andrews, *Amulets*, 43–44.

20 G. Pinch, *Egyptian Mythology: A Guide to the Gods, Goddesses, and Traditions of Ancient Egypt* (Oxford: Oxford University Press, 2004), 131–32.

21 Ikram and Dodson, *Mummy*, 138.

22 Andrews, *Amulets*, 44.

23 Pinch, *Egyptian Mythology*, 131–32.

24 Pinch, *Egyptian Mythology*, 131–32; Ikram and Dodson, *Mummy*, 18.

25 J. Allen, *The Ancient Egyptian Pyramid Texts* (Atlanta: Society of Biblical Literature, 2005), 74.

26 J. Wasserman, R.O. Faulkner, and O. Goelet, *The Egyptian Book of the Dead*, 2nd ed. (San Francisco: Chronicle Books, 1998), 119.

27 W. Russell, A.T. Storey, and P.V. Ponitz, "Radiographic Techniques in the Study of the Mummy," in *An X-Ray Atlas of the Royal Mummies*, ed. J.E. Harris and E.F. Wente (Chicago: University of Chicago Press, 1980), 172.

28 Z. Hawass et al., "Ancestry and Pathology in King Tutankhamun's Family," *JAMA* 303:7 (2010): 645; Z. Hawass, "The Discovery of the Mummy of Queen Hatshepsut," in Ola El-Aguizy Festschrift, *BIFAO*, forthcoming; Saleem and Hawass, "Multi-detector Computed Tomography."

Notes to Chapter 13

1 S.N. Saleem and Z. Hawass, "Multi-detector Computerized Tomography (MDCT) Study of Cosmetic Care and Beautification of Royal Ancient Egyptian Mummies Related to the 18th to 20th Dynasties," presentation at the Eighth World Congress on Mummies Studies, Rio de Janeiro, Brazil, August 8, 2013.

2 C.L. Brace et al., "Clines and Clusters versus 'Race': A Test in Ancient Egypt and the Case of a Death on the Nile," *Yearbook of Physical Anthropology* 36 (1993): 1–31; D.V. Poosha et al., "Family Resemblance for Cranio-facial Measurements in Velanti Brahmins from Andhra Pradesh, India," *Am J Phys Anthropol* 65:1 (September 1984): 15–22; B. Johannsdottir et al., "Heritability of Craniofacial Characteristics between Parents and Offspring Estimated from Lateral Cephalograms," *Am J Orthod Dentofacial Orthop* 127:2 (February 2005): 200–207.

3 B.O. Hughes and G.R. Moore, "Heredity, Growth, and the Dentofacial Complex," *The Angle Orthodontist* 11 (1941): 217–22.

4 C.L. Brace, "Region Does Not Mean 'Race': Reality versus Convention in Forensic Anthropology," *Journal of Forensic Science* 40 (1995): 171–75; S. Ousley, R. Jantz, and D. Fried, "Understanding Race and Human Variation: Why Forensic Anthropologists are Good at Identifying Race," *Am J Phys Anthropol* 139 (2009): 68–76.

5 C.A. Diop, *African Origins of Civilization* (Chicago: Lawrence Hill Books, 1974).

6 V. Lywood and A.J. Nelson, "The Face of the Mummy: Phenotypic Variability among Facial Reconstructions of Ancient Egyptian Mummies" (abstract), *CAPA Newsletter* 1 (2012): 36.

7 S.N. Saleem and Z. Hawass, "Subcutaneous Packing in Royal Egyptian Mummies Dated from the 18th to 20th Dynasties," *JCAT* (in press).

8 L.M. Berman, "Overview of Amenhotep III and His Reign," in *Amenhotep III: Perspectives on His Reign*, ed. D. O'Connor and E. Cline (Ann Arbor: University of Michigan Press, 1998), 5.

9 Saleem and Hawass, "Subcutaneous Packing."

10 Saleem and Hawass, "Subcutaneous Packing."

11 Hughes and Moore, "Heredity"; W.L. Wylie, "A Quantitative Method for Comparison of Craniofacial Patterns in Different Individuals," *Am J Anat* 74 (1944): 39–60.

12 W.M. Krogman and V. Sassouni, *A Syllabus in Roentgenographic Cephalometry* (Philadelphia: Philadelphia Center for Research in Child Growth, 1957).

13 J.E. Harris, C.J. Kowalski, and G.F. Walker, "Craniofacial Variation in the Royal Mummies," in *An X-Ray Atlas of the Royal Mummies*, ed. J.E. Harris and E.F. Wente (Chicago: University of Chicago Press, 1980), 346–57.

14 E.F. Wente, "Who Was Who among the Royal Mummies," *The Oriental Institute* 144 (Winter 1995): 1–6, revised July 3, 2007, http://oi.uchicago.edu/research/pubs/nn/win95_wente.html

15 M.G. Cavalcanti, S.S. Rocha, and M.W. Vannier, "Craniofacial Measurements Based on 3D-CT Volume Rendering: Implications for Clinical Applications," *Dentomaxillofac Radiol* 33:3 (May 2004): 170–76.

16 F. Cesarani et al., "Whole-Body Three-Dimensional Multidetector CT of 13 Egyptian Human Mummies," *AJR* 180:3 (2003): 597–606.

17 Lywood and Nelson, "The Face of the Mummy."

18 R. Taylor and P. Craig, "The Wisdom of Bones: Facial Approximation on the Skull," in *Computer-Graphic Facial Reconstruction*, ed. J.G. Clement and M.K. Marks (London:

Elsevier Academic Press, 2005), 33–56; L. Verzé, "History of Facial Reconstruction," *Acta Bio Medica* 80 (2009): 5–12.

19 M.M. Gerasimov, *The Face Finder* (New York: CRC Press, 1971).

20 B. Gatliff and C.C. Snow, "From Skull to Visage," *Journal of Biocommunications* 6 (1979): 27–30; K.T. Taylor, *Forensic Art and Illustration* (Boca Raton: CRC Press, 2001).

21 J. Prag and R. Neave, *Making Faces: Using Forensic and Archaeological Evidence* (London: British Museum Press, 1997).

22 C. Wilkinson, "Computerized Forensic Facial Reconstruction: A Review of Current Systems," *Forensic Science, Medicine, and Pathology* 1:3 (2005): 173–78; Verzé, "History."

23 A.J. Nelson et al., "The ROM/UWO Mummy Project: A Microcosm of Progress in Mummy Research," *Yearbook of Mummy Studies* 1 (2011): 127–32.

24 G. Quatrehomme et al., "Assessment of the Accuracy of Three-Dimensional Manual Craniofacial Reconstruction: A Series of 25 Controlled Cases," *Int J Legal Med* 121 (2007): 469–75.

25 Lywood and Nelson, "The Face of the Mummy."

Bibliography

Abdou, R. *Tarikh Misr al-qadima*. Vol. 2. Cairo: al-Majlis al-A ʿla li-l-Athar, 1993.

Ägyptisches Museum, Staatliche Museen Preußischer Kulturbesitz. Stuttgart: Belser, 1980.

Aldred, C. *Akhenaten and Nefertiti*. New York: The Brooklyn Museum, 1973.

———. *Akhenaten, King of Egypt*. London: Thames and Hudson, 1989.

———. "The Horizon of the Aten." *JEA* 62 (1976): 184.

Allen, J. "Akhenaten's 'Mystery' Coregent and Successor." *Amarna Letters* 1 (1991): 74–85.

———. "The Amarna Succession." In *Causing His Name to Live: Studies in Epigraphy and History in Memory of William Murnane*, edited by P. Brand and L. Cooper, 9–20. Culture and History of the Ancient Near East 37. Leiden: Brill, 2009. http://cassian.memphis.edu/history/murnane/Allen.pdf

———. *The Ancient Egyptian Pyramid Texts*. Atlanta: Society of Biblical Literature, 2005.

American Dental Association. "Eruption Charts." *JADA* 136 (2005): 1619. http://www.mouth-healthy.org/en/az-topics/e/eruption-charts

American Heritage Medical Dictionary. "Cosmetic." http://medical-dictionary.thefreedictionary.com/cosmetic

Andrews, C. *Amulets of Ancient Egypt*. London: British Museum Press, 1994.

Architectural Survey, University of Chicago, Oriental Institute. *The Excavation of Medinet Habu*. 5 vols. Chicago: University of Chicago Press, 1934–54.

Arnold, D. *The Royal Women of Amarna: Images of Beauty from Ancient Egypt*. New York: Metropolitan Museum of Art, 1996.

Aufderheide, A.C. *The Scientific Study of Mummies*. Cambridge: Cambridge University Press, 2003.

Baer, A.N., Z.A. Zahr, S. Khan, and M. Polydefkis. "Acroosteolysis in Diabetes Mellitus." *J Rheumatol* 39:12 (December 2012): 2364–65.

Bass, W.M. *Human Osteology: A Laboratory and Field Manual*. 5th ed. Columbia: Missouri Archaeological Society, 2005.

Beals, R.K., and L. Mason. "The Marfan Skull." *Radiology* 140:3 (1981): 723–25.

Bell, M. "An Armchair Excavation of KV55." *JARCE* 27 (1990): 97–137.

Belova, G.A. "TT320 and the History of the Royal Cache during the Twenty-first Dynasty." In *Egyptology at the Dawn of the Twenty-first Century I: Archaeology*, edited by Z. Hawass and L.P. Brock, 73–80. Cairo: American University in Cairo Press, 2004.

Belzoni, G.B. *Narrative of the Operations and Recent Discoveries in Egypt and Nubia*. London: John Murray, 1820.

Berman, L.M. "Overview of Amenhotep III and His Reign." In *Amenhotep III: Perspectives on His Reign*, edited by D. O'Connor and E. Cline, 1–26. Ann Arbor: University of Michigan Press, 1998.

Bianucci, R., G. Mattutino, R. Lallo, P. Charlier, H. Jouin-Spriet, A. Peluso, T. Higham, C. Torre, and E.R. Massa. "Immunological Evidence of *Plasmodium falciparum* Infection in an Egyptian Child Mummy from the Early Dynastic Period." *J Arch Sci* 35:7 (2008): 1880–85.

Bietak, M. "Comments on the 'Exodus.'" In *Egypt, Israel, Sinai: Archaeological and Historical Relationships in the Biblical Period*, edited by A.F. Rainey, 163–71. Tel Aviv: Tel Aviv University, 1987.

Biggerstaff, R.H. "Forensic Dentistry and the Human Dentition in Individual Age Estimation." *Dent Clin North Am* 21:1 (1977): 167–74.

Boas, F.E., and D. Fleischmann. "Evaluation of Two Iterative Techniques for Reducing Metal Artifacts in Computed Tomography." *Radiology* 259:3 (2011): 894–902.

Bogdonoff, M.D., J.K. Crellin, R. Good, J.P. McGovern, S.B. Nuland, and M.H. Saffon.

The Genuine Works of Hippocrates. Birmingham, UK: Classics of Medicine Library, 1985.

Böni, T., F.J. Rühli, and R.K. Chhem. "History of Paleoradiology: Early Published Literature, 1896–1921." *Can Assoc Radiol J* 55:4 (October 2004): 203–10.

Boyer, R.S., E.A. Rodin, T.C. Grey, and R.C. Connolly. "The Skull and Cervical Spine Radiographs of Tutankhamen: A Critical Appraisal." *AJNR* 24:61 (2003): 1142–47.

Brace, C.L. 1995. "Region Does Not Mean 'Race'—Reality versus Convention in Forensic Anthropology." *Journal of Forensic Science* 40 (1995): 171–75.

Brace, C.L., D.P. Tracer, L.A. Yaroch, J. Robb, K. Brandt, and A.R. Nelson. "Clines and Clusters versus 'Race': A Test in Ancient Egypt and the Case of a Death on the Nile." *Yearbook of Physical Anthropology* 36 (1993): 1–31.

Brand, P.J. *The Monuments of Seti I: Epigraphic, Historical, and Art Historical Analysis*. Probleme der Ägyptologie 16. Leiden: Brill, 2000.

Braunstein, E.M., S.J. White, W. Russell, and J.E. Harris. "Paleoradiologic Evaluation of the Egyptian Royal Mummies." *Skeletal Radiol* 17 (1988): 348–52.

Breasted, J.H. *Ancient Records of Egypt*. 5 vols. Chicago: University of Chicago Press, 1906–1907.

Brier, B. "The Mummy of Unknown Man E: A Preliminary Re-examination." *BEM* 3 (2006): 23–32.

———. *The Murder of Tutankhamun*. Berkeley: Berkeley Publishing Group, 1999.

———. "The Mystery of Unknown Man E." *Archaeology* 59 (2006): 36–42.

British Museum. "The Abbott Papyrus." http://www.britishmuseum.org/explore/highlights/highlight_objects/aes/t/the_abbott_papyrus.aspx

Brooks, S. "Skeletal Age at Death: The Reliability of Cranial and Pubic Age Indicators." *AJPA* 13 (1955): 567–97.

Brooks, S., and J.M. Suchey. "Skeletal Age Determination Based on the Os Pubis: A Comparison of the Acsádi-Nemeskéri and Suchey-Brooks Methods." *Hum Evol* 5:3 (1990): 227–38.

Bucaille, M. *Mummies of the Pharaohs: Modern Medical Investigations*. New York: St. Martin's Press, 1990.

Buikstra, J.E., and D.H. Ubelaker, eds. *Standards for Data Collection from Human Skeletal Remains*. Fayetteville: Arkansas Archeological Survey Research Series 44 (1994).

Capart, J., A.H. Gardiner, and B. van de Walle. "New Light on the Ramesside Tomb Robberies." *JEA* 22:2 (1936): 169–93.

Carter, H. "Report of Work Done in Upper Egypt (1902–1903)." *ASAE* 4 (1903): 176–77.

———. "Report of the Work Done in Upper Egypt, 1903–1904." *ASAE* 6 (1905): 112–19.

———. "A Tomb Prepared for Queen Hatshepsut Discovered by the Earl of Carnarvon (October 1916)." *ASAE* 16 (1916): 79–82.

Carter, H., and A.C. Mace. *The Tomb of Tut-Ankh-Amen*. 3 vols. London: Cassell & Co., 1927, repr. New York: Cooper Square Publishers, 1963.

Cavalcanti, M.G., S.S. Rocha, and M.W. Vannier. "Craniofacial Measurements Based on 3D-CT Volume Rendering: Implications for Clinical Applications." *Dentomaxillofac Radiol* 33:3 (May 2004): 170–76.

Černy, J. *A Community of Workmen at Thebes in the Ramesside Period*. Cairo: IFAO, 1973.

Cesarani, F., M.C. Martina, A. Ferraris, R. Grilletto, R. Boano, E.F. Marochetti, A.M. Donadoni, and G. Gandini. "Whole-body Three-Dimensional Multidetector CT of 13 Egyptian Human Mummies." *AJR* 180:3 (2003): 597–606.

Chapman, P.H., and R. Gupta. "The Mummified Head of Tomb 10A." In *The Secrets of Tomb 10A: Egypt 2000 BC*, edited by R.E. Freed, L.M. Berman, D.M. Doxey, and N.S. Picardo, 180–82. Boston: Museum of Fine Arts, 2009.

Chhem, R.K., and D.R. Brothwell. *Paleoradiology: Imaging Mummies and Fossils*. Berlin and Heidelberg: Springer, 2010.

Chhem, R.K., P. Schmit, and C. Fauré. "Did Ramesses II Really Have Ankylosing Spondylitis? A Reappraisal." *Can Assoc Radiol J* 55:4 (October 2004): 211–17.

Clayton, P. *The Complete Pharaohs*. Cairo: American University in Cairo Press, 2006.

Cline, E., and D. O'Connor, eds. *Ramesses III: The Life and Times of Egypt's Last Hero*. Ann Arbor: University of Michigan Press, 2012.

———. *Thutmose III: A New Biography*. Ann Arbor: University of Michigan Press, 2009.

Colombini, M.P., F. Modugno, F. Silvano, and M. Onor. "Characterization of the Balm of an Egyptian Mummy from the Seventh Century BC." *Studies in Conservation* 45 (2000): 19–29.

Connolly, K. "Is This Nefertiti—or a 100-year-old Fake?" *The Guardian*, May 2, 2009.

Connolly, R.C., R.G. Harrison, and S. Ahmed. "Serological Evidence for the Parentage of Tut'ankhamūn and Smenkharē'." *JEA* 62 (1976): 184–86.

David, R. "Mummification." In *Ancient Egyptian Materials and Technology*, edited by P.T. Nicholson and I. Shaw, 372–89. Cambridge: Cambridge University Press, 2000.

Davies, N. de G. *The Rock Tombs of El Amarna, Part 2: The Tombs of Panehesy and Meryra II*. London: Egypt Exploration Society, 1905.

———. *The Tomb of Ken-Amūn at Thebes*. New York: Metropolitan Museum of Art, repr. 1973.

Davies, N.M. *Ancient Egyptian Paintings*. Chicago: University of Chicago Press, 1936.

Davis, T. *The Tomb of Queen Tîye*. 2nd ed. San Francisco: KMT Communications, 1990.

Davis, T., G. Maspero, E. Ayrton, and G. Daressy. *The Tomb of Siphtah; The Monkey Tomb and the Gold Tomb*. London: Constable, 1908.

Davis, T., G. Maspero, and G. Daressy. *The Tombs of Harmhabi and Touatânkhamanou*. London: Constable, 1912.

Davis, T., G. Maspero, and P.E. Newberry. *The Tomb of Iouiyu and Touiyou*. London: Constable, 1907.

Davis, T., E. Naville, and H. Carter. *The Tomb of Hâtshopsîtû*. London: Constable, 1906.

Dawson, W.R., and P.H.K. Gray. *Catalogue of Egyptian Antiquities in the British Museum I: Mummies and Human Remains*. London: Trustees of the British Museum, 1968.

de Buck, A. "The Judicial Papyrus of Turin." *JEA* 23:2 (1937): 152–66.

De Paepe, A., R.B. Devereux, H.C. Dietz, R.C.M. Hennikam, and R.E. Pyeritz. "Revised Criteria for the Marfan Syndrome." *Am J Med Genet* 62:4 (1996): 417–26.

Derry, D.E. "Report upon the Two Human Fetuses Discovered in the Tomb of Tut-Ankh-Amen." In *The Tomb of Tut-Ankh-Amen 2*, edited by H. Carter and A.C. Mace, 167–69. London: Cassell and Company, 1933.

———. "An X-ray Examination of the Mummy of King Amenophis I." *ASAE* 34 (1934): 47–48.

Desroches-Noblecourt, C. *Ramses II: An Illustrated Biography*. Paris: Flammarion, 2007.

De Wit, C. *The Date and Route of the Exodus*. London: Tyndale Press, 1960.

Diop, C.A. *African Origins of Civilization*. Chicago: Lawrence Hill Books, 1974.

Dodson, A. *Amarna Sunset: Nefertiti, Tutankhamun, Ay, Horemheb, and the Egyptian Counter-Reformation*. Cairo: American University in Cairo Press, 2009.

———. "The Coregency Conundrum." *KMT* 35:2 (Summer 2014): 28–35.

———. "Were Nefertiti and Tutankhaten Coregents?" *KMT* 20:3 (Fall 2009): 41–49.

Dodson, A., and D. Hilton. *The Complete Royal Families of Ancient Egypt*. London: Thames & Hudson, 2004.

Dodson, A., and S. Ikram. *The Mummy in Ancient Egypt: Equipping the Dead for Eternity*. London: Thames & Hudson, 1998.

Dorairajan, N. "Inguinal Hernia—Yesterday, Today and Tomorrow." *Indian Journal of Surgery* 66:3 (June 2004): 137–39.

Dorman, P. *The Monuments of Senenmut: Problems in Historical Methodology*. London and New York: Kegan Paul International, 1988.

Eaton-Krauss, M. "Tutankhamun." *LÄ* 6, cols. 812–16.

Edgerton, W. "The Strikes in Ramses III's Twenty-ninth Year." *JNES* 10 (1951): 137–45.

Edwards, A. "Lying in State in Cairo." *Harper's New Monthly Magazine* 65 (July 1882): 185–204.

Epigraphic Survey, University of Chicago. *Medinet Habu*. 9 vols. Chicago: University of Chicago Press, 1930–2009.

Erichsen, W. *Papyrus Harris I : Hieroglyphische Transkription*. Brussels: Édition de la Fondation égyptologique Reine Élisabeth, 1933.

Erman, A. *Zur Erklärung des Papyrus Harris*. Berlin: Akademie der Wissenschaften, 1903.

Ertman, E. "The Eyes of Nefertiti." *Archaeology* 61:2 (March/April 2008): 28–32.

Eyre, C.J. "A Strike Text from the Theban Necropolis." In *Glimpses of Ancient Egypt: Studies in Honor of H.W. Fairman*, edited by J. Ruffle, G.A. Gaballa, and K. Kitchen, 80–91. Warminster: Aris and Phillips, 1979.

Fakhry, A. *Misr al-far'uniya*. 2nd ed. Cairo: Maktabat al-Anglu, 1960.

Feldtkeller, E., E.M. Lemmel, and A.S. Russell. "Ankylosing Spondylitis in the Pharaohs of Ancient Egypt." *Rheumatol Int* 23 (2003): 1–5.

Filer, J. "Anatomy of a Mummy." *Archaeology* 55:2 (March/April 2002): 26–29.

Fletcher, J. *The Search for Nefertiti.* New York: Harper Collins, 2004.

Forbes, D.C. "Akheperenre Djehutymes: The All-But-Forgotten Second Thutmose." *KMT* 11:2 (Summer 2000): 62–75.

———. "Circumstantial Evidence for an Amenhotep III/Amenhotep IV Coregency." *KMT* 35:2 (Summer 2014): 36–49.

———. *Tombs, Treasures, Mummies: Seven Great Discoveries of Egyptian Archaeology.* Sebastopol, CA: KMT Communications, Inc., 1998.

Forbes, D.C., S. Ikram, and J. Kamrin. "Tutankhamun's Ribs: A Proposed Solution to the Problem." *KMT* 18:1 (Spring 2007): 50–56.

Fouquet, D. *Les momies royales de Deir el-Bahari: Rapport addressé à M. Le Directeur Général des fouilles en Egypte.* Cairo: IFAO, 1890.

Frandsen, P.J. "Editing Reality: The Turin Strike Papyrus." In *Studies in Egyptology Presented to Miriam Lichtheim* 1, edited by S. Israelit-Groll, 166–99. Jerusalem: Magness Press, Hebrew University, 1990.

Franke, D. "Verwandschaftsbezeichnungen." *LÄ* 6, col. 1033.

Franklin, D. "Forensic Age Estimation in Human Skeletal Remains: Current Concepts and Future Directions." *Leg Med* 12:1 (January 2010): 1–7. Epub 2009 Oct 22.

Freed, R.E., Y.J. Markowitz, and S.H. D'Auria, eds. *Pharaohs of the Sun: Akhenaten, Nefertiti, Tutankhamun.* Boston: Museum of Fine Arts, 1999.

Fully, G., and H. Pineau. "Détermination de la stature au moyen du squelette." *Ann Méd Légale* 40 (1960): 145–54.

Gabolde, L. "La montagne thébaine garde encore des secrets." *Dossiers d'Archéologie*, 149–50 (1990): 56–59.

———. "Les Tombes d'Hatchepsout." *Egypte: Afrique et Orient* 17 (2000): 51–56.

Gabolde, M. "Baketaten fille de Kiya?" *BSEG* 16 (1992): 39.

———. *D'Akhenaton à Toutânkhamon.* Collection de l'Institut d'archéologie et d'histoire de l'antiquité, Université Lumière-Lyon 3. Lyon: Université Lumière 2, Institut d'archéologie et d'histoire de l'antiquité, 1998.

———. "Under a Deep Blue Starry Sky." In *Causing His Name to Live: Studies in Egyptian Epigraphy and History in Memory of William Murnane*, edited by P. Brand and L. Cooper, 109–20. Leiden: Brill, 2009. http://cassian.memphis.edu/history/murnane/M_Gabolde.pdf

Gardiner, A.H. *Egypt of the Pharaohs.* Oxford: Oxford University Press, 1961.

———. *Ramesside Administrative Documents.* Oxford: Griffith Institute, 1948.

Gatliff, B., and C.C. Snow. "From Skull to Visage." *Journal of Biocommunications* 6 (1979): 27–30.

Gerasimov, M.M. *The Face Finder.* New York: CRC Press, 1971.

Gertzen, T.L. "New Evidence for Nefertiti in Akhenaten's Regnal Year 16." *KMT* 24:1 (Spring 2013): 34.

Gibson, G. "How Tall was Thutmose III? An Investigation into the Nature of Information." *KMT* 11:1 (Spring 2000): 60–65.

Gilbert-Barness, E., and D. Debich-Spicer. *Embryo and Fetal Pathology: Color Atlas with Ultrasound Correlation.* Cambridge, UK: Cambridge University Press, 2004.

Goedicke, H. "Was Magic Used in the Harem Conspiracy against Ramesses III?" *JEA* 49 (1963): 71–92.

Görg, M. "Exodus." In *The Oxford Encyclopedia of Ancient Egypt* 1, edited by D. Redford, 489–90. Cairo: American University in Cairo Press, 2001.

Gostner, P., M. Monelli, P. Pernter, A. Graefen, and A. Zink. "New Radiological Approach for Analysis and Identification of Foreign Objects in Ancient and Historic Mummies." *J Arch Sci* 40:2 (2013): 1003–11.

Grabherr, S., C. Cooper, S. Ulrich-Bochsler, T. Uldin, S. Ross, L. Oesterhelweg, S. Bolliger, A. Christe, P. Schnyder, P. Mangin, and M.J. Thali. "Estimation of Sex and Age of 'Virtual Skeletons': A Feasibility Study." *Eur Radiol* 19:2 (February 2009): 419–29. Epub 2008 Sep 3.

Grandet, P. *Le Papyrus Harris I, BM 9999*. 3 vols. Cairo: IFAO, 1994–99.

Gray, P.H.K. "Notes Concerning the Position of Arms and Hands of Mummies with a View to Possible Dating of the Specimen." *JEA* 58 (1972): 200–204.

Griffith Institute, Diaries 4th Season. "Tutankhamun: Anatomy of an Excavation. Howard Carter's Diaries. The Fourth Excavation Season in the Tomb of Tutankhamun. September 23, 1925 to May 21, 1926."
http://www.griffith.ox.ac.uk/gri/4sea4not.html

Griffith Institute. "Tutankhamun: The Anatomy of an Excavation," photo p. 1566.
http//www.griffith.ox.ac.uk/gri/4tut.html

Griffith Institute. "Tutankhamun: Anatomy of an Excavation. The Howard Carter Archives." Database entries for fetus mummies.
http://www.griffith.ox.ac.uk/gri/carter/300-349.html

Grimal, N. *A History of Ancient Egypt*. Translated by Ian Shaw. Oxford and Cambridge, MA: Blackwell, 1992.

Grist, J. "The Identity of the Ramesside Queen Tyti." *JEA* 71 (1985): 71–81.

Guevara-Aquirre, J., and A.L. Rosenbloom. "Obesity, Diabetes and Cancer: Insight into the Relationship from a Cohort with Growth Hormone Receptor Deficiency." *Diabetologia* 58:1 (Jan. 2015): 37–42. doi: 10.1007/s00125-014-3397-3. Epub 2014 Oct 15.

Gupta, R., Y. Markowitz, L. Berman, and P. Chapman. "High-resolution Imaging of an Ancient Egyptian Mummified Head: New Insights into the Mummification Process." *AJNR* 29:4 (2008): 705–13.

Haller, J., D. Resnick, C.W. Miller, J.P. Schils, R. Kerr, D. Bielecki, D.J. Sartoris, and C.R. Gundry. "Diffuse Idiopathic Skeletal Hyperostosis: Diagnostic Significance of Radiographic Abnormalities of the Pelvis." *Radiology* 172 (1989): 835–39.

Harer, W.B., Jr. "An Explanation of King Tutankhamun's Death." *BEM* 3 (2006): 83–88.

———. "New Evidence for King Tutankhamen's Death: His Bizarre Embalming." *JEA* 97 (2011): 228–32.

———. "Was Tutankhamun Killed by a Hippo?" *Ancient Egypt* 72 (2012): 50–54.

Hari, R. *Horemheb et la reine Moutnedjemet; ou, la fin d'une dynastie*. Geneva: Impr. La Sirène, 1965.

Harris, J.E., C.J. Kowalski, and G.F. Walker. "Craniofacial Variation in the Royal Mummies." In *An X-Ray Atlas of the Royal Mummies*, edited by J.E. Harris and E.F. Wente, 346–57. Chicago: University of Chicago Press, 1980.

Harris, J.E., and K.R. Weeks. *X-Raying the Pharaohs*. New York: Charles Scribner's Sons, 1973.

Harris, J.E., and E.F. Wente. "Mummy of the 'Elder Lady' in the Tomb of Amenhotep II: Egyptian Museum Catalog Number 61070." *Science* (9 June 1978): 1149–51.

———. *An X-Ray Atlas of the Royal Mummies*. Chicago: University of Chicago Press, 1980.

Harris, J.E., E.F. Wente, C. F. Cox, I. El Nawaway, C.J. Kowalski, A.T. Storey, W.R. Russell, P.V. Ponitz, and G.F. Walker. "The Identification of the Elder Lady in the Tomb of Amenhotep II as Queen Tiye." *Delaware Medical Journal* 51:2 (1979): 89–93.

Harrison, R.G. "Postmortem on Two Pharaohs: Was Tutankhamun's Skull Fractured?" *Buried History* 4 (1971): 114–29.

Harrison, R.G., and A.B. Abdalla. "The Remains of Tutankhamun." *Antiquity* 46 (1972): 8–14.

Harrison, R.G., R.C. Connolly, and A. Abdalla. "Kinship of Smenkhkare and Tutankhamun Affirmed by Serological Micromethod: Kinship of Smenkhkare and Tutankhamen Demonstrated Serologically." *Nature* 224 (1969): 325–26.

Harrison, R.G, R.C. Connolly, S. Ahmed, A.B. Abdalla, and M. El Ghawaby. "A Mummified Foetus from the Tomb of Tutankhamun." *Antiquity* 53:207 (1979): 19–21.

Hoelauer, F. "Harem," In *The Oxford Encyclopedia of Ancient Egypt* 2, edited by D. Redford, 76–80. Cairo: American University in Cairo Press, 2001.

Hassan, S. *Misr al-qadima*. Vol. 8. Cairo: Maktabat al-Usra, 2000.

Hawass, Z. *Discovering Tutankhamun: From Howard Carter to DNA*. Cairo: American University in Cairo Press, 2013.

———. "The Discovery of the Mummy of Queen Hatshepsut." In Ola El-Aguizy Festschrift, *BIFAO*, forthcoming.

———. "The Egyptian Mummy Project." *KMT* 15:4 (Winter 2004–2005): 29–38.

———. *The Golden King: The World of Tutankhamun*. Cairo: American University in Cairo Press, 2006.

———. *King Tutankhamun: The Treasures of the Tomb*. New York: Thames & Hudson, 2007.

———. "King Tut's Family Secrets." *National Geographic Magazine*, September 2010, 34–59.

http://ngm.nationalgeographic.com/print/2010/09/tut-dna/hawass-text

———. "New Evidence for the Cause of Tutankhamun's Death." Bibliotheca Alexandrina. http://www.bibalex.org/archeology/attachments/lectures/201201221342049314.pdf

———. "Newly Discovered Scenes of Tutankhamun from Memphis and Rediscovered Fragments from Hermopolis." In *The Art and Culture of Ancient Egypt: Studies in Honor of Dorothea Arnold*, edited by O. Goelet and A. Oppenheim. *BES* 19 (2012), forthcoming.

———. "A Preliminary Report on the Excavation of the Valley of the Kings: Season 3 (2009–2010)." *ASAE*, forthcoming.

———. "Quest for the Mummy of Queen Hatshepsut." *KMT* 17:2 (Summer 2006): 40–43.

———. "The Scientific Search for Hatshepsut's Mummy." *KMT* 18:3 (Fall 2007): 20–25.

———. *Silent Images: Women in Pharaonic Egypt*. Cairo: American University in Cairo Press, 2008.

———. *Tutankhamun: All About the Golden King*. Cairo: American University in Cairo Press, forthcoming.

———. *Tutankhamun and the Golden Age of the Pharaohs*. Washington, D.C.: National Geographic, 2005.

Hawass, Z., and T. El Awady. "The Tunnel Inside the Tomb of Seti I (KV17): Secrets Revealed." *ASAE*, forthcoming.

Hawass, Z., Y.Z. Gad, Z. Ismail, R. Khairat, D. Fathalla, N. Hasan, A. Ahmed, H. Elleithy, M. Ball, F. Gaballah, S. Wasef, M. Fateen, H. Amer, P. Gostner, A. Selim, A. Zink, and C.M. Pusch. "Ancestry and Pathology in King Tutankhamun's Family." *JAMA* 303:7 (2010): 638–47.

Hawass, Z., S. Ismail, A. Selim, S.N. Saleem, D. Fathalla, S. Wasef, A.Z. Gad, R. Saad, S.

Fares, H. Amer, P. Gostner, Y.Z. Gad, C.M. Pusch, and A.R. Zink. "Revisiting the Harem Conspiracy and Death of Ramesses III: Anthropological, Forensic, Radiological, and Genetic Study." *BMJ* 345 (2012): e8268.

Hawass, Z., and S.N. Saleem. "Mummified Daughters of King Tutankhamun: Archeologic and CT Studies." *AJR* 197:5 (November 2011): W829–36.

———. "Reply." *AJR* 198:6 (2012): W630.

Hawass, Z., M. Shafik, F.J. Rühli, A. Selim, E. El-Sheikh, S. Abdel Fatah, H. Amer, F. Gaballa, A. Gamal Eldin, E. Egarter-Vigl, and P. Gostner. "Computed Tomographic Evaluation of Pharaoh Tutankhamun, ca. 1300 BC." *ASAE* 81 (2007): 159–74.

Hawass, Z., and A.G. Wagdy. "Excavations North-west of Amenhotep III Temple: Season 2010–11." *MDAIK* 70/71 (2014/2015), forthcoming.

Hawass, Z., A.G. Wagdy, and M.A. Badea. "The Discovery of the Missing Pieces of the Statue of Amenhotep III and Queen Tiye at the Egyptian Museum." *ASAE* 85 (2011): 165–76.

Hayes, W.C. "Egypt: Internal Affairs from Thutmosis I to the Death of Amenophis III." In *Cambridge Ancient History*, 3rd ed., vol. 2, part 1, ch. 9, edited by I.E.S. Edwards, C.J. Gadd, N.G.L. Hammond, and E. Sollberger, 313–416. Cambridge: Cambridge University Press, 1973.

Helck, W. "Kije." *MDAIK* 40 (1984): 159–67.

Hellier, C.A., and R.C. Connolly. "A Re-assessment of the Larger Fetus Found in Tutankhamen's Tomb." *Antiquity* 83:319 (2009): 165–73.

Herodotus. *The Histories*. Translated by A. de Sélincourt, rev. A.R. Burns. Harmondsworth: Penguin, 1972.

Hoffman, H., and S. D'Auria. "Mummies and Modern Medical Imaging." In *The Realm of Osiris: Mummies, Coffins, and Ancient Egyptian Funerary Art in the Michael C. Carlos Museum*, edited by P. Lacovara and B.T. Trope, 37–42.

Atlanta: Michael C. Carlos Museum, Emory University, 2001.

Hoffman, H., and P.A. Hudgins. "Head and Skull Base Features of Nine Egyptian Mummies: Evaluation with High-Resolution CT and Reformation Techniques. *AJR* 178:6 (2002): 1367–76.

Holm, S. "The Privacy of Tutankhamen—Utilising the Genetic Information in Stored Tissue Samples." *Theo Med Bioeth* 22 (2001): 437–49.

Hornung, E. *Echnaton: die Religion des Lichtes.* Zurich: Artemis and Winkler, 1995.

———. *Das Grab des Haremhab im Tal der Könige.* Bern: Francke Verlag, 1971.

———. *The Tomb of Pharaoh Seti I.* Zurich and Munich: Artemis Verlag, 1971.

Hübener, K.H., and W.M. Pahl. "Computertomographische Untersuchungen an altägyptischen Mumien." *Fortschr Geb Röntgenstr Nuklearmed* 135:8 (1981): 213–19.

Hughes, B.O., and G.R. Moore. "Heredity, Growth, and the Dentofacial Complex." *The Angle Orthodontist* 11 (1941): 217–22.

Huppertz, A., D. Wildung, B.J. Kemp, T. Nentwig, P. Asbach, F.M. Rasche, and B. Hamm. "Nondestructive Insights into Composition of the Sculpture of Egyptian Queen Nefertiti with CT." *Radiology* 25:1 (April 2009): 233–40.

Hussein, F., and J.E. Harris. 1988. "The Skeletal Remains from Tomb No. 55." In *Fifth International Congress of Egyptology, October 29–November 3, Cairo, 1988. Abstracts of Papers*, 140–41. Cairo: International Association of Egyptologists.

Ikram, S. "Some Thoughts on the Mummification of King Tutankhamun." *Institut des Cultures Méditerranéennes et Orientales de l'Académie Polonaise des Sciences, Études et Travaux* 26 (2013): 292–301.

Ikram, S., and A. Dodson. *The Mummy in Ancient Egypt.* Cairo: American University in Cairo

Press; London: Thames & Hudson Limited, 1998.

Iskander, Z. "Mummification in Ancient Egypt: Development, History and Techniques." In *An X-ray Atlas of the Royal Mummies*, edited by J.E. Harris and E.F. Wente, 1–26. Chicago: University of Chicago Press, 1980.

James, S. "Dueling Nefertitis? In the Valley of the King's Tomb of Amenhotep II." *KMT* 14:3 (Fall 2003): 22–30.

———. "End Paper." *KMT* (Fall 1993): 86–87.

Jansen, R.J., M. Poulus, W. Taconis, and J. Stoker. "High Resolution Spiral Computed Tomography with Multiplanar Reformatting, 3D Surface- and Volume Rendering: A Non-destructive Method to Visualize Ancient Egyptian Mummification Techniques." *Comput Med Imaging Graph* 26 (2002): 211–16.

Jasnow, R., and K.M. Cooney, eds. *Joyful in Thebes: Egyptological Studies in Honor of Betsy M. Bryan*. Atlanta: Lockwood Press, 2015 (forthcoming).

Johannsdottir, B., B.F. Thorarinsson, A. Thordarson, and T.E. Magnusson. "Heritability of Craniofacial Characteristics between Parents and Offspring Estimated from Lateral Cephalograms." *Am J Orthod Dentofacial Orthop* 127:2 (February 2005): 200–207.

Johnson, W.R. "Monuments and Monumental Art under Amenhotep III." In *Amenhotep III: Perspectives on His Reign*, edited by D. O'Connor and E.H. Cline, 63–94. Ann Arbor: University of Michigan Press, 1998.

Johnstone, E.M., C.E. Hutchinson, A. Vail, A. Chevance, and A.L. Herrick. "Acro-osteolysis in Systemic Sclerosis is Associated with Digital Ischaemia and Severe Calcinosis." *Rheumatology* (Oxford) 51:12 (December 2012): 2234–38.

Kate, B.R., and R.D. Mujumdar. "Stature Estimation from Femur and Humerus by Regression and Autometry." *Acta Anat* 94:2 (1976): 311–20.

Kemp, B. *The City of Akhenaten and Nefertiti: Amarna and Its People*. London: Thames & Hudson, 2012.

———. "The Harim Palace at Medinet el-Ghurab." *ZÄS* 105 (1978): 122–23.

King, M.R., G.M. Cooper, and D. DeNevi. *Who Killed King Tut? Using Modern Forensics to Solve a 3300-Year-Old Mystery*. Amherst, NY: Prometheus Books, 2004.

Kiss, C., M. Szilágyi, A. Paksy, and G. Poór. "Risk Factors for Diffuse Idiopathic Skeletal Hyperostosis: A Case-Control Study." *Rheumatology* 41 (2002): 27–30.

Kitchen, K.A. "A Long-Lost Portrait of Princess Neferurē' from Deir el-Baḥri." *JEA* 49 (1963): 38–40.

———. *Pharaoh Triumphant: The Life and Times of Ramesses II*. Warminster: Aris and Phillips, 1982.

———. *Ramesside Inscriptions: Historical and Biographical*. 7 vols. Oxford: Wiley-Blackwell, 1969–90.

Kozloff, A., B. Bryan, and L. Berman. *Egypt's Dazzling Sun: Amenhotep III and His World*. Cleveland: Cleveland Museum of Art, 1992.

Krogman, W.M., and V. Sassouni. *A Syllabus in Roentgenographic Cephalometry*. Philadelphia: Philadelphia Center for Research in Child Growth, 1957.

Laboury, D. "A propos de l'authenticité de la momie attribuée à Thoutmosis III (CG 61068)." *GM* 156 (1997): 73–79.

Lacau, P. *Stèles du Nouvel Empire*. Catalogue général des antiquités égyptiennes du Musée du Caire 45. Cairo: IFAO, 1909.

Lacovara, P., and B.T. Trope, eds. *The Realm of Osiris: Mummies, Coffins, and Ancient Egyptian Funerary Art in the Michael C. Carlos Museum*. Atlanta: Michael C. Carlos Museum, Emory University, 2001.

Leahy, A.M. "The Libyan Period in Egypt: An Essay in Interpretation." *Libyan Studies* 16 (1985): 51–65.

———, ed. *Libya and Egypt c. 1300–750 BC.* London: SOAS Centre of Near and Middle Eastern Studies and the Society for Libyan Studies, 1990.

Leblanc, C. "The Tomb of Ramesses II and Remains of His Funerary Treasure." *Egyptian Archaeology* 10 (1997): 11–13.

Leek, F.F. "How Old Was Tutankhamun?" *JEA* 63 (1977): 112–15.

———. *The Human Remains from the Tomb of Tutankhamun*. Oxford: Griffith Institute, 1972.

Loret, V. "Le tombeau d'Aménophis II et la cachette royale de Biban el-Molouk." *BIE* (3rd series) 9 (1899): 98–112.

Lovejoy, C.O., R.S. Meindl, R.P. Mensforth, and T.J. Barton. "Multifactoral Determination of Skeletal Age at Death: A Method and Blind Tests of Its Accuracy." *AJPA* 68:1 (1985): 1–14.

Luban, M. "Do We Have the Mummy of Nefertiti?" http://www.geocities.com/scribelist/do_we_have_.htm

———. "Is the Mummy 'Tuthmosis I' Really Hatshepsut?" *DE* 42 (1998): 69–84.

Luccichenti, G., F. Cademartiri, F.R. Pezzella, G. Runza, M. Belgrano, M. Midiri, U. Sabatini, S. Bastianello, and G.P. Krestin. "3D Reconstruction Techniques Made Easy: Know-how and Pictures." *Eur Radiol* 15:10 (October 2005): 2146–56. Epub 2005 Apr 5.

Lywood, V., and A.J. Nelson. "The Face of the Mummy: Phenotypic Variability among Facial Reconstructions of Ancient Egyptian Mummies" (abstract). *CAPA Newsletter* 1 (2012): 36.

MacKay, K., C. Mack, S. Brophy, and A. Calin. "The Bath Ankylosing Spondylitis Radiology Index (BASRI): A New, Validated Approach to Disease Assessment." *Arthritis & Rheumatism* 14:12 (December 1998): 2263–70.

Magid, D., R.E. Pyeritz, and E.K. Fishman. "Musculoskeletal Manifestations of the Marfan Syndrome: Radiologic Features." *AJR* 155:1 (1990): 99–104.

Mahoney, G., and C. Wilkinson. *Craniofacial Identification*. New York: Cambridge University Press, 2012.

Manuelian, P. der, and C. Loeben. "From Daughter to Father: The Recarved Egyptian Sarcophagus of Queen Hatshepsut and King Thutmose I." *JMFA* 5 (1993): 24–61.

Martin, G. *The Memphite Tomb of Horemheb, Commander-in-Chief of Tut'ankhamūn* 1: *The Reliefs, Inscriptions, and Commentary*. London: Egypt Exploration Society, 1990.

———. *The Royal Tomb at El-Amarna* 2: *The Reliefs, Inscriptions, and Architecture*. London: Egypt Exploration Society, 1989.

Maspero, G. *Les Momies Royales de Déir el-Baharî*. MMAF 3. Paris: Leroux, 1889.

———. *The Struggle of the Nations*. London: Society for Promoting Christian Knowledge, 1896.

Massare, C. "Anatomo-radiologie et vérité historique: à propos du bilan xéroradiographique de Ramsès II." *Bruxelles Medical* 59:3 (1979): 163–70.

Maystre, C. "Le tombeau de Ramsès II." *BIFAO* 38 (1939): 183–90.

McMichael, A.J. *Human Frontiers, Environments and Disease: Past Patterns, Uncertain Futures*. Cambridge: Cambridge University Press, 2001.

Meindl, R.S., and C.O. Lovejoy. "Ectocranial Suture Closure: A Revised Method for the Determination of Skeletal Age at Death Based on the Lateral-Anterior Sutures." *AJPA* 68:1 (1985): 57–66.

Michael C. Carlos Museum, Emory University. "Ramesses I: The Search for the Lost Pharaoh." www.carlos.emory.edu/RAMESSES/index.html

Müller, M.E., M. Allgöwer, R. Schneider, and H. Willenegger. *Manual der Osteosynthese*. Berlin: Springer, 1971.

Murnane, W.J. "The Return to Orthodoxy." In *Pharaohs of the Sun: Akhenaten, Nefertiti, Tutankhamun*, edited by R. Freed, Y. Markowitz, and S. D'Auria, 177–85. Boston: Museum of Fine Arts, 1999.

———. *Texts from the Amarna Period in Egypt*. Writings from the Ancient World 5. Atlanta: Society of Biblical Literature, 1995.

Naville, E. *The Temple of Deir el Bahari*. 7 vols. London: Egypt Exploration Fund, 1894–1908.

Nelson, A.J., R. Chhem, I.A. Cunningham, S.N. Friedman, G. Garvin, G. Gibson, P.V. Granton, D.W. Holdsworth, S. Holowka, F. Longstaffe, V. Lywood, N. Nguyen, R. Shaw, M. Trumpour, A.D. Wade, and C.D. White. "The ROM/UWO Mummy Project: A Microcosm of Progress in Mummy Research." *Yearbook of Mummy Studies* 1 (2011): 127–32.

Nicholson, P.T., and I. Shaw. *Ancient Egyptian Materials and Technology*. Cambridge: Cambridge University Press, 2000.

Nunn, J.F. *Ancient Egyptian Medicine*. London: British Museum, 1996.

———. "Disease." In *The Oxford Encyclopedia of Ancient Egypt* 1, edited by D. Redford, 398. Cairo: American University in Cairo Press, 2001.

O'Connor, D. "Thutmose III: An Enigmatic Pharaoh." In *Thutmose III: A New Biography*, edited by E. Cline and D. O'Connor, 1–38. Ann Arbor: University of Michigan Press, 2009.

O'Connor, D., and E. Cline. *Amenhotep III: Perspectives on His Reign*. Ann Arbor: University of Michigan Press, 1998.

Olivier, G., and H. Pineau. "Nouvelle détermination de la taille foetale d'après les longueurs diaphysaires des os longs." *Ann Méd Légale* 40 (1960): 141–44.

Olivieri, I., S. D'Angelo, M.S. Cutro, A. Padula, G. Peruz, M. Montaruli, E. Scarano, V. Giasi, C. Palazzi, and M.A. Khan. "Diffuse Idiopathic Skeletal Hyperostosis May Give the Typical Postural Abnormalities of Advanced Ankylosing Spondylitis." *Rheumatology* (Oxford) 46 (2007): 1709–11.

Olsen, Ø.E., R.T. Lie, R.S. Lachman, H. Maartmann-Moe, and K. Rosendahl. "Ossification Sequence in Infants Who Die During the Perinatal Period: Population-based References." *Radiology* 225:1 (2002): 240–44.

Osman, A. "Who Was Joseph? The Mummy of Patriarch Joseph in the Cairo Museum." http://www.dwij.org/forum/amarna/3_joseph.html

Ousley, S., R. Jantz, and D. Fried. "Understanding Race and Human Variation: Why Forensic Anthropologists are Good at Identifying Race." *Am J Phys Anthropol* 139 (2009): 68–76.

Panchbhai, A.S. "Dental Radiographic Indicators, a Key to Age Estimation." *Dentomaxillofac Radiol* 40:4 (2011): 199–212; doi:http://dx.doi.org/10.1259/dmfr/19478385

Papavramidou, N.S., and H. Christopoulou-Aletras. "Treatment of 'Hernia' in the Writings of Celsus (First Century AD)." *World J Surg* 29 (2005): 1343–47.

Partridge, R.B. *Faces of Pharaohs: Royal Mummies and Coffins from Ancient Thebes*. London: Rubicon Press, 1994.

Peden, A.J. *Egyptian Historical Inscriptions of the Twentieth Dynasty*. Jonsered, Sweden: Paul Åströms Förlag, 1994.

Peet, T.E. *The Great Tomb Robberies of the Twentieth Egyptian Dynasty*. Oxford: Clarendon Press, 1930.

Pendlebury, J.D.S. *The City of Akhenaten* 3. 2 vols. London: Egypt Exploration Society, 1951.

Petrie, W.M.F. *A History of Egypt*. 6 vols. London: Methuen and Co., 1896, repr. Michael S. Sanders, 1991.

———. *The Royal Tombs of the Earliest Dynasties, 1901*. Part 2. London: Egypt Exploration Fund, 1901.

———. *Tell el Amarna*. London: Methuen and Co., 1894.

Phenice, T.W. "A Newly Developed Visual Method of Sexing the Os Pubis." *Am J Phys Anthropol* 30:2 (1969): 297–301.

Piacentini, P. *La Valle di Re riscoperta: I giornali di scavo di Victor Loret (1898–1899) e altri inediti*. Milan: University of Milan, 2004.

———, ed. *Victor Loret in Egypt (1881–1899): From the Archives of the Milan University to the Egyptian Museum in Cairo*. Cairo: Supreme Council of Antiquities, 2008.

Piankoff, A. "La tombe de Ramsès 1er." *BIFAO* 56 (1957): 189–200.

Pinch, G. "Ancient Egyptian Magic." http://www.bbc.co.uk/history/ancient/egyptians/magic_01.shtml

———. *Egyptian Mythology: A Guide to the Gods, Goddesses, and Traditions of Ancient Egypt*. Oxford: Oxford University Press, 2004.

Pirelli, R. *The Queens of Ancient Egypt*. Cairo: American University in Cairo Press, 2008.

Poosha, D.V., P.J. Byard, M. Satyanarayana, J.P. Rice, and D.C. Rao. "Family Resemblance for Cranio-facial Measurements in Velanti Brahmins from Andhra Pradesh, India." *Am J Phys Anthropol* 65:1 (September 1984): 15–22.

Prag, J., and R. Neave. *Making Faces: Using Forensic and Archaeological Evidence*. London: British Museum Press, 1997.

Qteishat, W.A., G.H. Whitehouse, and N.E. Hawass. "Acro-osteolysis Following Snake and Scorpion Envenomation." *Br J Radiol* 58:695 (November 1985): 1035–39.

Quatrehomme, G., T. Balaguer, P. Staccini, and V. Alunni-Perret. "Assessment of the Accuracy of Three-dimensional Manual Craniofacial Reconstruction: A Series of 25 Controlled Cases." *Int J Legal Med* 121 (2007): 469–75.

Quibell, J. *Tomb of Yuaa and Thuiu*. Catalogue général des antiquités égyptiennes du Musée du Caire. Cairo: IFAO, 1908.

Raxter, M.H., C.B. Ruff, A. Azab, M. Erfan, M. Soliman, and A. El-Sawaf. "Stature Estimation in Ancient Egyptians: A New Technique Based on Anatomical Reconstruction of Stature." *AJPA* 136:2 (June 2008): 147–55.

Recheis, W., G.W. Weber, K. Schafer, H. Prossinger, R. Knapp, and H. Seidler. "New Methods and Techniques in Anthropology." *Coll Antropol* 23:2 (1999): 495–509.

Redford, D.B. *Akhenaten: The Heretic King*. Princeton: Princeton University Press, 1984.

———. "An Egyptological Perspective on the Exodus." In *Egypt, Israel, Sinai: Archaeological and Historical Relationships in the Biblical Period*, edited by A.F. Rainer, 137–61. Tel Aviv: Tel Aviv University Press, 1987.

———, ed. *The Oxford Encyclopedia of Ancient Egypt*. 3 vols. Cairo: American University in Cairo Press, 2001.

Redford, S. *The Harem Conspiracy: The Murder of Ramesses III*. Dekalb, IL: Northern Illinois University Press, 2008.

Reeves, N. *Akhenaten: Egypt's False Prophet*. London: Thames & Hudson, 2005.

———. *The Complete Tutankhamun: The King, the Tomb, the Royal Treasure*. London: Thames & Hudson, 1990.

———. "The Royal Family." In *Pharaohs of the Sun: Akhenaten, Nefertiti, Tutankhamun*, edited by R. Freed, Y. Markowitz, and S. D'Auria, 80–95. Boston: Museum of Fine Arts, 1999.

———. "Tuthmosis IV as 'Great-Grandfather' of Tut'ankhamūn." *GM* 56 (1982): 65–69.

———. *Valley of the Kings: The Decline of a Royal Necropolis*. London: Kegan Paul, 1990.

Reeves, N., and R.H. Wilkinson. *The Complete Valley of the Kings: Tombs and Treasures of Egypt's Greatest Pharaohs*. London: Thames & Hudson, 1996.

Reiser, E. *Der königliche Harim im alten Ägypten und seine Verwaltung*. Vienna: Verlag Notring, 1972.

Resnick, D., and G. Niwayama. "Entheses and Enthesopathy: Anatomical Pathological and Radiological Correlation." *Radiology* 146 (1983): 1–9.

———. "Radiographic and Pathologic Features of Spinal Involvement in Diffuse Idiopathic Skeletal Hyperostosis (DISH)." *Radiology* 119 (1976): 559–68.

Ritner, R.K. *The Mechanics of Ancient Egyptian Magical Practice*. SAOC 54. Chicago: Oriental Institute of the University of Chicago, 1993.

Roeder, G. *Amarna-Reliefs aus Hermopolis*. Hildesheim: Gerstenberg, 1969.

Roehrig, C.H., R. Dreyfus, and C.H. Keller, eds. *Hatshepsut: From Queen to Pharaoh*. New York: Metropolitan Museum of Art, 2005.

Rogers, J., I. Watt, and P. Dieppe. "Palaeopathology of Spinal Osteophytosis, Vertebral Ankylosis, Ankylosing Spondylitis, and Vertebral Hyperostosis." *Ann Rheum Dis* 44:2 (February 1985): 113–20.

Romer, J. "Tuthmosis I and the Bibân el-Molûk: Some Problems of Attribution." *JEA* 60 (1974): 119–33.

Roth, A.M. "Models of Authority: Hatshepsut's Predecessors in Power." In *Hatshepsut: From Queen to Pharaoh*, edited by C.H. Roehrig, 9–14. New York: Metropolitan Museum of Art, 2005.

Ruffer, M.A. *Studies in the Palaeopathology of Egypt*. Chicago: University of Chicago Press, 1921. http://www.ebooksread.com/authors-eng/marc-armand-ruffer/studies-in-the-palaeopathology-of-egypt-ffu/1-studies-in-the-palaeopathology-of-egypt-ffu.shtml

Rühli, F., and T. Böni. "Radiological Aspects and Interpretation of Post-mortem Artefacts in Ancient Egyptian Mummies from Swiss Collections." *Int J Osteoarchaeol* 10:2 (2000): 153–57.

Rühli, F.J., R.K. Chhem, and T. Böni. "Diagnostic Paleoradiology of Mummified Tissue: Interpretation and Pitfalls." *Can Assoc Radiol J* 55:4 (2004): 218–27.

Russell, W., A.T. Storey, and P.V. Ponitz. "Radiographic Techniques in the Study of the Mummy." In *An X-Ray Atlas of the Royal Mummies*, edited by J.E. Harris and E.F. Wente, 163–87. Chicago: University of Chicago Press, 1980.

Ryan, D.P. "Return to Wadi Biban el Moluk: The 2nd (1990) Season of the Valley of the Kings Project." *KMT* 2:1 (Spring 1991): 29–30.

———. "Who Is Buried in KV60? A Field Report." *KMT* 1 (1990): 34–39.

Saleem, S.N., and Z. Hawass. "Ankylosing Spondylitis or Diffuse Idiopathic Skeletal Hyperostosis (DISH) in Royal Egyptian Mummies of the 18th–20th Dynasties? CT and Archaeology Studies." *Arthritis and Rheumatology* 66:12 (December 2014), published online October 20, 2014 (doi:10.1002/art.38864).

———. "Multi-detector Computed Tomography Study of Amulets, Jewelry, and Other Foreign Objects in Royal Egyptian Mummies Dated to the 18th to 20th Dynasties." *JCAT* 38:2 (2013): 153–58. doi:10.1097/RCT.0b013e3182ab2221

———. "Multi-detector Computerized Tomography (MDCT) Study of Cosmetic Care and Beautification of Royal Ancient Egyptian Mummies Related to the 18th to 20th Dynasties." Presentation at the Eighth World Congress on Mummies Studies, Rio de Janeiro, Brazil, August 8, 2013.

———. "Multi Detector CT of Royal Ancient Egyptian Mummies: An Approach to Study." Presentation at Radiological Society of North America (RSNA), Chicago, November 25–30, 2012.

———. "Mummification of Fetuses in Ancient Egypt: Anthropology and Multi-detector Computed Tomography Study (MDCT)." Presentation at American Anthropology Association (AAA) annual meeting, Chicago, November 22, 2013.

———. "Subcutaneous Packing in Royal Egyptian Mummies Dated from the 18th to 20th Dynasties." *JCAT* (in press.)

———. "Variability in Brain Treatment during Mummification of Royal Egyptians Dated to the 18th–20th Dynasties: MDCT Findings Correlated with the Archaeologic Literature." *AJR* 200:4 (April 2013): W 336–44. doi:10.2214/AJR.12.9405.

———. "Variability in Cranial Mummification of Royal Ancient Egyptians (18th–20th Dynasties): A Multi-detector Computed Tomography Study." The Eighth World Congress on Mummies Studies, Rio de Janeiro, Brazil, August 8, 2013.

Saleh, M., and H. Sourouzian. *Official Catalogue of the Egyptian Museum, Cairo.* Mainz: Philipp von Zabern, 1987.

Sallares, R., and S. Gomzi. "Biomolecular Archaeology of Malaria." *Anc Biomol* 3 (2001): 195–213.

Sandars, N.K. *The Sea Peoples: Warriors of the Eastern Mediterranean.* London: Thames & Hudson, 1978.

Sandison, A.T., and E. Tapp. "Disease in Ancient Egypt." In *Mummies, Disease, and Ancient Cultures,* 2nd ed., edited by A. Cockburn, E. Cockburn, and T.A. Reyman, 38–58. Cambridge, UK: Cambridge University Press, 1998.

Scheuer, J.L., J.H. Musgrave, and S.P. Evans. "The Estimation of Late Fetal and Perinatal Age from Limb Bone Length by Linear and Logarithmic Regression." *Ann Hum Biol* 7:3 (1980): 257–65.

Scheuer, L., and S. Black. *Developmental Juvenile Osteology.* San Diego: Academic Press, 2000.

Schneider, H.D. "Horemheb." In *The Oxford Encyclopedia of Ancient Egypt* 2, edited by D. Redford, 114–16. Cairo: American University in Cairo Press, 2001.

Schour, I., and M. Massler. "The Development of the Human Dentition." *JADA* 28 (1941): 1153–60.

Seipel, W. "Research on Mummies in Egyptology: An Overview." In *Human Mummies: A Global Survey of Their Status and the Techniques of Their Conservation,* edited by K. Spindler, H. Wilfing, E. Rastbichler-Zissernig, D. zur Nedden, and H. Nothdurfter, 41–45. Vienna: Springer, 1996.

Serpico, M., and R. White. "Resins, Amber and Bitumen." In *Ancient Egyptian Materials and Technology,* edited by P.T. Nicholson and I. Shaw, 430–74. Cambridge: Cambridge University Press, 2000.

Shafik, M., A. Selim, I. El Sheikh, and Z. Hawass. "Computed Tomography of King Tut-Ankh-Amen." *The Ambassadors Online Magazine* 11:23 (2008): Selected Study 3. http://ambassadors.net/archives/issue23/selectedstudy3.htm

Shaw, I., and P. Nicholson. *The Dictionary of Ancient Egypt.* London: British Museum, 1995.

Sigmund, G., and M. Minas. "The Trier Mummy Paï-es-tjau-em-aui-nu: Radiological and Histological Findings." *Eur Radiol* 12:7 (2002): 1854–62.

Silverman, D.P., J. Wegner, and J.H. Wegner. *Akhenaten and Tutankhamun: Revolution and Restoration.* Philadelphia: University of Pennsylvania Museum of Archaeology and Anthropology, 2006.

Simpson, W.K., ed. *The Literature of Ancient Egypt.* New Haven: Yale University Press, 1972.

Smith, G.E. "The Body of Queen Tii." *Nature* 76 (1907): 615–16.

———. "On the Mummies in the Tomb of Amenhotep II." *BIE* 51, series 1 (1907): 221–28.

———. "Queen Teie." *The Times*, October 15, 1907, Letter to the Editor.

———. *The Royal Mummies*. Catalogue général des antiquités égyptiennes du Musée du Caire. Cairo: IFAO, 1912, repr. London: Duckworth, 2000.

Smith, R.W., and D. Redford. *The Akhenaten Temple Project I: Initial Discoveries*. Warminster: Aris & Phillips, 1976.

Soto-Heim, P., P. Le Floch-Prigent, and M. Laval-Jeantet. "Scanographie d'une momie égyptienne antique de nourisson et de deux fausses momies de nouveau-nés." *Bull Mém Soc Anthrop Paris*, 14th series, vol. 2 (1985): 115–40.

Sourouzian, H. "Beyond Memnon: Buried More than 3,300 Years, Remnants of Amenhotep III's Extraordinary Mortuary Temple at Kom el-Hettan Rise from Beneath the Earth." *ICON Magazine* (Summer 2004): 10–17.

Sousa, R. "The Heart Amulet in Ancient Egypt: A Typological Study." In *Proceedings of the Ninth International Congress of Egyptologists* 1, edited by J.-C. Goyon and C. Cardin, 713–21. Dudley, MA: Peeters, 2007.

———. "The Meaning of the Heart Amulets in Egyptian Art." *JARCE* 43 (2007): 59–70.

Spalinger, A. "Some Notes on the Libyans of the Old Kingdom and Later Historical Reflexes." *JSSEA* 9 (1979): 125–60.

Stemplé, N., Y. Huten, C. Fondacci, T. Lang, M. Hassan, and C. Nessmann. "Fetal Bone Age Revisited: Proposal of a New Radiographic Score." *Pediatr Radiol* 25:7 (1995): 551–55.

Stierlin, H. *Le Buste de Nefertiti—une Imposture de l'Egyptologie?* Gollion, Switzerland: Infolio, 2009.

Strouhal, E. "Queen Mutnodjmet at Memphis: Anthropological and Paleopathological Evidence." In *L'Égyptologie en 1979: Axes prioritaires de recherches* 2, 317–22. Paris: Éditions du Centre national de la recherche scientifique, 1982.

Swales, J.D. "Tutankhamun's Breasts." *The Lancet* 301:7796 (27 January 1973): 201.

Taylor, G.M., P. Rutland, and T. Molleson. "A Sensitive Polymerase Chain Reaction Method for the Detection of *Plasmodium* Species DNA in Ancient Human Remains." *Anc Biomol* 1 (1997): 193–203.

Taylor, K.T. *Forensic Art and Illustration*. Boca Raton: CRC Press, 2001.

Taylor, R., and P. Craig. "The Wisdom of Bones: Facial Approximation on the Skull." In *Computer-Graphic Facial Reconstruction*, edited by J.G. Clement and M.K. Marks, 33–56. London: Elsevier Academic Press, 2005.

Thomas, A.J. "The Other Woman at Akhetaten, Royal Wife Kiya." *Amarna Letters* 3 (1994): 73–81.

Thomas, E. *The Royal Necropoleis of Thebes*. Princeton: privately published, 1966.

Tyldesley, J. *Hatchepsut: The Female Pharaoh*. New York: Viking, 1996.

———. *Nefertiti: Egypt's Sun Queen*. New York: Penguin, 1998.

Utsinger, P.D. "Diffuse Idiopathic Skeletal Hyperostosis." *Clin Rheum Dis* 11 (1985): 325–51.

Valentin, F.M., and T. Bedman. "Proof of a 'Long Coregency' between Amenhotep III and Amenhotep IV Found in the Chapel of Vizier Amenhotep Huy (Asasif Tomb 28), West Luxor." *KMT* 35:2 (Summer 2014): 17–27.

Van der Perre, A. "Nefertiti's Last Documented Reference (for Now)." In *In the Light of Amarna: One Hundred Years of the Nefertiti Discovery*, edited by F. Seyfried, 195–97. Berlin: Ägyptisches Museum und Papyrussammlung, Staatliche Museen zu Berlin, 2013.

———. "The Year 16 Graffito of Akhenaten in Dayr Abu Hinnis: A Contribution to the Study of the Later Years of Nefertiti." *Journal of Egyptian History* 7:1 (2014): 67–108.

van Dijk, J. "The Amarna Period and Later New Kingdom." In *The Oxford History of Ancient Egypt*, edited by I. Shaw, 265–307. Oxford: Oxford University Press, 2000.

———. "The Death of Meketaten." In *Causing His Name to Live: Studies in Egyptian Epigraphy and History in Memory of William J. Murnane*, edited by P. Brand and L. Cooper, http://www.jacobusvandijk.nl/docs/Meketaten.pdf, 83–88. Leiden: Brill, 2009.

———. "Kiya Revisited." In *Seventh International Congress of Egyptologists, Cambridge, 3–9 September 1995, Abstracts of Papers*, ed. C. Eyre, 50. Oxford: Oxford Books, 1995.

———. "New Evidence on the Length of the Reign of Horemheb." *JARCE* 44 (2008): 193–200.

van Dijk, J., and M. Eaton-Krauss. "Tutankhamun and Memphis." *MDAIK* 42 (1986): 35–41.

Vergnieux, R. "Recherches sur les monuments thébains d'Amenhotep IV à l'aide d'outils informatiques: Méthodes et résultats." *CSEG* 4 (1999).

Verzé, L. "History of Facial Reconstruction." *Acta Bio Medica* 80 (2009): 5–12.

Wade, A.D., G.J. Garvin, J.H. Hurnanen, L.L. Williams, B. Lawson, A.J. Nelson, and D. Tampieri. "Scenes from the Past: Multidetector CT of Egyptian Mummies of the Redpath Museum." *Radiographics* 32:4 (2012): 1235–50.

Wade, A.D., and A.J. Nelson. "Evisceration and Excerebration in the Egyptian Mummification Tradition." *J Arch Sci* 40:12 (2013): 4198–4206.

Wade A.D, A.J. Nelson, and G.J. Garvin. "A Synthetic Radiological Study of Brain Treatment in Ancient Egyptian Mummies." *HOMO—Journal of Comparative Human Biology* 62:4 (2011): 248–69.

Wasserman, J., R.O. Faulkner, and O. Goelet. *The Egyptian Book of the Dead.* 2nd ed. San Francisco: Chronicle Books, 1998.

Weeks, K.R., ed. *KV5: A Preliminary Report on the Excavation of the Tomb of the Sons of Ramesses II in the Valley of the Kings.* Rev. ed. Cairo: American University in Cairo Press, 2006.

Weigall, A. *Histoire de l'Égypte ancienne.* Paris: Payot, 1949.

Wente, E.F. "Age at Death of Pharaohs of the New Kingdom, Determined from Historical Sources." In *An X-Ray Atlas of the Royal Mummies*, edited by J.E. Harris and E.F. Wente, 234–85. Chicago: University of Chicago Press, 1980.

———. "Who Was Who among the Royal Mummies." *The Oriental Institute* 144 (Winter 1995): 1–6. Revised July 3, 2007. http://oi.uchicago.edu/research/pubs/nn/win95_wente.html

Whitehouse, W.M. "Radiologic Findings in the Royal Mummies." In *An X-Ray Atlas of the Royal Mummies*, edited by J.E. Harris and E.F. Wente, 286–327. Chicago: University of Chicago Press, 1980.

Wilkinson, C. "Computerized Forensic Facial Reconstruction: A Review of Current Systems." *Forensic Science, Medicine, and Pathology* 1:3 (2005): 173–78.

Wilkinson, R.H. *Reading Egyptian Art: A Hieroglyphic Guide to Ancient Egyptian Painting and Sculpture.* New York: Thames & Hudson, 1992.

———. *Tausret: Forgotten Queen and Pharaoh of Egypt.* Oxford: Oxford University Press, 2012.

Wilson, E. "Finding Pharaoh." *Century Magazine* 34:1 (May 1887): 3–10.

Wylie, W.L. "A Quantitative Method for Comparison of Craniofacial Patterns in Different Individuals." *Am J Anat* 74 (1944): 39–60.

Index

Ramesses XI 29, 30, 175
Re 63, 65, 147, 187
rectum, of Thuya 73, 232, 245
Reeves, Nicholas 130
resin 55, 107, 195, 197, 198, 199, 202, 203, 205,
    207, 209, 211, 212, 215, 224, 251; Amenhotep
    III 75, 76, 121, 197, 198, 211, 213, 225, 226,
    227, 228, 229, 249; Elder Lady of KV35 (Tiye)
    77, 78, 213, 226, 227, 228, 229; KV21 B 139,
    140; Merenptah 167, 168, 169, 171, 173, 174,
    197, 201–202, 213, 216, 225, 226, 227, 228,
    229; Ramessses II 6, 162, 164, 166, 197, 201–
    202, 203, 205, 206, 211, 226, 227, 228;
    Ramesses III 180, 184, 187, 190, 197, 201–202,
    203, 210, 225, 226, 227, 228, 229; Seti I 154,
    157, 158, 159–60, 197, 198, 203, 205, 209, 211,
    218, 225, 226, 227, 228, 229, 239; 'Thutmose I'
    50, 227, 243, 248; Thutmose II 52, 197, 205,
    226, 227, 229; Thutmose III 53, 206, 227, 228,
    229; Thuya 71, 72, 73, 197, 201–202, 206, 212,
    226, 227, 228; Tutankhamun 40, 104, 105, 204,
    227; Unknown Man E 188; Unknown Woman
    B 46; Younger Lady of KV35 (mother of
    Tutankhamun) 82, 226, 227, 228; Yuya 68, 70,
    71, 197, 201–202, 203, 205, 225, 226, 227, 228,
    229
resorption, alveolar: Amenhotep III 75; Elder
    Lady of KV35 (Tiye) 78, 79; KV60 A 59;
    Merenptah 169; Ramesses II 162; Ramesses
    III 181; Seti I 157; Yuya 70
restorations, multiple 220
'royal position' of arms: KV21 B 135; KV60 A
    (Hatshepsut) 135; Merenptah 196; Ramesses II
    196; Ramesses III 196; Seti I 196; Thutmose II
    196; Thutmose III 53, 196; Tiye 135
Ryan, Donald 40, 48, 51, 56, 57, 58, 133–34

sacroiliac joint 172; Amenhotep III 75;
    Merenptah 169, 172; Ramesses II 162, 172;
    Ramesses III 183; Seti I 157; Thutmose II 52
Sadat, Anwar 3, 5, 33
sandals 233

Saqqara 33, 89, 143, 145
sarcophagi: Amenhotep II 37, 39, 40; KV20 46,
    60; Merenptah 150; Mutnodjmet 143;
    Thutmose I 39; Tiye 84; Yuya 66
sawdust 198, 199, 209, 220; Ramesses III 184,
    227; Ramesses V 199; Thuya 73
SCA see Supreme Council of Antiquities (SCA)
scarabs 31, 56; heart 66, 239
Schaden, Otto 130
Schmorl's nodes 78, 140
scoliosis: fetus 317b 108; Marfan's Disease 124, 125,
    126; Ramesses II 162; Thuya 72, 73, 125;
    Tutankhamun 93, 95; Younger Lady of KV35 82
scrotum 214, 215; Merenptah 169, 171, 174, 216,
    230; Ramesses II 164; Ramesses III 184;
    'Thutmose I' 230; Thutmose II 230; Yuya 70,
    71, 215, 230
seeds 205, 224; in mummy of Ramesses II 161–
    62, 166, 211, 226, 229, 250
Selim, Ashraf 7, 8, 49, 54, 55, 59, 60, 67, 97, 109,
    125, 131, 132, 150
Senisoneb 47
Seqenenre 33, 46
Seth 147, 187, 241, 242
Sethnakht 36, 37, 166, 175, 179
Seti I 31, 147, 160; mummy of 2, 33, 125, 150,
    151, 154–60, 187, 196, 197, 198, 201, 203,
    205, 206, 207, 209, 211, 212, 213, 214, 216,
    220, 222, 225, 226, 227, 228, 229, 230, 232,
    234, 236, 239, 241, 243, 249–50; tomb of 2,
    30, 35, 147
Seti II 37, 150; mummy of 41, 173; tomb of 35,
    40, 51, 91
Shaded Surface Display (SSD) 19
sheepskin 188–89
Siamun 159
silver 66, 242
Siptah 37, 150, 173, 199
Sitamun 66, 67, 121, 132
Sitkamose, Queen 173
Sitre-In 40, 49, 56, 61; see also KV60 B mummy
Smendes I 159